Pulmonary Diseases: Diagnosis and Treatment

Pulmonary Diseases: Diagnosis and Treatment

Editor: Beatrice Gunther

AMERICAN
MEDICAL PUBLISHERS
www.americanmedicalpublishers.com

AMERICAN
MEDICAL PUBLISHERS
www.americanmedicalpublishers.com

Cataloging-in-Publication Data

Pulmonary diseases : diagnosis and treatment / edited by Beatrice Gunther.
p. cm.
Includes bibliographical references and index.
ISBN 978-1-63927-463-5
1. Lungs--Diseases. 2. Lungs--Diseases--Diagnosis. 3. Lungs--Diseases--Treatment. I. Gunther, Beatrice.
RC756 .P85 2022
616.24--dc23

American Medical Publishers,
41 Flatbush Avenue,
1st Floor, New York,
NY 11217, USA

ISBN 978-1-63927-463-5 (Hardback)

Contents

Preface

I am honored to present to you this unique book which encompasses the most up-to-date data in the field. I was extremely pleased to get this opportunity of editing the work of experts from across the globe. I have also written papers in this field and researched the various aspects revolving around the progress of the discipline. I have tried to unify my knowledge along with that of stalwarts from every corner of the world, to produce a text which not only benefits the readers but also facilitates the growth of the field.

Pulmonology is a specialty which is concerned with the management of the diseases of the respiratory tract. It include asthma, pneumonia, emphysema, tuberculosis and chest infections. The diagnosis of a pulmonary condition can be rigorous and may involve measurement of respiratory rate, inspection of signs of clubbing or cyanosis in hands, palpation of the trachea and the cervical lymph nodes, auscultation of the lung fields for unusual breath sounds, etc. Pulmonary clinical procedures include various pulmonary tests and procedures, such as spirometry, pulmonary function tests, scintigraphy, chest X-rays, bronchoscopy with broncho alveolar lavage, etc. Radiographic imaging is used to visualize the vasculature of the heart and the lungs. Inhalatory medicine such as steroids and bronchodilators, and oral medicine comprising of leukotriene antagonists and antibiotics are commonly used for the management of pulmonary conditions. This book presents some path-breaking studies in various pulmonary diseases. It outlines the diagnosis and treatment of such conditions in detail. Scientists and students actively engaged in pulmonology will find this book full of crucial and unexplored concepts.

Finally, I would like to thank all the contributing authors for their valuable time and contributions. This book would not have been possible without their efforts. I would also like to thank my friends and family for their constant support.

Editor

1

Clinical utility of blood neutrophil-lymphocyte ratio in Japanese COPD patients

Kaori Sakurai[1], Shotaro Chubachi[1*], Hidehiro Irie[1], Akihiro Tsutsumi[1], Naofumi Kameyama[1], Takashi Kamatani[1], Hidefumi Koh[2], Takeshi Terashima[3], Hidetoshi Nakamura[4], Koichiro Asano[5] and Tomoko Betsuyaku[1]

Abstract

Background: Neutrophil-to-lymphocyte ratio (NLR) is a biomarker of inflammation in chronic obstructive pulmonary disease (COPD) patients. But, a meaningful threshold and the longitudinal changes are unknown. We aimed to investigate the association between NLR and the clinical characteristics of COPD patients and to determine a meaningful threshold and the longitudinal changes for NLR.

Methods: Keio University and its affiliate hospitals conducted an observational COPD cohort study over 3 years. We performed a blood examination and a pulmonary function test. Blood examination was completed at baseline and annually thereafter, at a time when the disease was stable. Two hundred seventy-four patients who had at least 3 blood examinations over 3 years were included.

Results: Baseline NLR was correlated with baseline C-reactive protein (CRP) ($r = 0.18$, $p = 0.003$) and SAA ($r = 0.34$, $p < 0.001$). We defined an NLR score of 2.7 as the arbitrary cut-off value based on upper quartile points. COPD patients with NLR ≥ 2.7 were older ($p = 0.037$), had a lower BMI ($p = 0.005$) and a lower %FEV1 ($p = 0.0003$) compared to patients with NLR < 2.7. Receiver-operating-characteristic (ROC) curves showed the optimal cutoff for the baseline NLR in the predicting moderate/severe exacerbation to be 2.7, which was same as the upper quartile points. Follow-up analysis over 3 years revealed that the differences in the trends of NLR among the three groups based on the categories of exacerbations (moderate or severe, mild, no exacerbation) were significant ($p = 0.006$).

Conclusions: NLR is associated with COPD severity and exacerbations. For predicting exacerbations, we estimated the threshold of NLR to be 2.7 at baseline.

Keywords: COPD, NLR, Acute exacerbation, Comorbidity

Background

Chronic obstructive pulmonary disease (COPD) is common worldwide and is a major health-care concern [1]. COPD is characterized by low-grade chronic systemic inflammation [2], and several biomarkers such as C-reactive protein (CRP) [3, 4], IL-6 [4, 5] and surfactant protein D (SPD) [6] have been reported to be associated with increased risk of death in COPD patients. Although many biomarkers of systemic inflammation have recently been evaluated to identify some features of COPD [7, 8], excessive costs and technical factors prevent their clinical use.

Recently, blood neutrophil-to-lymphocyte ratio (NLR) has been shown to be a valuable predictor of inflammatory conditions and is used for risk stratification of different diseases such as acute coronary syndrome [9], pancreatitis [10], sepsis and infectious conditions [11]. This index is a rapid, easy and cost-effective method which is a calculated index derived from a routine complete blood count test in clinical practice [12]. NLR

* Correspondence: bachibachi472000@live.jp
[1]Division of Pulmonary Medicine, Department of Medicine, Keio University School of Medicine, 35 Shinanomachi, Shinjuku-ku, Tokyo 160-8582, Japan
Full list of author information is available at the end of the article

has been reported to be higher in exacerbated COPD patients than in stable patients [13] and is associated with severity of COPD [14, 15]. As with other inflammatory markers, NLR has been reported to vary with time [16, 17]. However, annual time-series data of individual NLR, its distribution and a meaningful threshold in COPD remain to be investigated.

Comorbidities and extrapulmonary manifestations have important contributions to disease expression, disease burden, and survival in COPD patients [18]. Several comorbidities such as heart disease, hypertension, and diabetes [19] are also associated with systemic inflammation. However, the association between these comorbidities and NLR in COPD patients has not been elucidated.

We have been conducting a multicenter, observational cohort study, called the Keio COPD Comorbidity Research (K-CCR), to comprehensively examine the comorbidities of COPD in Japan [20–22].

The specific aims of this study are to determine (a) whether NLR is a biomarker that can reflect the severity of airflow limitation and certain other characteristics of COPD patients, (b) if it can predict future exacerbations and (c) if it is associated with any comorbidities. We thus monitored NLR and other known blood biomarkers in Japanese COPD patients over 3 years to evaluate its stability as a biomarker in patients at steady state and investigated its association with a variety of clinical aspects of COPD.

Methods

Study population

The overall design of the K-CCR has been previously published [20, 22, 23]. In brief, this study was a 3-year, prospective observational study that enrolled 572 men and women aged 40–91 years who had been diagnosed with COPD ($n = 440$) or as being at risk for COPD ($n = 132$) by pulmonary physicians from April 2010 to December 2012 [20, 22, 23]. For the purpose of this study, only data from the patients with spirometrically confirmed COPD (FEV1/forced vital capacity (FVC) < 0.7) who had undergone at least 3 blood examinations over 3 years and were not receiving any oral steroid treatments ($n = 274$) were selected and analyzed (Fig. 1). All patients were clinically stable and had no exacerbations and no acute infections for at least 1 month prior to recruitment [20, 22, 23]. The ethics committees of the Keio University and its affiliated hospitals approved the study protocol. Each patient provided written, informed consent to analyze and present their data. All aspects of the study conformed to the principles of the Declaration of Helsinki adopted by the 59th WMA General Assembly, Seoul, Republic of Korea, October 2008.

Assessment of clinical parameters

Complete medical and smoking histories, as well as information regarding the current pharmacologic treatments, were obtained on enrolment and annually thereafter [20, 22]. All patients were assessed by spirometry and chest computed tomography (CT) imaging. On the CT images, the extent of emphysema was quantified as the ratio of low attenuation area (LAA %) and the percentage of airway wall area (WA %) using a custom-made software (AZE Ltd., Tokyo, Japan) [22, 23]. Independent investigators judged the number and severity of exacerbations based on the reviews of physicians' medical records, as previously reported [22, 24]. Mild COPD exacerbation was defined as worsening of symptoms that were self-managed (by measures such as an increase in salbutamol use) and resolved without systemic corticosteroids or antibiotics [24]. Moderate COPD exacerbation was defined by the requirement for treatment with systemic corticosteroids and/or antibiotics [24]. Severe COPD exacerbation was defined as one that required hospitalization, including an emergency admission for 24 h [24]. Comorbid diagnoses were established by clinical history and examination findings based on a review of available medical records [20, 21, 23, 24].

Evaluation of neutrophil-to-lymphocyte ratio (NLR) and other inflammatory markers

Blood samples were collected at baseline and annually thereafter, at a time when the disease was stable. The total numbers of white blood cells (WBCs), neutrophils, and lymphocytes were measured at each participating center. NLR was defined as the absolute neutrophil count divided by the absolute lymphocyte count [9]. Serum C-reactive protein (CRP) levels were measured using a Hitachi Ltd. LABOSPECT 008 devise. Serum amyloid A (SAA) is an acute-phase protein similar to CRP, and its levels were evaluated by latex agglutination immunoassay. The annual rates of change in NLR were measured over 3 years. Excel (Microsoft Inc., Redmond, WA, USA) was used to calculate the derived slope between each of the above measures and the date of data collection [22, 25].

Questionnaires on health-related quality of life

All patients were clinically stable and had no exacerbations for at least 1 month before study enrollment and on the day of the annual examination [22]. The Japanese version of COPD assessment test (CAT) [26, 27] and the St. George's Respiratory Questionnaire (SGRQ) in Japanese were used for the assessment of COPD-specific health status [28–30]. All of the questionnaires were completed by the patients themselves at home [20].

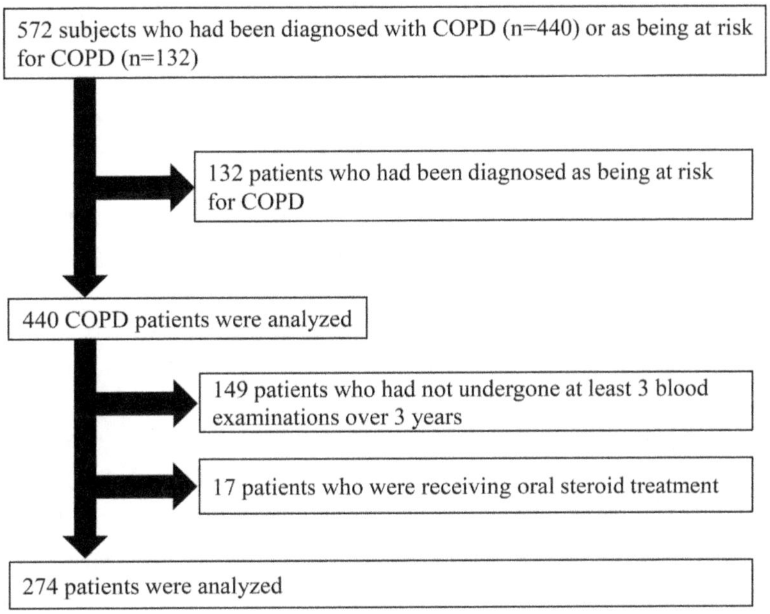

Fig. 1 Process of patient selection in this study. Data from only those COPD patients with spirometrically confirmed COPD (FEV1/forced vital capacity (FVC) < 0.7) who had undergone at least 3 blood examinations over 3 years and were not receiving any oral steroid treatments ($n = 274$) were analyzed. COPD, chronic obstructive pulmonary disease

Statistical analysis

Data are presented as the mean ± standard deviation (SD) or as median (interquartile range (IQR)). Data were compared between two groups using the student *t*-test, Mann-Whitney U test, and χ^2 test. Data were compared among three or more groups using Kruskal-Wallis test and Steel-Dwass test. Correlations between continuous variables were evaluated using the Pearson's correlation coefficient. Univariate and multivariate logistic regression analyses were performed in order to assess the effects of factors on increasing NLR. Receiver operating characteristics (ROC) curves were constructed to assess the areas under the curves (AUCs). We investigated the optimal cutoff value by maximizing the Youden index. The data of NLR over 3 years were only used in the analysis of the annual rates of change in NLR, and in the comparison of the average of NLR among the three groups over 3 years. Differences in rates of change over time and in NLR among the 3 groups classified based on the severity of exacerbation were estimated using mixed-effects modeling with Bonferroni correction [22]. For all tests, two-sided p values < 0. 05 were considered significant. Data were analyzed using the JMP 13 software (SAS Institute, Cary, NC, USA). A mixed-effect model was applied using SPSS 23 (IBM Corporation, Armonk, NY, USA).

Results

Characteristics of the study population

Table 1 shows the baseline clinical characteristics of the study patients. The mean age of the 274 COPD patients was 72.2 ± 7.9 years, and 9.6% of them were current smokers. At baseline, 23.0%, 48.9%, 22.3%, and 5.8% were diagnosed as COPD grade 1, 2, 3, and 4, respectively based on the Global Initiative for Chronic Obstructive Lung Disease (GOLD) classification [31]. Baseline NLR significantly increased with the severity of COPD grade (1.9 (1.4–2.4) vs. 2.1 (1.5–2.6) vs. 2.3 (2.0–3.0) vs. 2.7 (1.9–5.3), $p = 0.002$) (Table 2).

Comparison of patient characteristics based on baseline NLR

NLR data showed a non-normal distribution. The median baseline NLR was 2.1(1.6–2.7). Baseline characteristics of patients according to the baseline NLR are shown in Table 3. The cut-off value of NLR was arbitrarily defined based on the upper quartile points as 2.7. COPD patients with NLR ≥ 2.7 ($n = 66$) were older (74.0 ± 7.1 years vs. 71. 6 ± 8.1 years, $p = 0.037$), had a lower BMI (22.0 ± 3.4 vs. 23.2 ± 2.9, $p = 0.005$) and a lower % FEV_1 (55.8 ± 21.3% vs. 66.5 ± 20.4%, $p = 0.0003$) compared to patients with NLR < 2.7 ($n = 199$). Baseline NLR did not differ between current smokers and past smokers (2.12 ± 0.24 vs. 2.38 ± 0.08, $p = 0.30$). On CT images, LAA% of the patients with NLR ≥ 2.7 tended to be higher than that of the others (18.4 (6.4–28.7) % vs. 11.3 (5.0–23.3) %, $p = 0.093$), while WA% did not differ between the two groups (54.9 (46.4–59.8) % vs. 52.4 (47.4–57.7) %, $p = 0.416$). The COPD patients with NLR ≥ 2.7 exhibited a significantly higher total CAT score (13.9 ± 7.7 vs. 11.5 ± 8.0, $p = 0.039$) and SGRQ total score (36.2 ± 19.1 vs. 24.8 ± 18.0, $p < 0.001$) compared to the others.

Table 1 Baseline clinical characteristics of the study patients

	COPD
Number	274
Gender, female, *n* (%)	17 (6.2)
Age, years	72.2 ± 7.9
Smoking Index, pack-years	55.2 ± 29.7
Current smokers, *n* (%)	26 (9.6)
BMI, kg/m^2	22.9 ± 3.1
FEV_1/FVC, %	52.4 ± 12.3
% FEV_1, %	63.3 ± 21.1
GOLD grade 1/2/3/4, *n* (%)	63/134/61/16 (23.0/48.9/22.3/5.8)
Baseline CAT score	12.2 ± 8.0
LAMA, *n* (%)	170 (62.0)
LABA, *n* (%)	136 (49.6)
ICS, *n* (%)	93 (33.9)
Dose of ICS[a], μg/day, median	500
WBC, *n*	6208 ± 1566
Neutrophil, %	60.3 ± 8.9
Neutrophil, *n*	3797 ± 1320
Lymphocyte, %	29.2 ± 8.2
Lymphocyte, *n*	1770 ± 553
NLR	2.1(1.6–2.7)
Eosinophil, %	3.4 ± 2.6
Eosinophil, *n*	204 ± 150

Data are shown as mean ± SD and median (interquartile range)
COPD chronic obstructive pulmonary disease, *BMI* body mass index, *FEV_1* forced expiratory volume in one second, *FVC* forced vital capacity, *% FEV_1* ratio of predicted FEV_1, *GOLD* Global Initiative for Chronic Obstructive Lung Disease, *CAT* COPD assessment test, *LAMA* long-acting muscarinic antagonist, *LABA* long-acting β_2 agonist, *ICS* inhaled corticosteroids, *WBC* white blood cell, *NLR* Neutrophil-to-Lymphocyte ratio
[a]Dose of inhaled corticosteroid is shown as fluticasone propionate equivalent

Relationship between NLR and other inflammatory markers

Baseline NLR showed a weak but significant correlation with baseline CRP ($r = 0.18$, $p = 0.003$) and SAA ($r = 0.34$, $p < 0.001$). Similarly, baseline absolute neutrophil count also correlated significantly with baseline CRP ($r = 0.24$, $p < 0.001$) and baseline SAA ($r = 0.31$, $p < 0.001$), but the baseline absolute lymphocyte count did not show correlation with the other inflammatory markers. The absolute neutrophil count showed no correlation with the absolute lymphocyte count ($r = 0.08$, $p = 0.214$). These results imply that the absolute neutrophil count has a bigger impact on the value of NLR as systemic inflammation.

Table 2 Comparison of the baseline NLR stratified by the GOLD COPD grade

GOLD COPD grade	NLR
1	1.9 (1.4–2.4)
2	2.1 (1.5–2.6)
3	2.3 (2.0–3.0)*
4	2.7 (1.9–5.3)

Data are shown as median (interquartile range). *P*-values among the four groups; $p = 0.002$, *$p = 0.008$ vs. grade 1
GOLD Global Initiative for Chronic Obstructive Lung Disease, *COPD* chronic obstructive pulmonary disease, *NLR* Neutrophil-to-Lymphocyte ratio

Table 3 Patient characteristics based on baseline NLR

	NLR < 2.7	NLR ≥ 2.7	*p*-value
Number	199	66	
Gender, female, *n* (%)	14 (7.0)	3 (4.6)	0.474
Age, years	71.6 ± 8.1	74.0 ± 7.1	0.037
Smoking Index, pack-years	53.7 ± 28.8	59.9 ± 33.8	0.159
Current smokers, *n* (%)	21 (10.7)	4 (6.1)	0.270
BMI, kg/m^2	23.2 ± 2.9	22.0 ± 3.4	0.005
FEV_1/FVC, (%)	53.8 ± 11.8	48.9 ± 13.3	0.005
% FEV_1, (%)	66.5 ± 20.4	55.8 ± 21.3	0.0003
LAA%, (%)	11.3 (5.0–23.3)	18.4 (6.4–28.7)	0.093
WA%, (%)	52.4 (47.4–57.7)	54.9 (46.4–59.8)	0.416
Baseline CAT score	11.5 ± 8.0	13.9 ± 7.7	0.039
SGRQ total score	24.8 ± 18.0	36.2 ± 19.1	< 0.001
LAMA, *n* (%)	120 (60.3)	44 (66.7)	0.356
LABA, *n* (%)	94 (47.2)	40 (60.6)	0.060
ICS, *n* (%)	63 (31.7)	28 (42.4)	0.111
Dose of ICS[a], μg/day, median	500	500	0.980
Eosinophil, (%)	3.6 ± 2.6	2.9 ± 2.4	0.080
Eosinophil, *n*	209 ± 149	188 ± 153	0.318

Data are shown as mean ± SD and median (interquartile range)
COPD chronic obstructive pulmonary disease, *NLR* Neutrophil-to-Lymphocyte ratio, *BMI* body mass index, *FEV_1* forced expiratory volume in one second, *FVC* forced vital capacity, *% FEV_1* ratio of predicted FEV_1, *LAA%* ratio of low attenuation area, *WA%* ratio of airway wall area, *CAT* COPD assessment test, *SGRQ* St. George's Respiratory Questionnaire, *LAMA* long-acting muscarinic antagonist, *LABA* long-acting β_2 agonist, *ICS* inhaled corticosteroids, *CRP* C-reactive protein, *SAA* serum amyloid A
[a]Dose of inhaled corticosteroid is shown as fluticasone propionate equivalent

Determinant factors of NLR

Univariate logistic regression analysis showed that high age, % $FEV_1 < 50\%$, low BMI (BMI < 18.5), high CRP and high SAA were all significantly associated with NLR ≥ 2.7 (Additional file 1: Table S1). We then performed a multivariate logistic regression analysis including the associating factors that reached significance in the univariate analysis. Because of the significant correlations between SAA and CRP ($r = 0.84$, $p < 0.001$), SAA was excluded from the multivariate analysis. % $FEV_1 < 50\%$, low BMI, and high CRP were found to be independent determinant factors of NLR ≥ 2.7 (Table 4). These results imply that NLR is multifactorial, and is independently associated with severe airflow limitation, advanced age, and low BMI. Also, it is reflective of other systemic inflammation markers.

Table 4 Predictors of high NLR (NLR ≥ 2.7) by multivariate logistic regression analysis

	Odds ratio (95% CI)	*P*-value
Age	1.04 (0.99–1.08)	0.063
BMI < 18.5	2.95 (1.22–7.09)	0.016
% FEV_1 < 50%	2.35 (1.25–4.41)	0.008
CRP	1.89 (1.08–3.28)	0.008

NLR Neutrophil-to-Lymphocyte ratio, *BMI* body mass index, *FEV_1* forced expiratory volume in one second, *% FEV_1* ratio of predicted FEV_1, *CRP* C-reactive protein

Comparison of comorbidity prevalence according to the baseline NLR

Prevalence of comorbidity in the study patients according to the baseline NLR is shown in Table 5. The prevalence of arteriosclerosis obliterans, cancer and cataract were tended to be higher in the NLR ≥ 2.7 group than in the NLR < 2.7 group (arteriosclerosis obliterans; 0.5% vs. 3.0%, $P = 0.096$, caner; 18.4% vs. 28.7%, $p = 0.072$, cataract; 38.7% vs. 53.3%, $p = 0.081$). There were no statistical differences in the prevalence of cardiovascular disease, hypertension, diabetes. These results imply that NLR is not influenced by comorbidities in COPD patients.

Table 5 Prevalence of comorbidity in the study patients according to the baseline NLR

n (%)	NLR < 2.7	NLR ≥ 2.7	p-value
Benign prostatic hyperplasia	30 (15.3)	10 (15.2)	0.976
Tuberculosis	17 (8.7)	5 (7.6)	0.781
Arteriosclerosis obliterans	1 (0.5)	2 (3.0)	0.096
Aortic aneurysm	7 (3.6)	2 (3.0)	0.835
Arrhythmia	23 (11.7)	6 (9.1)	0.554
Heart failure	13 (6.6)	2 (3.0)	0.276
Coronary artery disease	23 (11.7)	8 (12.1)	0.933
Peptic ulcer disease	13 (6.6)	4 (6.1)	0.870
Dyslipidemia	35 (17.9)	10 (15.2)	0.614
Diabetes mellitus	30 (15.3)	8 (12.1)	0.525
Hypertension	71 (36.2)	23 (34.9)	0.840
Interstitial pneumonia	38 (26.8)	12 (35.3)	0.322
Pneumothorax	10 (5.1)	3 (4.6)	0.857
Hyperuricemia	16 (8.2)	6 (9.1)	0.814
Cerebral infarction	11 (5.6)	5 (7.6)	0.565
Asthma (Asthma COPD overlap)	38 (19.5)	16 (24.2)	0.410
Depression	15 (7.7)	9 (14.1)	0.124
Cancer	36 (18.4)	19 (28.7)	0.072
Cataract	58 (38.7)	24 (53.3)	0.081

NLR Neutrophil-to-Lymphocyte ratio, *COPD* chronic obstructive pulmonary disease

Longitudinal changes in NLR over 3 years

Overall, time-dependent changes in NLR showed a slight increase over 3 years ($p = 0.003$) (Fig. 2a). The distribution of the annual rate of change in NLR (ΔNLR score/year) over 3 years is shown in Fig. 2b. The median ΔNLR score/year was 0.05 (− 0.15–0.25).

Relationship between NLR and COPD exacerbation over 3 years

Based on the degree of exacerbations defined in our previous paper [24], the COPD subjects were classified into 3 groups: without exacerbations ($n = 86$), only mild exacerbations ($n = 52$), and moderate or severe exacerbations ($n = 74$). Among the 3 groups, the median baseline NLR was significantly higher in the moderate/severe exacerbation group compared to the exacerbation-free group but it was not significantly different when compared to the mild exacerbation group (2.4 (1.8–3.2) vs. 2.0 (1.5–2.4) and 2.0(1.4–2.7), $p = 0.010$ and 0.104, respectively) (Fig. 3a). Univariate logistic regression analysis showed that the baseline NLR ≥ 2.7 (OR; 2.89, $p = 0.001$), Age (OR; 1.05, p = 0.01), $\%FEV_1 < 50$ (OR; 3.23, $p = 0.0002$) and LAA% (OR; 1.05, $p = 0.0004$) were significant predictors of moderate/severe exacerbation (Additional file 1: Table S2). Multivariate logistic regression analysis was performed using risk factors that reached significance on univariate analyses. Because of the significant negative correlations between $\%FEV_1$ and LAA% ($r = -0.47$, $p < 0.0001$), LAA% were excluded from multivariate analysis. The baseline NLR ≥ 2.7 was an independent risk factor for moderate exacerbations over 3 years (OR; 2.22, $p = 0.025$) (Additional file 1: Table S3). ROC curves showed that the optimal cutoff for the baseline NLR for predicting moderate/severe exacerbations was 2.7 (AUC 62.3, sensitivity 37.8%, specificity 83.3%) (Fig. 3b). Follow-up analysis over 3 years revealed that there was a significant difference in the average value of NLR among the three groups ($p = 0.006$), but the trends of NLR were comparable among the three groups over 3 years ($p = 0.476$) (Fig. 4).

Comparison of receiver-operator curves for NLR, neutrophil and lymphocyte counts, and other biomarkers to stratify the severity of airflow limitation and predict future exacerbations

The area under ROC for NLR to predict future exacerbation was 63.4% (95% CI 55.0–71.7) and the baseline low % FEV_1 ($\%FEV_1 < 50\%$) was 64.2% (95% CI 56.9–71.6), and both seemed to be better than the baseline absolute neutrophil and lymphocyte counts alone, CRP and SAA, implying that NLR was a superior predictor of the severity of airflow limitations and future exacerbations compared to the neutrophil and lymphocyte counts alone (Table 6).

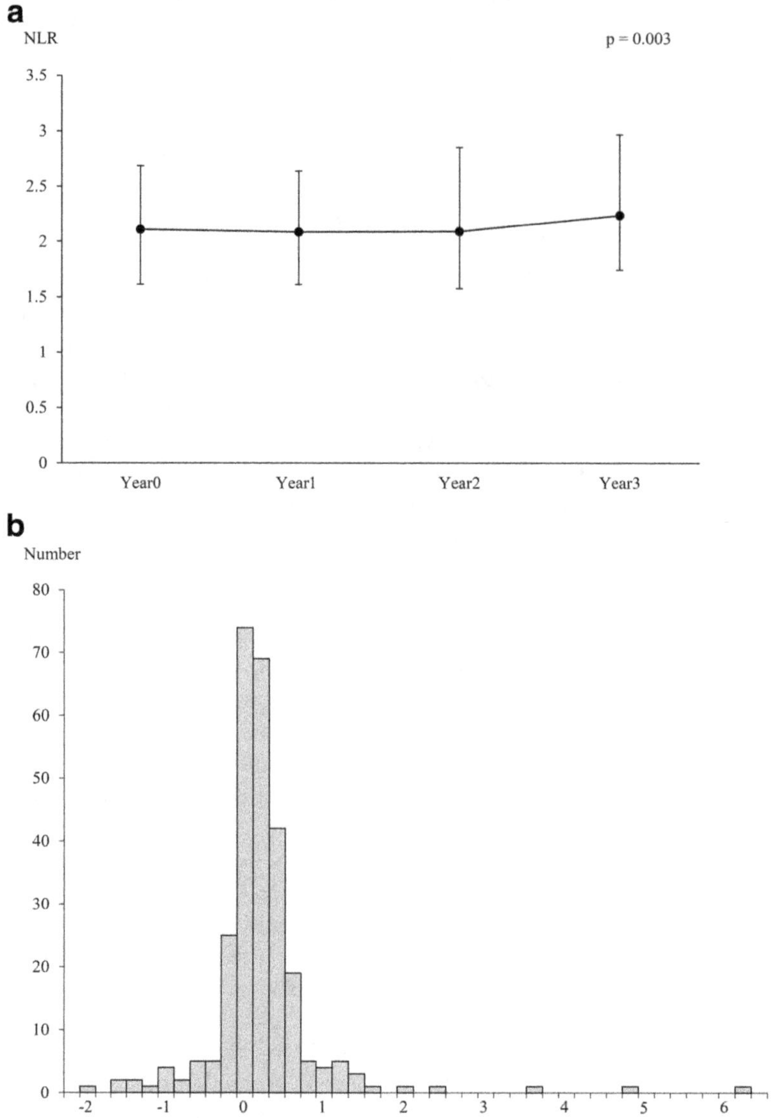

Fig. 2 Longitudinal changes in NLR. **a** Time-dependent changes in NLR. **b** The distribution of the annual rate of change in NLR (ΔNLR score/year) over 3 years. NLR, Neutrophil-to-Lymphocyte ratio; ΔNLR, the rate of change in NLR

Discussion

Mechanism of the relationship between NLR and COPD severity

Consistent with a previous report [14], in this study, we found that NLR was associated with COPD severity and exacerbations. Several studies have reported the appropriate thresholds to predict the natural history of systemic diseases other than COPD. In this study, we revealed the appropriate cut-off value of NLR as 2.7 to predict COPD severity and future exacerbations [32, 33]. The mechanisms underlying these relationships are unknown, but there could be several explanations. Firstly, it is well known that, even after smoking cessation, inflammation in the lungs continue, especially in patients with advanced COPD [34], suggesting that the persistent inflammatory response in the lungs could lead to neutrophil recruitment and activation [35]. When activated, neutrophils release a variety of serine- and metalloproteinases, which contribute to the development and progression of emphysema [36]. It has been shown that sputum neutrophilia is increased in advanced COPD and is associated with severity of airflow limitation [37]. Blood neutrophilia is a hallmark of current smokers [38] and is also a predictor of mortality in COPD patients [4]. Secondly, a relationship between bacterial colonization and exacerbations is increasingly recognized [39]. Thus, in some patients with COPD, the disturbed flora may continue to activate the innate immune

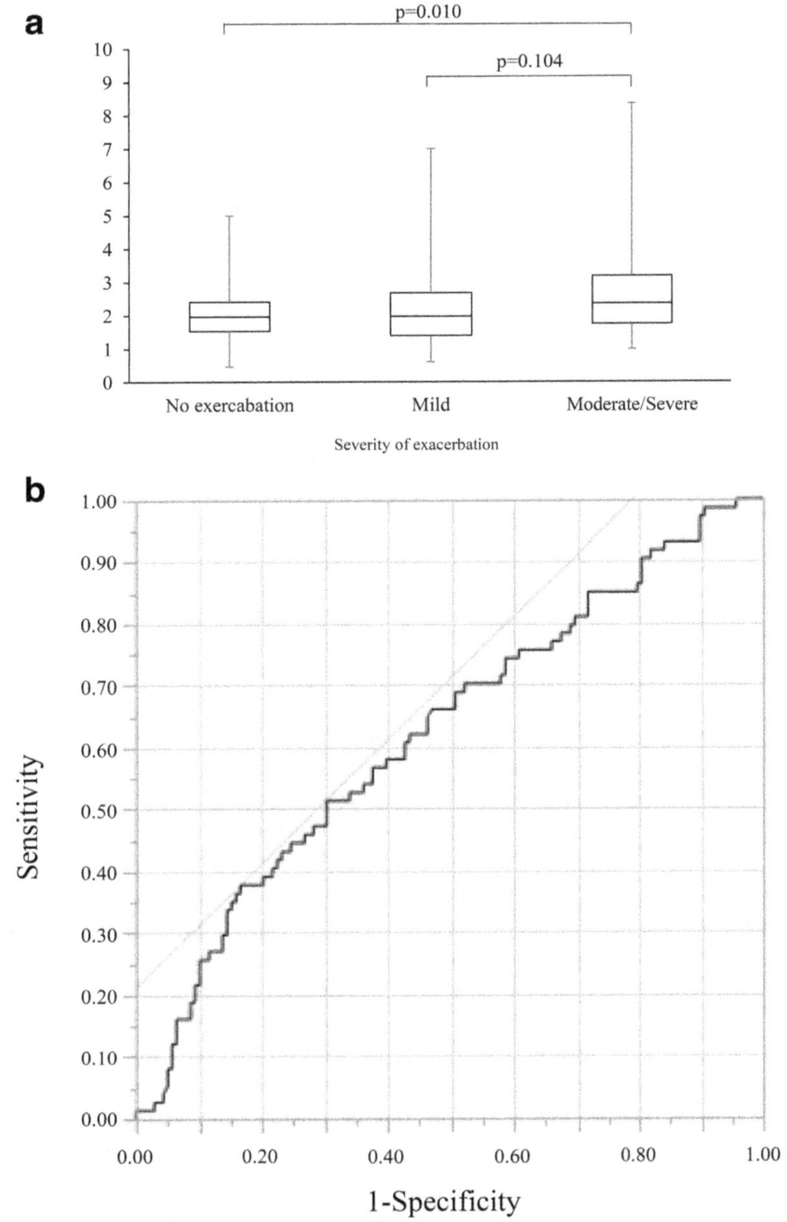

Fig. 3 Relationship between NLR and COPD exacerbation. **a** Comparison of median baseline NLR based on the severity of exacerbation over 3 years. **b** ROC curves of median baseline NLR in the predicting moderate or severe exacerbation. Data were compared among three groups using Steel-Dwass test. NLR, Neutrophil-to-Lymphocyte ratio

responses, perpetuating lung inflammation and blood neutrophilia. We would like to emphasize that most of the participants in this study were not current smokers. Thirdly, blood lymphopenia is associated with age [40] and poor nutritional status [41], which could also be applicable to a subset of COPD patients. Taken together, NLR along with age and nutritional status could be reflective of the systemic inflammatory condition. Weak correlations between NLR and other biomarkers might be caused by multifactorial determinants of NLR.

NLR and COPD comorbidities

It should be noted that this is the first study to assess the relationships between NLR and COPD comorbidities. Chronic systemic inflammation which is a characteristic of most comorbidities is believed to be a key factor that links COPD with its comorbidities [42]. In the ECLIPSE cohort, most COPD patients with heart disease had elevated IL-6, IL-8, and fibrinogen, while those with hypertension had elevated fibrinogen and those with diabetes had elevated CRP [19]. In our study, these comorbidities were not associated with NLR. It

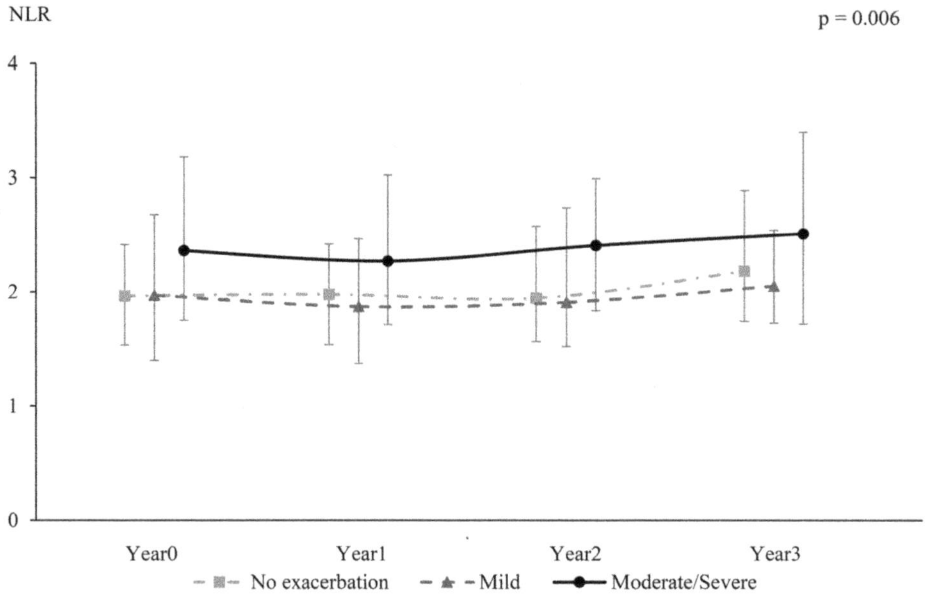

Fig. 4 Trend in NLR changes over 3 years. The trend of NLR changes in the none, mild and moderate/severe exacerbations groups was significantly different ($p = 0.006$). Moderate/severe exacerbation vs exacerbation-free, $p = 0.014$; Moderate/severe exacerbation vs mild exacerbation, $p = 0.022$. NLR, Neutrophil-to-Lymphocyte ratio

would, therefore, be unreliable to predict the presence of comorbidities by the serum inflammatory markers in COPD patients.

Clinical usefulness of NLR

NLR is a new addition to the list of inflammatory markers and has got special attention in the recent years. The value for NLR is obtained by dividing the absolute neutrophil count by the absolute lymphocyte count in peripheral blood samples. Moreover, this test is quite inexpensive, usually not requiring a proper setup and can be used as a screening and drug monitoring tool in population on a large scale [43].

Table 6 Comparison of the areas under ROC for NLR and other biomarkers to predict future exacerbations and low % FEV_1 (% $FEV_1 < 50\%$)

Exacerbation	AUC (95% CI)
NLR	63.4 (55.0–71.7)
Neutrophil count	55.2 (46.3–64.2)
Lymphocyte count	59.2 (50.8–67.6)
Eosinophil count	51.2 (41.9–60.6)
CRP	54.3 (45.2–63.4)
SAA	59.4 (50.5–68.3)
% $FEV_1 < 50\%$	AUC (95% CI)
NLR	64.2 (56.9–71.6)
Neutrophil count	55.3 (47.3–63.2)
lymphocyte count	59.8 (52.3–67.3)
Eosinophil count	51.5 (43.4–59.6)
CRP	55.5 (47.7–63.5)
SAA	57.7 (49.8–65.6)

NLR Neutrophil-to-Lymphocyte ratio, *CRP* C-reactive protein, *SAA* serum amyloid A

Strategies to prevent exacerbations include targeting risk factors, addressing comorbid conditions, and giving bronchodilator therapies which include long-acting β2-agonists (LABAs) or long-acting muscarinic antagonists (LAMAs) used alone or in combination with each other or with an inhaled corticosteroid [ICS]) [44, 45]. A number of studies have shown that the higher the blood eosinophil count, higher is the risk of exacerbation [46] and greater is the exacerbation reduction response to inhaled corticosteroids [47, 48]. In this study, although NLR was a predictor of exacerbations, blood eosinophilia was not a risk factor. This may be because the prescription rate of ICS was high in our populations than in the other cohort studies. One previous report has shown that the count and percent of blood eosinophils were not associated with the exacerbation frequency in COPD patients after carefully excluding the Asthma–COPD overlap syndrome (ACOS) patients [49]. ICS may be insufficient to prevent exacerbations in COPD patients with a high NLR, and a new prophylactic therapy should be considered. NLR may be a simple and inexpensive biomarker for detecting a neutrophilic endotype, and this endotype may be indicative of the new pharmacological strategy for treating the exacerbation. In addition to the usual care, azithromycin and roflumilast are likely candidates for prophylactic therapy in these patients. Azithromycin and roflumilast treated patients had lower sputum proline-glycine-proline (PGP) levels and showed a reduction in other markers of neutrophilic inflammation [50, 51].

Limitations of this study

Our study had several limitations. First, although NLR was associated with exacerbations over 3 years, outcomes such as hospital admissions, emergency room visits, and mortality remain to be evaluated. Sørensen et al. reported that NLR was associated with higher mortality in moderate to very severe COPD patients [52], but it is unknown whether this result can be applied to milder COPD patients in our study. Second, blood NLR may not accurately reflect the lung inflammation of COPD patients. Low sensitivity of NLR to predict future exacerbations and airflow limitation severity may be caused by this reason. It would be preferable if we could compare blood NLR and biomarkers or cell fractionation of bronchoalveolar lavage and sputum. Third, COPD patients of the KCCR cohort study had few women (6.2%) and were older compared to subjects of other clinical studies in Western countries. Therefore, the results may not apply to women and younger COPD patients.

Conclusions

The present study demonstrates that NLR is associated with COPD severity and exacerbations, but not with systemic comorbidity in COPD patients. For predicting exacerbations, we estimated the threshold of NLR to be 2.7 at baseline. This information could be useful in the phenotyping of COPD patients, and their careful monitoring in clinical settings. Appropriate interventions for these patients should be considered in future.

Abbreviations

%FEV_1: Ratio of predicted FEV_1; BMI: Body mass index; CAT: COPD assessment test; COPD: Chronic obstructive pulmonary disease; CRP: C-reactive protein; FEV_1: Forced expiratory volume in one second; FVC: Forced vital capacity; GERD: Gastroesophageal reflux disease; GOLD: Global Initiative for Chronic Obstructive Lung Disease; HAD-A: Seven items for anxiety of hospital anxiety and depression; HAD-D: Seven items for depression of hospital anxiety and depression; ICS: Inhaled corticosteroids; LAA%: Ratio of low attenuation area; LABA: Long-acting β_2 agonist; LAMA: Long-acting muscarinic antagonist; NLR: Neutrophil-to-Lymphocyte ratio; SAA: Serum amyloid A; SGRQ: St. George's Respiratory Questionnaire; WA%: Ratio of airway wall area; ΔNLR: Rate of change in NLR

Acknowledgements

The authors acknowledge Chiyomi Uemura for helping with data collection. The authors acknowledge all the members of the K-CCR group who participated in this study, including Saiseikai Utsunomiya Hospital, Eiju General Hospital, Tokyo Saiseikai Central Hospital, Sano Public Welfare General Hospital, Nihon Kokan Hospital, Saitama Social Insurance Hospital, Kawasaki City Ida Hospital, Saitama City Hospital, Tokyo Medical Center, Tokyo Dental College Ichikawa General Hospital, Tokyo Electric Power Company Hospital and the International Medical Welfare College Shioya Hospital.

Authors' contributions

KS participated in the design of the study, performed the statistical analyses, and was a major contributor in writing the manuscript. SC planned the study design and contributed to interpretation of results. HN, KA, and TB conceived the study, participated in its design and coordination, and helped draft the manuscript. HI, AT, NK, TK, HK, and TT contributed to collection of data and interpretation of results. All authors read and approved the final manuscript. TB was the guarantor of is this study.

Consent for publication

Each patient provided written informed consent to analyze and publish his/her data.

Competing interests

The authors declare that they have no competing interests.

Author details

[1]Division of Pulmonary Medicine, Department of Medicine, Keio University School of Medicine, 35 Shinanomachi, Shinjuku-ku, Tokyo 160-8582, Japan. [2]Department of Medicine, Tachikawa Hospital, Tokyo, Japan. [3]Division of Pulmonary Medicine, Department of Internal Medicine, Tokyo Dental College, Chiba, Japan. [4]Department of Respiratory Medicine, Saitama Medical University, Saitama, Japan. [5]Division of Pulmonary Medicine, Department of Medicine, Tokai University School of Medicine, Kanagawa, Japan.

References

1. Rabe KF, Watz H. Chronic obstructive pulmonary disease. Lancet. 2017;389(10082):1931–40.
2. Barnes PJ. Inflammatory mechanisms in patients with chronic obstructive pulmonary disease. J Allergy Clin Immunol. 2016;138(1):16–27.
3. Dahl M, Vestbo J, Lange P, Bojesen SE, Tybjaerg-Hansen A, Nordestgaard BG. C-reactive protein as a predictor of prognosis in chronic obstructive pulmonary disease. Am J Respir Crit Care Med. 2007;175(3):250–5.
4. Celli BR, Locantore N, Yates J, Tal-Singer R, Miller BE, Bakke P, Calverley P, Coxson H, Crim C, Edwards LD, et al. Inflammatory biomarkers improve clinical prediction of mortality in chronic obstructive pulmonary disease. Am J Respir Crit Care Med. 2012;185(10):1065–72.
5. Mehrotra N, Freire AX, Bauer DC, Harris TB, Newman AB, Kritchevsky SB, Meibohm B, Health ABCS. Predictors of mortality in elderly subjects with obstructive airway disease: the PILE score. Ann Epidemiol. 2010;20(3):223–32.
6. Calfee CS, Ware LB, Glidden DV, Eisner MD, Parsons PE, Thompson BT, Matthay MA, National Heart B. Lung institute acute respiratory distress syndrome N: use of risk reclassification with multiple biomarkers improves mortality prediction in acute lung injury. Crit Care Med. 2011;39(4):711–7.
7. Bozinovski S, Hutchinson A, Thompson M, Macgregor L, Black J, Giannakis E, Karlsson AS, Silvestrini R, Smallwood D, Vlahos R, et al. Serum amyloid a is a biomarker of acute exacerbations of chronic obstructive pulmonary disease. Am J Respir Crit Care Med. 2008;177(3):269–78.

8. Yonchuk JG, Silverman EK, Bowler RP, Agusti A, Lomas DA, Miller BE, Tal-Singer R, Mayer RJ. Circulating soluble receptor for advanced glycation end products (sRAGE) as a biomarker of emphysema and the RAGE axis in the lung. Am J Respir Crit Care Med. 2015;192(7):785–92.
9. Tamhane UU, Aneja S, Montgomery D, Rogers EK, Eagle KA, Gurm HS. Association between admission neutrophil to lymphocyte ratio and outcomes in patients with acute coronary syndrome. Am J Cardiol. 2008;102(6):653–7.
10. Azab B, Jaglall N, Atallah JP, Lamet A, Raja-Surya V, Farah B, Lesser M, Widmann WD. Neutrophil-lymphocyte ratio as a predictor of adverse outcomes of acute pancreatitis. Pancreatology. 2011;11(4):445–52.
11. Yoon NB, Son C, Um SJ. Role of the neutrophil-lymphocyte count ratio in the differential diagnosis between pulmonary tuberculosis and bacterial community-acquired pneumonia. Ann Lab Med. 2013;33(2):105–10.
12. Taylan M, Demir M, Kaya H, Selimoglu Sen H, Abakay O, Carkanat AI, Abakay A, Tanrikulu AC, Sezgi C. Alterations of the neutrophil-lymphocyte ratio during the period of stable and acute exacerbation of chronic obstructive pulmonary disease patients. Clin Respir J. 2017;11(3):311–7.
13. Gunay E, Sarinc Ulasli S, Akar O, Ahsen A, Gunay S, Koyuncu T, Unlu M. Neutrophil-to-lymphocyte ratio in chronic obstructive pulmonary disease: a retrospective study. Inflammation. 2014;37(2):374–80.
14. Lee H, Um SJ, Kim YS, Kim DK, Jang AS, Choi HS, Kim YH, Kim TE, Yoo KH, Jung KS. Association of the neutrophil-to-lymphocyte ratio with lung function and exacerbations in patients with chronic obstructive pulmonary disease. PLoS One. 2016;11(6):e0156511.
15. Furutate R, Ishii T, Motegi T, Hattori K, Kusunoki Y, Gemma A, Kida K. The neutrophil to lymphocyte ratio is related to disease severity and exacerbation in patients with chronic obstructive pulmonary disease. Intern Med. 2016;55(3):223–9.
16. Cho KM, Park H, Oh DY, Kim TY, Lee KH, Han SW, Im SA, Kim TY, Bang YJ. Neutrophil-to-lymphocyte ratio, platelet-to-lymphocyte ratio, and their dynamic changes during chemotherapy is useful to predict a more accurate prognosis of advanced biliary tract cancer. Oncotarget. 2017;8(2):2329–41.
17. Jin F, Han A, Shi F, Kong L, Yu J. The postoperative neutrophil-to-lymphocyte ratio and changes in this ratio predict survival after the complete resection of stage I non-small cell lung cancer. Onco Targets Ther. 2016;9:6529–37.
18. Vanfleteren L, Spruit MA, Wouters EFM, Franssen FME. Management of chronic obstructive pulmonary disease beyond the lungs. Lancet Respir Med. 2016;4(11):911–24.
19. Miller J, Edwards LD, Agusti A, Bakke P, Calverley PM, Celli B, Coxson HO, Crim C, Lomas DA, Miller BE, et al. Comorbidity, systemic inflammation and outcomes in the ECLIPSE cohort. Respir Med. 2013;107(9):1376–84.
20. Miyazaki M, Nakamura H, Chubachi S, Sasaki M, Haraguchi M, Yoshida S, Tsuduki K, Shirahata T, Takahashi S, Minematsu N, et al. Analysis of comorbid factors that increase the COPD assessment test scores. Respir Res. 2014;15:13.
21. Chubachi S, Sato M, Kameyama N, Tsutsumi A, Sasaki M, Tateno H, Nakamura H, Asano K, Betsuyaku T, Keio CCRG. Identification of five clusters of comorbidities in a longitudinal Japanese chronic obstructive pulmonary disease cohort. Respir Med. 2016;117:272–9.
22. Irie H, Chubachi S, Sato M, Tsutsumi A, Nakachi I, Miyao N, Nishio K, Nakamura H, Asano K, Betsuyaku T. Characteristics of patients with increasing COPD assessment test scores within 3 years. Respir Med. 2017;131:101–8.
23. Chubachi S, Nakamura H, Sasaki M, Haraguchi M, Miyazaki M, Takahashi S, Tanaka K, Funatsu Y, Asano K, Betsuyaku T, et al. Polymorphism of LRP5 gene and emphysema severity are associated with osteoporosis in Japanese patients with or at risk for COPD. Respirology. 2015;20(2):286–95.
24. Sato M, Chubachi S, Sasaki M, Haraguchi M, Kameyama N, Tsutsumi A, Takahashi S, Nakamura H, Asano K, Betsuyaku T. Impact of mild exacerbation on COPD symptoms in a Japanese cohort. Int J Chron Obstruct Pulmon Dis. 2016;11:1269–78.
25. Parr DG, Stoel BC, Stolk J, Stockley RA. Validation of computed tomographic lung densitometry for monitoring emphysema in alpha1-antitrypsin deficiency. Thorax. 2006;61(6):485–90.
26. Jones PW, Harding G, Berry P, Wiklund I, Chen WH, Kline Leidy N. Development and first validation of the COPD Assessment Test. Eur Respir J. 2009;34(3):648–54.
27. Kwon N, Amin M, Hui DS, Jung KS, Lim SY, Ta HD, Thai TTL, Yunus F, Jones PW. Validity of the COPD assessment test translated into local languages for Asian patients. Chest. 2013;143(3):703–10.
28. Hajiro T, Nishimura K, Tsukino M, Ikeda A, Koyama H, Izumi T. Analysis of clinical methods used to evaluate dyspnea in patients with chronic obstructive pulmonary disease. Am J Respir Crit Care Med. 1998;158(4):1185–9.
29. Hajiro T, Nishimura K, Tsukino M, Ikeda A, Koyama H, Izumi T. Comparison of discriminative properties among disease-specific questionnaires for measuring health-related quality of life in patients with chronic obstructive pulmonary disease. Am J Respir Crit Care Med. 1998;157(3 Pt 1):785–90.
30. Jones PW, Quirk FH, Baveystock CM, Littlejohns P. A self-complete measure of health status for chronic airflow limitation. The St. George's Respiratory Questionnaire. Am Rev Respir Dis. 1992;145(6):1321–7.
31. Global strategy for the diagnosis, management, and prevention of chronic obstructive pulmonary disease. http://goldcopd.org/gold-2017-global-strategy-diagnosis-management-prevention-copd/. Accessed 28 Feb 2018.
32. Park CH, Han DS, Jeong JY, Eun CS, Yoo KS, Jeon YC, Sohn JH. The optimal cut-off value of neutrophil-to-lymphocyte ratio for predicting prognosis in adult patients with Henoch-Schonlein Purpura. PLoS One. 2016;11(4):e0153238.
33. Luo G, Liu C, Cheng H, Jin K, Guo M, Lu Y, Long J, Xu J, Ni Q, Chen J, et al. Neutrophil-lymphocyte ratio predicts survival in pancreatic neuroendocrine tumors. Oncol Lett. 2017;13(4):2454–8.
34. Rutgers SR, Postma DS, ten Hacken NH, Kauffman HF, van Der Mark TW, Koeter GH, Timens W. Ongoing airway inflammation in patients with COPD who do not currently smoke. Thorax. 2000;55(1):12–8.
35. Kido T, Tamagawa E, Bai N, Suda K, Yang HH, Li Y, Chiang G, Yatera K, Mukae H, Sin DD, et al. Particulate matter induces translocation of IL-6 from the lung to the systemic circulation. Am J Respir Cell Mol Biol. 2011;44(2):197–204.
36. Demedts IK, Morel-Montero A, Lebecque S, Pacheco Y, Cataldo D, Joos GF, Pauwels RA, Brusselle GG. Elevated MMP-12 protein levels in induced sputum from patients with COPD. Thorax. 2006;61(3):196–201.
37. O'Donnell RA, Peebles C, Ward JA, Daraker A, Angco G, Broberg P, Pierrou S, Lund J, Holgate ST, Davies DE, et al. Relationship between peripheral airway dysfunction, airway obstruction, and neutrophilic inflammation in COPD. Thorax. 2004;59(10):837–42.
38. Schwartz J, Weiss ST. Cigarette smoking and peripheral blood leukocyte differentials. Ann Epidemiol. 1994;4(3):236–42.
39. Patel IS, Seemungal TA, Wilks M, Lloyd-Owen SJ, Donaldson GC, Wedzicha JA. Relationship between bacterial colonisation and the frequency, character, and severity of COPD exacerbations. Thorax. 2002;57(9):759–64.
40. McNerlan SE, Alexander HD, Rea IM. Age-related reference intervals for lymphocyte subsets in whole blood of healthy individuals. Scand J Clin Lab Invest. 1999;59(2):89–92.
41. Fraker PJ, Lill-Elghanian DA. The many roles of apoptosis in immunity as modified by aging and nutritional status. J Nutr Health Aging. 2004;8(1):56–63.
42. Fabbri LM, Rabe KF. From COPD to chronic systemic inflammatory syndrome? Lancet. 2007;370(9589):797–9.
43. Bhat T, Teli S, Rijal J, Bhat H, Raza M, Khoueiry G, Meghani M, Akhtar M, Costantino T. Neutrophil to lymphocyte ratio and cardiovascular diseases: a review. Expert Rev Cardiovasc Ther. 2013;11(1):55–9.
44. Vestbo J, Hurd SS, Agusti AG, Jones PW, Vogelmeier C, Anzueto A, Barnes PJ, Fabbri LM, Martinez FJ, Nishimura M, et al. Global strategy for the diagnosis, management, and prevention of chronic obstructive pulmonary disease: GOLD executive summary. Am J Respir Crit Care Med. 2013;187(4):347–65.
45. Pavord ID, Jones PW, Burgel PR, Rabe KF. Exacerbations of COPD. Int J Chron Obstruct Pulmon Dis. 2016;11 Spec Iss:21–30.
46. Vedel-Krogh S, Nielsen SF, Lange P, Vestbo J, Nordestgaard BG. Blood eosinophils and exacerbations in chronic obstructive pulmonary disease. The Copenhagen general population study. Am J Respir Crit Care Med. 2016;193(9):965–74.
47. Pavord ID, Lettis S, Locantore N, Pascoe S, Jones PW, Wedzicha JA, Barnes NC. Blood eosinophils and inhaled corticosteroid/long-acting beta-2 agonist efficacy in COPD. Thorax. 2016;71(2):118–25.

48. Pascoe S, Locantore N, Dransfield MT, Barnes NC, Pavord ID. Blood eosinophil counts, exacerbations, and response to the addition of inhaled fluticasone furoate to vilanterol in patients with chronic obstructive pulmonary disease: a secondary analysis of data from two parallel randomised controlled trials. Lancet Respir Med. 2015;3(6):435–42.
49. Song JH, Lee CH, Kim JW, Lee WY, Jung JY, Park JH, Jung KS, Yoo KH, Park YB, Kim DK. Clinical implications of blood eosinophil count in patients with non-asthma-COPD overlap syndrome COPD. Int J Chron Obstruct Pulmon Dis. 2017;12:2455–64.
50. O'Reilly PJ, Jackson PL, Wells JM, Dransfield MT, Scanlon PD, Blalock JE. Sputum PGP is reduced by azithromycin treatment in patients with COPD and correlates with exacerbations. BMJ Open. 2013;3(12):e004140.
51. Wells JM, Jackson PL, Viera L, Bhatt SP, Gautney J, Handley G, King RW, Xu X, Gaggar A, Bailey WC, et al. A randomized, placebo-controlled trial of roflumilast. Effect on proline-glycine-proline and neutrophilic inflammation in chronic obstructive pulmonary disease. Am J Respir Crit Care Med. 2015;192(8):934–42.
52. Sorensen AK, Holmgaard DB, Mygind LH, Johansen J, Pedersen C. Neutrophil-to-lymphocyte ratio, calprotectin and YKL-40 in patients with chronic obstructive pulmonary disease: correlations and 5-year mortality - a cohort study. J Inflamm (Lond). 2015;12:20.

2

The first case of multiple pulmonary granulomas with amyloid deposition in a dental technician; a rare manifestation as an occupational lung disease

Taizou Hirano[1,2], Tadahisa Numakura[1,2*], Hiroshi Moriyama[3], Ryoko Saito[4], Yutaka Shishikura[1,2], Jun Shiihara[2,5], Hisatoshi Sugiura[1] and Masakazu Ichinose[1]

Abstract

Background: Occupational lung diseases, such as pneumoconiosis, are one of the health problems of dental workers that have been receiving increasing interest. Pulmonary amyloidosis is a heterogenous group of diseases, and can be classified into primary (idiopathic) and secondary (associated with various inflammatory diseases, hereditary, or neoplastic). To date, the development of pulmonary amyloidosis in dental workers has not been reported.

Case presentation: A 58-year-old Japanese female presented with chest discomfort and low-grade fever that has persisted for 2 months. She was a dental technician but did not regularly wear a dust mask in the workplace. Chest X ray and computed tomography revealed multiple well-defined nodules in both lungs and fluorodeoxyglucose (FDG)-positron emission tomography revealed abnormal FDG uptake in the same lesions with a maximal standardized uptake value (SUV [max]) of 5.6. We next performed thoracoscopic partial resection of the lesions in the right upper and middle lobes. The histological examination of the specimens revealed granuloma formation with foreign body-type giant cells and amyloid deposition that was confirmed by Congo red staining and direct fast scarlet (DFS) staining that produce apple-green birefringence under crossed polarized light. Because there were no other causes underlying the pulmonary amyloidosis, we performed electron probe X-ray microanalysis (EPMA) of the specimens and the result showed silica deposition in the lesions. Based on these results, we finally diagnosed the patient with pulmonary granulomas with amyloid deposition caused by chronic silica exposure. Afterward, her symptoms were improved and the disease has not progressed for 2 years since proper measures against additional occupational exposure were implemented.

Conclusions: Our case presented three important clinical insights: First, occupational exposure to silica in a dental workplace could be associated with the development of amyloid deposition in lung. Second, EPMA was useful to reveal the etiology of amyloid deposition in the lungs. Last, proper protection against silica is important to prevent further progression of the disease. In conclusion, our case suggested that occupational exposure to silica should be considered when amyloid deposition of unknown etiology is found in the lungs of working or retired adults.

Keywords: Dental technician, Amyloid deposition, Pulmonary granulomas, Silica

* Correspondence: tnumakura@rm.med.tohoku.ac.jp
[1]Department of Respiratory Medicine, Tohoku University Graduate School of Medicine, 1-1 Seiryou-machi, Aoba-ku, Sendai 980-8574, Japan
[2]Department of Respiratory Medicine, Hiraka General Hospital, Yokote, Japan
Full list of author information is available at the end of the article

Background

Occupational and environmental lung diseases are a broad group of pulmonary disorders caused by the inhalation of harmful dusts, chemicals, or proteins [1] and are one of the health problems among dental workers receiving increasing interest [2, 3]. Working with dental abrasives and polishing materials can result in chronic exposure to various harmful materials such as silica, alloys, and acrylic plastics [2–5]. Pneumoconiosis is a well-known pulmonary disease in dental workers [2–5]. Although various types of pneumoconioses have been reported [2–6], to our knowledge, the development of pulmonary amyloidosis has not been reported. Here, we describe the first reported case of a dental worker who developed multiple granulomas with amyloid deposition in the lung, which may have resulted from long-term exposure to silica in the workplace.

Case presentation

A 58-year-old Japanese woman presented with chest discomfort and low-grade fever that had persisted for 2 months. She was a dental technician but did not regularly wear a dust mask in the workplace. She previously had a smoking history of 2 pack/year and no medical history. On admission, her body temperature was 37 °C. Physical examination results were almost normal. The laboratory examinations were also normal including blood smear differentials, C-reactive protein, serological tests for autoimmune disorders and malignant and hematological disorders, and serological tests for infectious diseases (Table 1). Chest X ray and computed tomography revealed multiple well-defined nodules in both lungs (Fig. 1a and b) and fluorodeoxyglucose (FDG)-positron emission tomography revealed abnormal FDG uptake in the same lesions with a maximal standardized uptake value (SUV [max]) of 5.6 (Fig. 1c). Then, we performed thoracoscopic partial resection of the lesions in the right upper and middle lobes (Fig. 2a). Histological examination of the specimens revealed foreign body-type giant cells and mild and focal chronic inflammatory changes with the infiltration of lymphocytes and plasma cells together with eosin-positive deposits (Fig. 2b). The deposits were direct fast scarlet (DFS) staining positive and produced an apple-green birefringence under crossed polarized light (Fig. 2d and e). Congo-red staining was also positive (Fig. 2f). Based on these results, we concluded that the substance in the lesion was compatible with amyloid. Although we diagnosed the patient with pulmonary amyloidosis, there was no obvious underlying causes that could typically cause pulmonary amyloidosis, including rheumatoid arthritis, primary Sjögren's syndrome or multiple myeloma. We also excluded plasma cell neoplasm and multicentric Castleman's disease because there was no infiltration of atypical plasma cells nor formation of multicentric lymphoid follicles in the lesions. Consequently, we focused on her occupational history and performed electron probe X-ray microanalysis (EPMA) of the specimens to evaluate the cause of pulmonary amyloidosis. EPMA of the specimens revealed the deposition of silica throughout the granulomatous lesions as well as among giant cells (Fig. 2g and h). From these results, we finally diagnosed the patient with multiple lung granulomas with amyloid deposition caused by chronic silica exposure. Afterward, her symptoms improved and the disease has not progressed for 2 years since proper measures against additional occupational exposure were implemented.

Discussion and conclusions

Occupational lung diseases are caused by exposure to various toxic materials in the workplace environment. The inhaled dust particles are deposited around terminal bronchiole to their neighborhood alveoli due to their size and air speed causing lung injury and inflammation by the released oxidants, enzymes, growth factors, and other inflammatory cytokines [1]. Dental workers are exposed to various types of dusts such as silica, aluminum oxide and heavy metals when polishing and grinding prosthetics and during casting operations. Such exposure can increase the risk of occupational lung disease [2–6]. Silica, which was identified in our case, is associated with a variety of occupational lung diseases including silicosis, tuberculosis, obstructive lung disease, and lung cancer. Thus, Japan Society for Occupational Health recommends that the maximum allowable concentration (MAC) of silica is less than 0.03 mg/m^3 [7]. However, the concentration of silica in the workplace environment of dental workers sometimes exceeds the MAC. For example, one study showed that the concentration of silica in the air of the work environment of dental workers to be as high as 0.051 mg/m^3 [6]. The most common occupational lung disease caused by silica exposure is pneumoconiosis [8, 9]. Most cases develop without symptoms, whereas cough, shortness of breath and fever may develop in severe cases [8, 9]. Although various types of pneumoconioses have been reported, the development of pulmonary amyloidosis in dental workers has not been reported according to our PubMed search.

Amyloidosis is a heterogeneous group of diseases characterized by the deposition of Congo red and DFS positive amyloid fibrils in the extracellular matrix of organs such as lung [10, 11]. Radiological findings of pulmonary amyloidosis can be typically classified into several clinical types, such as showing a diffuse alveolar septal pattern, single or multiple pulmonary nodules and tracheobronchial amyloidosis [10, 11]. The diagnosis of pulmonary amyloidosis sometimes requires surgical lung biopsy to confirm the histopathological findings with Congo red staining, which produces an apple-green birefringence

Table 1 Results of laboratory examinations on admission

Blood count	
WBC	5800/μl
Neut	56.7%
Eos	3.6%
Bas	1.0%
Mo	4.9%
Ly	33.8%
RBC	430×10^4/μl
Hb	13.0 g/dl
Plt	28.4×10^4/μl
Arterial blood gas (room air)	
pH	7.427
PaO_2	94.5 Torr
$PaCO_2$	36.8 Torr
HCO_3^-	23.7 mEq/l
BE	−0.3 mEq/l
Blood chemistry	
TP	8.2 g/dl
Alb	5.0 g/dl
T-bil	0.3 mg/dl
AST	16 IU/l
ALT	16 IU/l
LDH	178 IU/l
ALP	242 IU/l
γGTP	16 IU/l
BUN	17.8 mg/dl
Cre	0.6 mg/dl
Na	143 mEq/l
K	4.0 mEq/l
Cl	108 mEq/l
Ca	9.9 mg/dl
Serum	
CRP	0.02 mg/dl
IgG	1952 mg/dl
IgA	309 mg/dl
IgM	95 mg/dl
IgG4	25 mg/dl
CEA	1.96 ng/ml
CA19-9	2.0 U/ml
ANA	x 40
Anti CCP antibody	< 0.6 U/ml
anti SS-Aantibody	negative
Anti SS-B antibody	negative
Serum amyloid A	2.9 μg/ml
s-IL-2R	412 IU/ml
β-D glucan	< 5.0 pg/ml
Cryptococcus antigen	negative
Aspergillus antigen	negative
Candida antigen	negative
T-SPOT	negative
Serum protein electrophoresis	
M protein	negative
Urine protein electrophoresis	
Bence-Jones protein	negative

Neut neutrophil, *UA* uric acid, *CRP* C-reactive protein, *CEA* carcinoembryonic antigen, *CA19-9* carbohydrate antigen 19-9, *CCP* cyclic citrullinated peptide, *s-IL-2R* soluble interluekin 2 receptor

under crossed polarized light. Pulmonary amyloidosis can be classified into primary (idiopathic) and secondary (associated with various inflammatory diseases, hereditary, or neoplastic) [9, 10]. In the present case, there was no obvious cause underlying the pulmonary amyloidosis. Therefore, taking into account the patient's occupation and the histological findings of foreign body-type giant cell granulomas in the lung, we performed EPMA for further evaluation.

EPMA with a wavelength dispersive spectrometer (WDS) is a method of mineralogical analysis that can qualitatively and semi-quantitatively analyze the chemical composition of solid materials found in human tissue histology [12]. Takada et al. analyzed 162 cases of suspected occupational and environmental lung diseases by EPMA-WDS, and concluded that EMPA-WDS was useful to confirm the causes of various occupational and environmental lung diseases [12]. Although it is unknown whether the inhaled silica was a direct cause of the pulmonary amyloidosis, our histological as well as EPMA findings (Fig. 2) suggest that the chronic exposure to silica in a dental office could be associated with chronic inflammation, resulting in the development of amyloid deposition in the lung. Furthermore, a recent scientific report demonstrating that exposure to silica could increase the production of Congo-philic amyloid deposition in *C. elegans* also supported our findings [13]. Because there is no proven specific treatment for such patients, clarifying the occupational cause is key to prevention with effective occupational safety measures, such as good ventilation in the laboratory and personal protective devices, to avoid further progression of the disease.

In summary, we report the first case of a dental worker who developed multiple granulomas with amyloid deposition in the lungs likely caused by silica exposure in the workplace. Our case presented three important clinical insights: First, chronic exposure to silica in dental workplace could be associated with the development of amyloid deposition in lung. Second, EPMA was useful

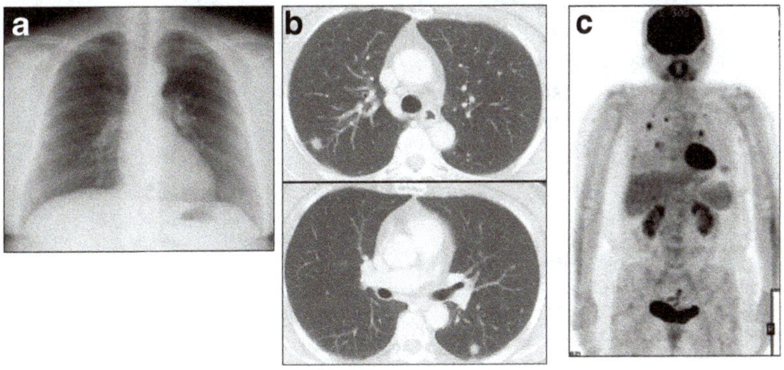

Fig. 1 a, b Chest X ray (**a**) and chest computed tomography on admission (**b**) revealed multiple well-defined nodules in both lungs. **c** Fluorodeoxyglucose (FDG)-positron emission tomography revealed abnormal FDG uptake in the same lesions with a maximal standardized uptake value (SUV [max]) of 5.6

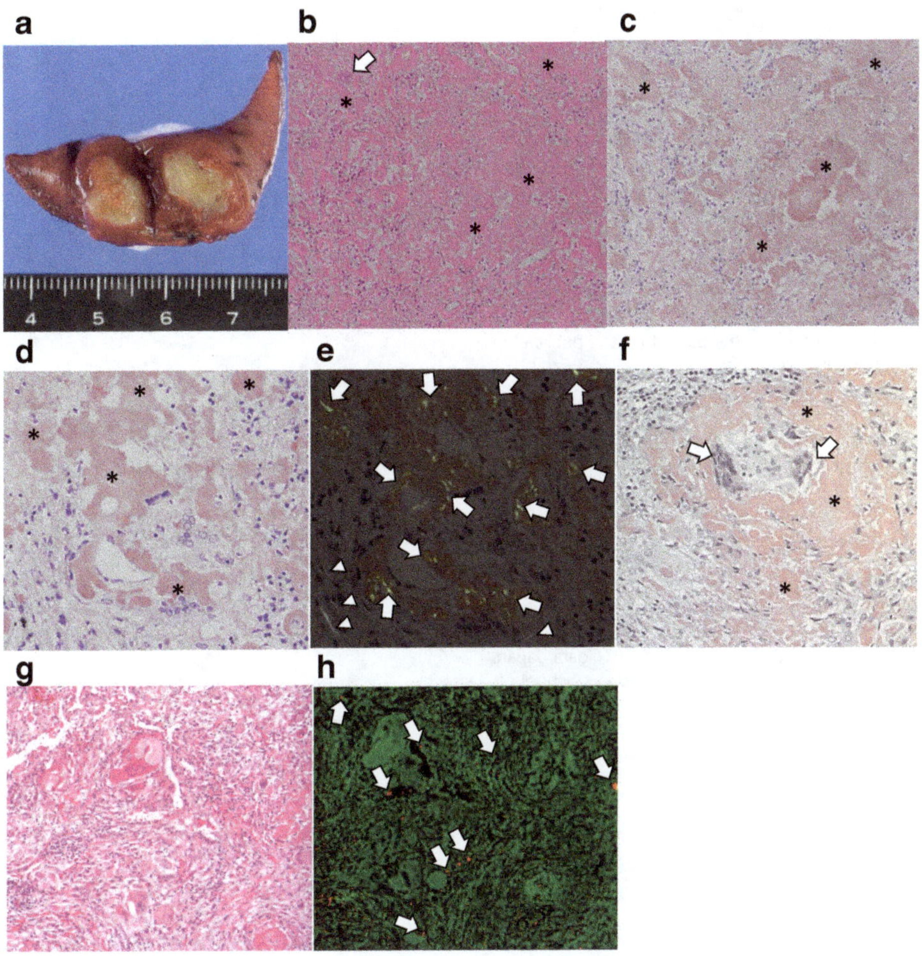

Fig. 2 Histopathological findings of the lung nodules. **a** Macroscopic examination of a white hard nodule in the right middle lobe. **b** Low-magnification image of a hematoxylin and eosin (HE) stained specimen revealed granuloma formation with foreign body-type giant cells (arrow) and mild and focal chronic inflammatory changes with eosin-positive deposits (asterisk). **c** and **d** The images of direct fast scarlet (DFS) staining revealed that the deposits were DFS positive (asterisk) (**c**, at lower-magnification, and **d**, at higher-magnification). **e** The DFS staining-positive lesions produced an apple-green birefringence under crossed polarized light (arrows) (× 100). The collagen fibrils appeared white (arrow heads). **f** The deposits were Congo red positive (asterisk). Foreign body-type giant cells were detected (arrows) (× 100). **g** and **h** A representative photograph of HE stained specimen (**g**) and its image of electron probe X-ray microanalysis (EPMA) (**h**). A two-dimension EPMA-wavelength dispersive spectrometer (WDS) image of an elemental map corresponding to the area shown in (**h**), showing orange dots indicating silica (Si) accumulated in giant cells (arrows). The distribution of amino nitrogen was colored green (**h**)

to reveal the unknown etiology of amyloid deposition in lung. Last, proper protection against silica is important to prevent further progression of the disease. In conclusion, occupational exposure to silica should be considered when amyloid deposition of unknown etiology is found in the lungs of working or retired adults.

Abbreviations

EPMA: Electron probe X-ray microanalysis; FDG-PET: Fluorodeoxyglucose (FDG)-positron emission tomography (PET); HE: Hematoxylin and eosin; MAC: Maximum allowable concentrations; SUV [max]: Maximal standardized uptake value; WDS: Wavelength dispersive spectrometer

Acknowledgements

We very much appreciate Mr. Brent K. Bell for critical reading of the manuscript.

Funding

This work was funded by the Japan Society for the Promotion of Science (grant number; 17H04180, 16 K15453).

Authors' contributions

TH, TN, YS, JS, HS and MI performed clinical, functional and laboratory assessments. HM performed the EMS analysis. RS performed and interpreted the histopathological examinations. All authors significantly contributed to the data interpretation and manuscript preparation. All authors read and approved the final manuscript.

Consent for publication

Written informed consent was obtained from the patient for the publication of this case report and all accompanying images.

Competing interests

The authors declare that they have no competing interests.

Author details

[1]Department of Respiratory Medicine, Tohoku University Graduate School of Medicine, 1-1 Seiryou-machi, Aoba-ku, Sendai 980-8574, Japan. [2]Department of Respiratory Medicine, Hiraka General Hospital, Yokote, Japan. [3]Department of Respiratory Medicine, Nishi-Niigata Chuo National Hospital, Niigata, Japan. [4]Department of Anatomic Pathology, Tohoku University Graduate School of Medicine, Sendai, Japan. [5]Department of Respiratory Medicine, Saitama Medical Center Jichi Medical University, Saitama, Japan.

References

1. William SB. Occupational respiratory diseases. New Engl J Med. 2000;342: 406–13.
2. Malhotra P, Sarkar PK, Sriram PS. An 84-year-old man with acute dyspnea and chronic radiographic findings. Chest. 2013;144:1076–9.
3. Kuehn B. Dentists at risk of lung disease? JAMA. 2018;319(16):1650. https://doi.org/10.1001/jama.2018.4585.
4. Ardekani A, Ayatollahi J, Ayatollahi F, Bahrololoomi R, Ayatollahi J, Ayatollahi A, et al. Occupational hazards to dental staff. Dent Res J (Isfahan). 2012;9:2–7.
5. Orriol R, Ferrer J, Tura JM, Xaus C, Coloma R. Sicca syndrome and silicoproteinosis in a dental technician. Eur Respir J. 1997;10:731–4.
6. Torbica N, Krstev S. World at work: dental laboratory technicians. Occup Envirion Med. 2006;63:145–8.
7. The Japan Society for Occupational Health. Recommendation of occupational health limits (2013-2014). J Occup Health. 2013;55:422–41.
8. Greenberg MI, Waksman J, Curtis J. Silicosis: a review. Dis Mon. 2007;53:394–416.
9. Leung CC, Yu IT, Chen W. Silicosis. Lancet. 2012;26:2008–18.
10. Khoor A, Colby TV. Amyloidosis of the lung. Arch Pathol Lab Med. 2017;141: 247–54.
11. Gillmore JD, Hawkins PN. Amyloidosis and the respiratory tract. Thorax. 1999;54:444–51.
12. Takada T, Moriyama H, Suzuki E. Elemental analysis of occupational and environmental lung diseases by electron probe microanalyzer with wavelength dispersive spectrometer. RespirInvestig. 2014;52:5–13.
13. Scharf A, Gührs K-H, von Mikecz A. Anti-amyloid compounds protect from silica nanoparticle-induced neurotoxicity in the nematode *C. elegans*. Nanotoxicology. 2016;10:426–35.

3

Mixed pneumonic plague and nosocomial MDR-bacterial infection of lung

Voahangy Andrianaivoarimanana[1], Eric Bertherat[2], Rojo Rajaonarison[3], Tiana Rakotondramaro[4], Christophe Rogier[5,6] and Minoarisoa Rajerison[1*]

Abstract

Background: Plague is a life-threatening disease caused by the bacterium, *Yersinia pestis*. Madagascar is the leading country for human plague cases worldwide. Human plague is a serious disease, particularly in its septicaemic and pneumonic forms. We report a case of pneumonic plague co-infected by a MDR-*Stenotrophomonas maltophilia*.

Case presentation: A 24 year-old man originated from Soavinandriana, a plague focus, felt uneasy and developed high fever with chills. He started treatment by himself, by private medical care and by a traditional healer for nine days moving several times from place to place. His condition had deteriorated when he presented to a district hospital with a syndrome of dyspnea, bronchial rale and altered state of consciousness. Two days later, plague diagnosis, performed as a last resort, revealed a positive F1 antigen on rapid diagnostic test. Additional tests (pla PCR and plague serology) evidenced a *Y. pestis* infection. However, streptomycin treatment did not achieve a complete recovery as the course of disease was complicated by the presence of MDR-*S. maltophilia* in his lung. This opportunistic infection could have been favored by an immunosuppression due to *Y. pestis* pulmonary infection and probably been acquired during his stay at a District Hospital. He was treated with a combination of ciprofloxacin and gentamycin and recovered fully.

Conclusions: Pneumonic plague infection may promote another virulent or avirulent bacterial infection particularly when it is not initially suspected. However, coinfection is rarely described and its occurrence frequency is unknown. In middle or low resources areas, which is the case of most plague endemic countries, control and prevention of infections in health facilities is not optimal. Co-infection with an opportunistic pathogen agent, such as *S. maltophilia*, is a risk which must not be disregarded as demonstrated by this case report. When deciding of a national control strategy, it should be taken into account in the choice of the first line treatment.

Keywords: *Yersinia pestis*, *Stenotrophomonas maltophilia*, Pneumonia, Madagascar

Background

Plague is a rapidly progressing disease in humans caused by the bacterium, *Yersinia pestis* [1]. Transmission of bubonic plague to human occurs after the bite of an infectious flea. Less frequently, infection may also occur by inhalation of infectious respiratory droplets spread from a patient suffering from pneumonic plague. In that case, the fatality rate is almost 100% if the patient is left untreated. Pneumonic plague severity is due to *Y. pestis* ability to evade the host immune system and also to the rapid establishment, by *Y. pestis* infection, of a permissive environment for microbial proliferation in the lung [2]. According to the World Health Organization (WHO), 3248 cases of human plague have been reported between 2010 and 2015 by 11 countries from Africa, the Americas and Asia. During this period, Madagascar accounted for 74% of all cases reported worldwide with 18% of case fatality rate, making this island the most affected country in the world [3]. Since its introduction in Madagascar in 1898, plague is endemic within a large

* Correspondence: mino@pasteur.mg
[1]Plague Unit- Institut Pasteur de Madagascar, BP1274 Ambatofotsikely, 101 Antananarivo, Madagascar
Full list of author information is available at the end of the article

area in the central and in the northern highlands above 800 m in elevation [4]. Although plague is mainly a rural disease, some sporadic cases may occur particularly in the urban setting [5]. In Madagascar, methods for plague diagnosis includes F1 antigen RDT, serology, bacteriological culture on selective media at 26–28 °C, and *Y. pestis* identification by biochemical profile using API20E kit and by bacteriophage lysis test [3]. Antibiotics susceptibility of each isolated strain is surveyed. Molecular biology is not used routinely. As per the Plague National Control Program (PNCP), specific treatment of pneumonic plague requires streptomycin injection during 8 days. However, this therapeutic strategy may fail in presence of MDR- *Y. pestis* [6] or mixed infection involving other MDR-pathogen. Here, we describe the features and medical history of a case of pneumonic plague complicated by a MDR-*Stenotrophomonas maltophilia* co-infection in a patient who travelled in different locations before reaching the capital Antananarivo as well as the case-management. *S. maltophilia* is an aerobic gram-negative bacillus which is an opportunistic and nosocomial pathogen causing blood-stream infections and pneumonia with considerable morbidity in immunocompromised patients [7, 8].

Case presentation

On December 30, 2013, a 24 year-old man developed high fever with chills and took self-medication of trimethoprim-sulfamethoxazole (2x80mg-2x400mg respectively) and antipyretic [9]. Later the same day, he sought private medical care and received antimalarial treatment (3 quinine injections). Two days earlier, he transported on his motorcycle a sick person who died later for unknown reasons. He lived in the village of Ambohimanana within the District of Soavinandriana (Fig. 1, Site 1), one of the plague foci of the central highlands of Madagascar. In the absence of improvement, he visited a traditional healer at Andoharanokely- Faratsiho (Fig. 1, Site 2) on December 31, and received herbal medicines and massage for 5 days. His condition continued to decline with severe asthenia and fever. The traditional healer authorized him to get a treatment by modern medicine. On January 7, 2014, an agent of a first-level health center (Fig. 1, Site 2) gave him primary

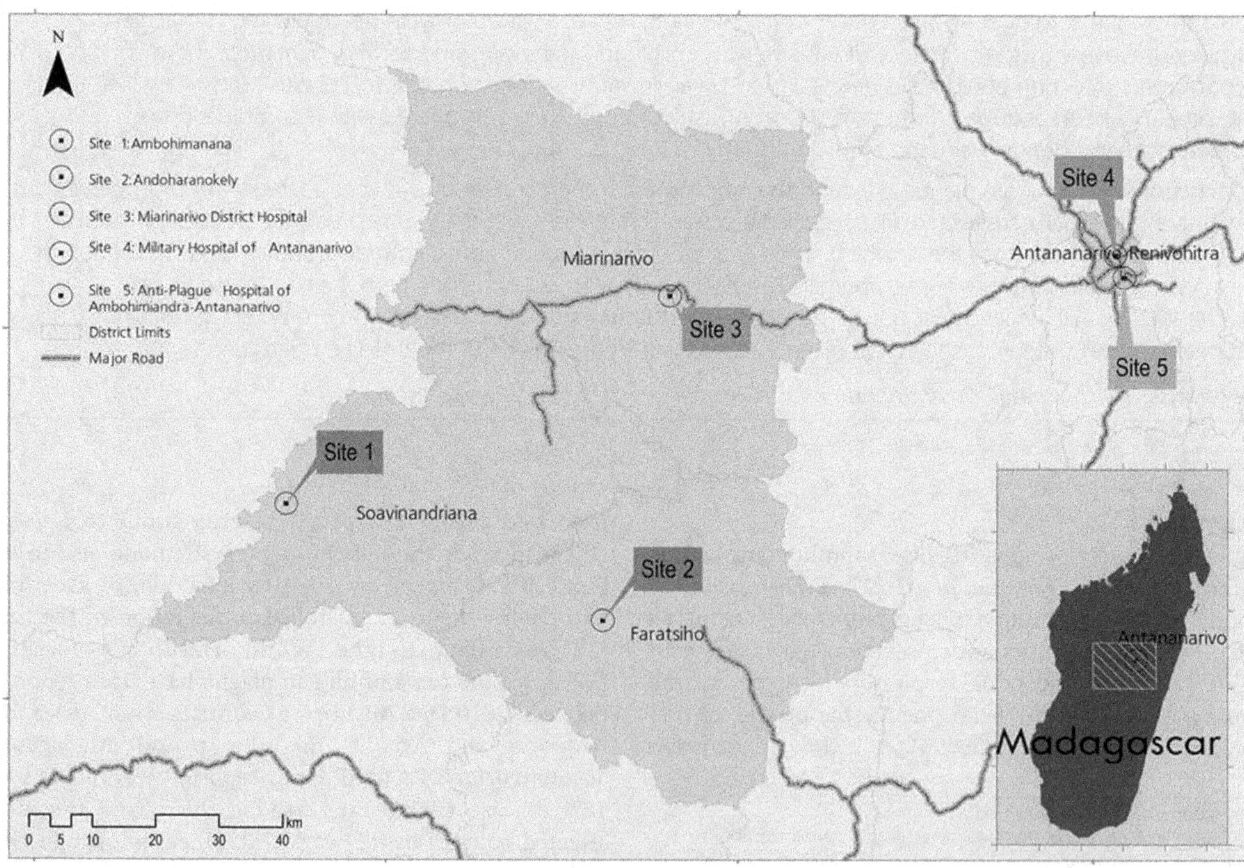

Fig. 1 Map emphasizing on the patient's itinerary. Site 1 Ambohimanana-Soavinandriana: patient's village; Site 2 Andoharanokely-Faratsiho: Traditional healer's village; Site 3 Miarinarivo District Hospital; Site 4 Military Hospital of Antananarivo; Site 5 Anti-Plague Hospital of Ambohimiandra-Antananarivo

available treatment (betalactam, antipyretic, bronchodilator and a prokinetic agent) and evacuated him to Miarinarivo District Hospital (MDH) (Fig. 1, Site 3) for a syndrome of dyspnea, bronchial rale and altered state of consciousness. On his admission to MDH on January 8, 2014, he had a temperature of 39.5 °C and a heart rate of 120 b/min. The chest radiograph showed right pleural effusion and left radio-opacities of the lower lobe (Fig. 2a). Rapid diagnostic test (RDT) for malaria and Widal-Felix serology for typhoid fever were both negative. Acid-fast bacilli from two sputa cultures were also negative. Therefore, he was treated for pneumonia with ceftriaxone (1 g) intravenously (IV).

Considering the fact that he was living in a known plague region, RDT for *Y. pestis* F1 antigen [10] was performed on sputum as a differential diagnosis the next day and was markedly positive, suggesting a pneumonic plague infection. Intramuscular streptomycin treatment was immediately initiated after the diagnosis according to the PNCP of the Malagasy Ministry of Health: 0,5 g every 3 h for 2 days followed by 0,5 g every 4 h for 2 days and 1 g twice a day for 4 days. This sputum sample was sent to the Central Laboratory for Plague at Institut Pasteur de Madagascar for bacteriological confirmation [11] but did not yield *Y. pestis* strain; instead *Citrobacter freundii* was identified. After completing an 8-day course of streptomycin treatment, the patient's condition remained stable without signs of recovery. Therefore, on January 17, 2014, he was discharged from the hospital by his family against medical advice and sought treatment at the Military Hospital of Antananarivo (MHA) (Fig. 1, Site 4). On his admission at MHA on January 18, 2014 at 11:30 a.m., a second chest radiograph revealed an enlargement of left opacities and appearance of right nodular opacity, but a decrease of right pleural effusion (Fig. 2b). His status has still altered and marked with asthenia, anorexia, weight loss, greyish complexion, colored conjunctiva with a temperature of 38.5 °C. During physical examination, he had a cough with purulent sputum associated with a mean abundance of hemoptysis, dyspnea, bilateral crackles and breath-sounds rales. The examination of lymph nodes was normal. Biological analysis showed a rise in the level of C-reactive protein (12 mg/ml) revealing an inflammatory syndrome. In addition, the second sputum sample collected remained positive for *Y. pestis* F1 antigen. In order to limit exposure to the disease, the patient was transferred to the Anti-Plague Hospital of Ambohimiandra-Antananarivo (APHAA) (Fig. 1, Site 5) the same day at 01:00 p.m. Once admitted, he was isolated in an individual room. Given the positive result of *Y. pestis* F1 antigen and the absence of patient's health improvement, another therapeutic scheme was initiated and consisted of a combination of IV ciprofloxacin (400 to 600 mg twice per day for 6 days) and IV gentamycin (3 mg/kg per day, for 6 days). Bacteriological culture of the second sputum sample also failed to isolate *Y. pestis*, however growing colonies on cefsulodin-irgasan-novobiocin medium were identified as *S. maltophilia* on API20E biochemical strip. Antibiotic susceptibility test using a disk diffusion method as per the Clinical and Laboratory Standards Institute guidelines showed that *S. maltophilia* isolate was sensitive to trimethoprim-sulfamethoxazole, ciprofloxacin and chloramphenicol, but was resistant to tetracycline, streptomycin, gentamycin and ampicillin. Strain *Escherichia coli* ATCC®25,922 was used as control. Moreover, plague ELISA serology testing in paired serum samples (Ethical Committee authorization 068- MSANPE of July 29, 2011) performed at a 7-day interval showed a three-fold rise in anti-F1 immunoglobulin G titer [12] and PCR test targeting *Y. pestis* plasminogen activator (pla) gene [13] was positive on all sputum samples.

The suggested bi-therapy treatment led to the patient's condition improvement and recovery. Upon discharge, on January 27, 2014, his third chest X-ray demonstrated a decrease of right opacity and left pleural effusion (Fig. 2c).

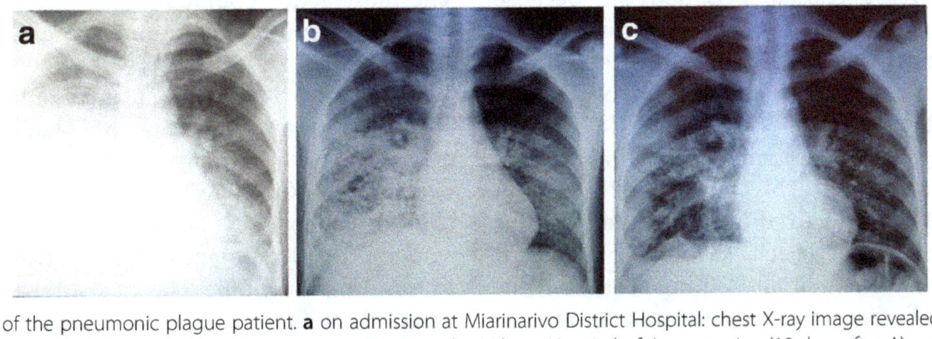

Fig. 2 Chest X-ray of the pneumonic plague patient. **a** on admission at Miarinarivo District Hospital: chest X-ray image revealed right pleural effusion and radio-opacities of left lower lobe, (**b**) On presentation to the Military Hospital of Antananarivo (10 days after A): enlargement of left opacities and appearance of right nodular opacity, decrease of right pleural effusion, and (**c**) Upon discharge at Anti-plague Hospital of Ambohimiandra- Antananarivo (9 days after B), decrease of right opacity and left pleural effusion

Discussion

Madagascar is one of the most active plague regions in the world and was the origin of a natural multi-drug resistant strain of *Y. pestis* [6]. Incidence has declined in the last 2 years but there has been an increase in the overall case-fatality rate (23% in 2015) associated with the high frequency of pneumonic form (23.3%) [3]. Within 24–36 h after the onset of symptoms, pneumonic plague progresses to an irreversible and lethal syndrome that cannot be effectively treated [14]. Indeed, most pneumonic plague patients succumb in less than 3 days without prompt and adequate treatment. For the present case, which is most likely a primary pneumonic infection, the early doses of trimethoprime-sulfamethoxazole self-administered might have induced a latent phase in pneumonic plague infection, a delayed infection course which allowed the patient to survive despite a delay of plague treatment. It was demonstrated that the most common indications for self-medication were pain, fever and cough [9]. In addition, antibiotic medication rapidly clears the sputum of plague bacilli, so that a patient is generally not infective within hours after initiation of effective antibiotic treatment [15]. In this report, clinical presentation and epidemiological evidence (residence in a plague endemic area) are consistent with a pneumonic plague infection. Additionally, laboratory results met the criterion of the WHO standard case definition for a "Confirmed plague case" [5]. It is noteworthy that F1 antigen is specific to *Y. pestis* [16], temperature-stable and is excreted in large amount in samples from plague infected people [10]. The failure of *Y. pestis* isolation by bacterial culture is not uncommon if antibiotic treatment was administered before sampling [17, 18]. Positive results of F1 antigen RDT on all sputum samples showed that *Y. pestis* F1 antigen could persist and be detected several days after the beginning of treatment, when the plague bacillus is no longer viable [10, 17, 19]; for this case, F1 antigen persisted for 10 days after the beginning of treatment and 20 days after disease onset. Due to the failure of the culture, sensitivity of *Y. pestis* to streptomycin was not tested; however a resistance is doubtful because the patient would have likely succumbed to pneumonic plague infection if the complete streptomycin treatment was not effective. The isolation of MDR-*S. maltophilia* from his sputum collected at MDH suggested that the patient had a mixed infection with *Y. pestis* and *S. maltophilia.* This nosocomial infection has probably been acquired during his stay at this hospital and may have been favored by patient immunocompromised condition. Without other medical information, his immune response maybe attenuated by the course of his disease or by malnutrition with a notable weight loss. However, it has been shown that pulmonary infection by *Y. pestis* may establish a permissive environment for proliferation of usually nonpathogenic bacteria [2]. In middle or low resources areas, which is the case of most plague endemic countries, control and prevention of infections in health facilities is not optimal. Co-infection with an opportunistic pathogen agent is a risk which must not be disregarded. Indeed, *S. maltophilia* is an important emergent opportunistic pathogen, causing lung colonization or pulmonary infections among immunosuppressed patients. According to available clinical information, distinction between *S. maltophilia* colonization and infection can be confusing [20]. His chest X-ray, 10 days after MDH admission, showed right nodular opacity (Fig. 2b) and might be evocative of *S. maltophilia* colonization or infection of a severely impaired host [21, 22].

S. maltophilia infection/colonization management is often problematic due to its inherent resistance to multiple broad-spectrum antibiotic agents [21]. Thus, for the presenting case, the initial streptomycin treatment was effective for *Y. pestis* infection but not for *S. maltophilia*. The use of ciprofloxacin in secondary bi-therapy allowed the recovery of the patient and this antibiotic is also recommended as an alternative treatment for *S. maltophilia* infection [23]. Indeed, recent study also supported the broader use of oral ciprofloxacin for treatment of human plague including pneumonic form. Its bactericidal activity is comparable to that of streptomycin, and its mode of administration is less restrictive; more acceptable for exposed population [24]. In addition, a wide range of antibiotics was already in vitro tested for their susceptibility to geographically diverse strains of *Y. pestis* which provide alternatives for plague treatment [25]. Another study had also investigated the susceptibility patterns of *Y. pestis* strains from diverse sources to 12 antimicrobial agents and showed that a large panel of *Y. pestis* remained susceptible not only to drugs traditionally used to treat plague (streptomycin, doxycycline and chloramphenicol), but also to newer agents (broad-spectrum cephalosporins and quinolones). The most active compounds against *Y. pestis* included ceftriaxone and trimethoprim-sulfamethoxazole, quinolones [26].

The severe pneumonic plague outbreak which occurred in urban context in Madagascar recently [27] questioned the pertinence of maintaining streptomycin as the first line treatment. The challenge of the clinical diagnosis in the context of an urban outbreak associated to the intense circulation of other potential causes of pneumonia could justify the choice of an antibiotic with a broader spectrum. This case report suggests that the possibility of mixed infection, especially in a nosocomial context, must be part of this strategic discussion.

To date, coinfection involving pneumonic plague and other pulmonary infections has been rarely described. Indeed, Quan et al. reported the recovery of *Y. pestis* and other respiratory pathogens from mammals and ectoparasites but not in human during plague investigations [28]. However in 2004, two cases of confirmed infection for plague and leptospirosis have been observed in the Democratic Republic of Congo, both of which can cause severe pulmonary manifestations [29]. To our knowledge, this study is the first describing a co-infection with *Y. pestis* and *S. maltophilia* in Madagascar and emphasizes on the complicated management of such pneumonic infections.

Conclusion

In conclusion, although mixed infection of lung with *Y. pestis* and *S. maltophilia* is rare, a combined therapy should be discussed when the condition of a plague patient does not improve under an appropriate treatment with streptomycin. The availability of plague alternative treatments is also crucial to improve the patient's outcome and need to be implemented in the PNCP of the Malagasy Ministry of Health thus a new plague therapeutic scheme is currently under evaluation.

This situation has been considered to be an important alert and allowed the establishment of a contingency plan to counteract plague epidemics, particularly the occurrence of the pneumonic form in urban areas where the transmission risk at national and international levels is high.

Abbreviations

APHAA: Anti-Plague Hospital of Ambohimiandra-Antananarivo; MDH: Miarinarivo District Hospital; MHA: Military Hospital of Antananarivo; PNCP: Plague National Control Program

Acknowledgements

We thank all the health workers involved in the care of this patient, the staff of the Plague Unit for technical assistance, and Dr. Tendro Tondrasoa Ramaharitra for the patient's itinerary mapping. Sincere thanks to Prof. Michel Simonet for critical review of the manuscript.

Funding

This work was supported by the Institut Pasteur de Madagascar. There was no role of the funding body in the writing of the manuscript.

Authors' contributions

VA analyzed clinical data, literature search, wrote the manuscript, EB provided advice on the management of the event and reviewed the manuscript, RR and TR collected and interpreted data, CR provided advice on the management of the event, literature search, reviewed the manuscript, MR analyzed clinical data, investigated the case and wrote the manuscript. All authors read and approved the final version of the report.

Consent for publication

Written informed consent was obtained from the patient for publication of this Case report and any accompanying images. A copy of the signed consent is available to the Editors on request.

Competing interests

The authors declare that they have no competing interests.

Author details

[1]Plague Unit- Institut Pasteur de Madagascar, BP1274 Ambatofotsikely, 101 Antananarivo, Madagascar. [2]Department of Infectious Hazard Management, World Health Organization, Avenue Appia 20, CH-1211, 27 Geneva, Switzerland. [3]Centre Hospitalier Anti-pesteux d'Ambohimiandra, 101 Antananarivo, Madagascar. [4]Centre Hospitalier de District de Miarinarivo, Antananarivo, Madagascar. [5]Institut Pasteur de Madagascar, BP1274 Ambatofotsikely, 101 Antananarivo, Madagascar. [6]Present address: Service de Santé des Armées, Direction Centrale, Division Expertise et Stratégie Santé de Défense, 60 Boulevard du Général Martial Valin – CS21623, 75509 Paris Cedex 15, France.

References

1. Stenseth NC, Atshabar BB, Begon M, Belmain SR, Bertherat E, Carniel E, et al. Plague: past, present, and future. PLoS Med. 2008;5:e3.
2. Price PA, Jin J, Goldman WE. Pulmonary infection by *Yersinia pestis* rapidly establishes a permissive environment for microbial proliferation. Proc Natl Acad Sci U S A. 2012;109:3083–8.
3. World Health Organization. Plague around the world, 2010–2015. Wkly Epidemiol Rec. 2016;91:89–93.
4. Brygoo ER. Epidemiologie de la peste à Madagascar. Arch Inst Pasteur Madagascar. 1966;35:9–147.
5. World Health Organization. International meeting on preventing and controlling plague: the old calamity still has a future. Wkly Epidemiol Rec. 2006;81:278–84.
6. Galimand M, Guiyoule A, Gerbaud G, Rasoamanana B, Chanteau S, Carniel E, et al. Multidrug resistance in *Yersinia pestis* mediated by a transferable plasmid. N Engl J Med. 1997;337:677–80.
7. Khardori N, Elting L, Wong E, Schable B, Bodey GP. Nosocomial infections due to *Xanthomonas maltophilia* (*Pseudomonas maltophilia*) in patients with cancer. Rev Infect Dis. 1990;12:997–1003.
8. Looney WJ, Narita M, Mühlemann K. *Stenotrophomonas maltophilia*: an emerging opportunist human pathogen. Lancet Infect Dis. 2009;9:312–23.
9. Sendrasoa FA, Razanakoto NH, Ranaivo IM, Andrianasolo RL, Randria MJDD, Antibiotic RRA. Antimalarial Selfmedication in Antananarivo, Madagascar. Int J Infect Dis Ther. 2016;1:1–5.
10. Chanteau S, Rahalison L, Ralafiarisoa L, Foulon J, Ratsitorahina M, Ratsifasoamanana L, et al. Development and testing of a rapid diagnostic test for bubonic and pneumonic plague. Lancet. 2003;361:211–6.
11. Rasoamanana B, Rahalison L, Raharimanana C, Chanteau S. Comparison of Yersinia CIN agar and mouse inoculation assay for the diagnosis of plague. Trans R Soc Trop Med Hyg. 1996;90:651.
12. Rasoamanana B, Leroy F, Boisier P, Rasolomaharo M, Buchy P, Carniel E, et al. Field evaluation of an immunoglobulin G anti-F1 enzyme-linked immunosorbent assay for serodiagnosis of human plague in Madagascar. Clin Diagn Lab Immunol. 1997;4:587–91.
13. Hinnebusch J, Schwan TG. New method for plague surveillance using polymerase chain reaction to detect Yersinia pestis in fleas. J Clin Microbiol. 1993;31:1511–4.
14. Pechous RD, Sivaraman V, Stasulli NM, Goldman WE. Pneumonic plague: the darker side of Yersinia pestis. Trends Microbiol. 2016;24:190–7.
15. Butler TC. Plague and other Yersinia infections. In: Greenough WB, editor. Current topics in infectious disease. New York: Plenum Medical Book Company; 1983.
16. Perry RD, Fetherston JD. *Yersinia pestis*–etiologic agent of plague. Clin Microbiol Rev. 1997;10:35–66.

17. Bertherat E, Thullier P, Shako JC, England K, Koné ML, Arntzen L, et al. Lessons learned about pneumonic plague diagnosis from two outbreaks, Democratic Republic of the Congo. Emerg Infect Dis. 2011;17:778–84.
18. Begier EM, Asiki G, Anywaine Z, Yockey B, Schriefer ME, Aleti P, et al. Pneumonic plague cluster, Uganda, 2004. Emerg Infect Dis. 2006;12:460–7.
19. Ratsitorahina M, Chanteau S, Rahalison L, Ratsifasoamanana L, Boisier P. Epidemiological and diagnostic aspects of the outbreak of pneumonic plague in Madagascar. Lancet. 2000;355:111–3.
20. Nicodemo AC, Garcia Paez JI. Antimicrobial therapy for *Stenotrophomonas maltophilia* infections. Eur J Clin Microbiol Infect Dis. 2007;26:229–37.
21. Fujita J, Yamadori I, Xu G, et al. Clinical features of *Stenotrophomonas maltophilia* pneumonia in immunocompromised patients. Respir Med. 1996; 90:35–8.
22. Pathmanathan A, Waterer GW. Significance of positive *Stenotrophomonas maltophilia* culture in acute respiratory tract infection. EurRespir J. 2005;25: 911–4.
23. Samonis G, Karageorgopoulos DE, Maraki S, Levis P, Dimopoulou D, Spernovasilis NA, et al. *Stenotrophomonas maltophilia* infections in a general hospital: patient characteristics, antimicrobial susceptibility, and treatment outcome. PLoS One. 2012;7:e37375.
24. Apangu T, Griffith K, Abaru J, Candini G, Apio H, Okoth F, et al. Successful treatment of human plague with oral ciprofloxacin. Emerg Infect Dis. 2017; 23(3):553–55.
25. Heine HS, Hershfield J, Marchand C, Miller L, Halasohoris S, Purcell BK, et al. In vitro antibiotic susceptibilities of Yersinia pestis determined by broth microdilution following CLSI methods. Antimicrob Agents Chemother. 2015; 59:1919–21.
26. Wong JD, Barash JR, Sandfort RF, Janda JM. Susceptibilities of *Yersinia pestis* strains to 12 antimicrobial agents. Antimicrob Agents Chemother. 2000;44: 1995–6.
27. Roberts L. Echoes of Ebola as plague hits Madagascar. Science. 2017;358:430–1.
28. Quan TJ, Tsuchiya KR, Carter LG. Isolation of pathogens other than *Yersinia pestis* during plague investigations. J Wildl Dis. 1979;15:505–10.
29. Bertherat E, Mueller MJ, Shako JC, Picardeau M. Discovery of a leptospirosis cluster amidst a pneumonic plague outbreak in a miners' camp in the Democratic Republic of the Congo. Int J Environ Res Public Health. 2014;11: 1824–33.

Heparin-binding protein in sputum as a marker of pulmonary inflammation, lung function, and bacterial load in children with cystic fibrosis

Gisela Hovold[1], Victoria Palmcrantz[2], Fredrik Kahn[1], Arne Egesten[3] and Lisa I. Påhlman[1*]

Abstract

Background: Cystic fibrosis (CF) is associated with bacterial pulmonary infections and neutrophil-dominated inflammation in the airways. The aim of this study was to evaluate the neutrophil-derived protein Heparin-binding protein (HBP) as a potential sputum marker of airway inflammation and bacterial load.

Methods: Nineteen CF patients, aged 6–18 years, were prospectively followed for 6 months with sputum sampling at every visit to the CF clinic. A total of 41 sputum samples were collected. Sputum-HBP was analysed with ELISA, neutrophil elastase activity with a chromogenic assay, and total bacterial load with RT-PCR of the 16 s rDNA gene. Data were compared to lung function parameters and airway symptoms.

Results: HBP and elastase correlated to a decrease in FEV_1%predicted compared to the patients´ individual baseline pulmonary function (ΔFEV_1), but not to bacterial load. Area under the receiver operating characteristic curve values for the detection of > 10% decrease in ΔFEV_1 were 0.80 for HBP, 0.78 for elastase, and 0.54 for bacterial load.

Conclusions: Sputum HBP is a promising marker of airway inflammation and pulmonary function in children with CF.

Keywords: Cystic fibrosis, Sputum, Inflammation, Airway infection, Lung function, Children

Background

Cystic fibrosis (CF) is associated with persistent bacterial infection and neutrophil-dominated inflammation in the respiratory tract [1]. Several bacterial species cause airway infection in CF, for example *Staphylococcus aureus,* Non-typable *Haemophilus influenzae* (Nt*Hi*), *Burkholderia cepacia complex,* and *Pseudomonas aeruginosa,* and it is well described that exacerbations contribute to the progressive lung destruction and pulmonary function decline that is a hallmark of CF [2, 3]. Many bacterial species show increasing resistance to antibiotics, and there is therefore a need for robust biomarkers to monitor airway inflammation and infection. Such biomarkers could prevent unnecessary use of antibiotics that promote development of bacterial resistance.

Heparin-binding protein (HBP) is stored in the secretory and azurophilic granules of neutrophils, and is released upon cell activation [4]. HBP is a multi-functional pro-inflammatory mediator that for example activates immune cells, has broad antibacterial activity, and induces vascular leakage [5, 6]. Plasma HBP has been described as a promising predictor of the progression into severe sepsis and septic shock [7]. HBP levels also increase in cerebrospinal fluid during bacterial meningitis [8] and in urine during urinary tract infection [9], suggesting its use as a biomarker indicating bacterial infection. Recently, HBP was described as a useful biomarker in broncho-alveolar lavage fluid for the detection of pulmonary infection in lung transplant recipients [10].

The aim of the present study was to evaluate if HBP levels in sputum from children with CF can be used as a

* Correspondence: Lisa.Pahlman@med.lu.se
[1]Department of Clinical Sciences Lund, Division of Infection Medicine, BMC B14, Lund University, Skåne University Hospital, Tornavägen 10, SE-22184 Lund, Sweden
Full list of author information is available at the end of the article

biomarker for pulmonary inflammation and bacterial load. Neutrophil elastase was analysed for comparison and as a marker reflecting neutrophil load in the airways.

Methods

Study population

CF patients, 6 to 18 years of age, at the paediatric CF centre of Skåne University Hospital in Lund, were eligible for inclusion in the study. Patients under shared care with other clinics were excluded. At each visit to the clinic, the subjects donated an expectorated or induced sputum sample to the study, and their lung function was evaluated with spirometry. Sputum was induced by administering individually tailored hypertonic saline (median 5%, range 3–7%), followed by airway clearance techniques such as positive expiratory pressure (PEP) and forced expiration technique (FET). Sputum was collected during or directly after airway clearance. The procedure was supervised by a physiotherapist. Forced expiratory volume in one second in % of predicted (FEV1%predicted) and forced expiratory flow between 25 and 75% of expired forced vital capacity in % of predicted (FEF%predicted) were determined from predicted values according to Zapletal [11]. A mean of the two best values of FEV_1%predicted or FEF%predicted from the previous year were used as baseline to calculate the change in FEV_1%predicted (ΔFEV_1) or change in FEF%predicted (ΔFEF), respectively, at the time of sampling. At start of *iv* antibiotic treatment, a blood sample was also donated to the study.

Sputum cultures were analysed at the department of Medical Microbiology, Laboratory medicine, Skåne University Hospital, according to approved conventional methods in the routine laboratory [12]. Information about pulmonary symptoms such as dyspnoea, cough, fever, increased mucus, or change in sputum colour, was extracted from the medical journal. The sample collection was performed from January to June 2015.

A written informed consent was obtained from all participants and/or their guardian. The study was approved by the Medical Ethic Committee (Institutional Review Board) of Lund University (reference number 2011/434).

Sample preparation

All sputum samples were taken care of within two hours of sampling. One aliquot of the sample was mixed with an equal volume of Saliva Preservation Solution (Norgen Biotek Corporation, Canada) and frozen at – 80 °C until further processing. The remaining portion of the sample was homogenized by mixing sputum 1:1 (*w*/*v*) with 0.1% dithiothreitol (DTT) in PBS. The samples were incubated at 37 °C for 20 min with intermittent mixing, followed by centrifugation at 3000 rpm for 10 min. The cell-free supernatants were collected and stored at – 80 °C until further analyses.

Blood samples were centrifuged at 3000 rpm for 10 min. Plasma was collected and stored at – 80 °C until analyses. All plasma samples were centrifuged and frozen within one hour from sampling.

Quantification of HBP

HBP concentrations were analysed with ELISA as previously described [4]. All samples were assayed in duplicates.

Neutrophil elastase activity

Ten μl of liquefied sputum sample was mixed with 90 μl of HEPES buffer (0.1 M HEPES, 0.5 M NaCl; pH 7.5), supplemented with 5 mM EDTA, 2 μg/ml of E64 (Sigma, St. Louis, MO) and 1 μg/ml of Pepstatin A (Sigma-Aldrich, St. Louis, MO) in a 96-wells plate. Neutrophil elastase (Sigma-Aldrich) in 2-fold dilutions from a 2 U/ml stem solution was used as a standard. Fifty μl of the chromogenic substrate N-methoxysuccinyl-Ala-Ala-Pro-Val p-nitroanilide (Sigma-Aldrich) was added to each well to a final concentration of 0.5 mM. The plates were incubated at 37 °C and the absorbance at 415 nm was determined every 10 min to measure enzyme kinetics. All samples were analysed in duplicates.

Nucleic acid extraction and real-time PCR

Sputum samples were homogenized with DTT as described above. DNA extraction was performed with a Sputum DNA isolation kit (cat. #46200, Norgen Biotek Corporation) according to the manufacturer's protocol.

Total bacterial load was quantified with real-time PCR of 16 s rDNA, using the following primer pair: forward: TGCCAGCAGCCGCGGTAA, reverse: AGGCCCGGG AACGTATTCAC. One μl of DNA template was added to 19 μl master mix containing SYBR® Green (cat. #172–5121, Bio-Rad, Hercules, CA), sterile water, and the forward and reverse primers. Expression was analyzed using the iTaq™ Universal SYBR® Green Supermix (Bio-Rad). Known amounts of *Staphylococcus aureus* DNA in 10-fold dilutions were analyzed in parallel and used as a standard. Amplification was performed at 54 °C for 35 cycles in an iCycler Thermal Cycler (Bio-Rad, Hercules, CA) and DNA concentrations were calculated from the standard curve.

Statistics

Statistical calculations were done using the GraphPad Prism 7 software (GraphPad Software, San Diego, CA) and R (R Core Team 2017, R Foundation for Statistical Computing, Vienna, Austria) using R Studio (RStudio, Inc., Boston, MA) with installed packages nlme, mgcv, r2glmm, geepack and MuMln (https://cran.r-project.org/web/packages/r2glmm/index.html) [13, 14] (https://cran.r-project.org/web/packages/MuMIn/index.html).

Comparisons between unpaired groups were made with the non-parametric Mann-Whitney U test, and with Wilcoxon matched-pairs signed rank test for paired observations. Correlations were done with Spearman rank coefficient. Cut-off values for the calculation of sensitivity, specificity and predictive values were chosen based on receiver operator characteristics data.

To account for possible dependency due to repeated measurements from the same patient, we used mixed model with random effects and generalised estimating equation (GEE) models with subjects as the random components. The linear relationship between biomarkers and lung function was confirmed using a mixed additive model with random effects. To assess the relative importance of each variable in the mixed model, a semi-partial r-square was calculated according to Jaeger et al. [15]. Two-tailed $P < 0.05$ and 95% confidence intervals (CIs) that did not overlap 1.0 were regarded as statistically significant.

Results

Patient characteristics

A total of 22 patients suffering from CF (aged 6–18 years) were eligible and enrolled in the study. The study participants had a median age of 9 years, and male sex was the dominating gender (Table 1). The participants were followed with consecutive sputum sampling during a six months period, from January to June 2015. Three patients were unable to donate a sputum sample during the study period and were therefore excluded (Fig. 1). The remaining 19 patients donated a total of 50 sputum samples. Nine sputum samples were excluded as no lung function evaluation had been performed at the time of sampling. This left 41 sputum samples from 17 patients, with a median of 2 samples per patient (range 1–4 samples). 83% of sputum samples were induced with sodium chloride. Samples collected from the same patient were obtained with a median of 37 days apart (range 7–176 days). Another 6 samples were excluded from DNA analyses, as they contained small volumes of sputum that only allowed HBP and elastase measurements.

Staphylococcus aureus and *Pseudomonas aeruginosa* were the most commonly found bacterial species in sputum cultures (32 and 24%, respectively). Thirty-six % of sputum samples were collected during on-going symptoms from the respiratory tract (dyspnoea, cough, fever, increased mucus, or change in sputum colour). Nine samples were collected at start of intravenous antibiotic treatment. Six of these treatments were initiated to eradicate *P. aeruginosa* and the remaining to treat exacerbations.

HBP, elastase and bacterial load in sputum

Sputum concentrations of HBP and elastase, but not bacterial load, were significantly increased in samples collected in the presence of respiratory symptoms (Fig. 2). To account for the possibility of bias due to repeated measures from the same patient, logistic regression with general estimating equation (GEE) models was performed using the logarithmic values of HBP, elastase

Table 1 Patient characteristics

Median age (IQR)[a]	9 (8–11)
Male gender; % (*n*)	71 (12)
CFTR mutation; % (n)	
- ΔF508/ΔF508	59 (10)
- Others	41 (7)
Pancreas insufficiency; % (n)	100 (17)
No of samples/patient; median (IQR)	2 (2–3)
Induced sputum; % (*n*)	83 (34)
Pseudomonas colonization[b]; % (*n*)	
- Never infected	24 (4)
- Free of infection	6 (1)
- Intermittent infection	53 (9)
- Chronic infection	18 (3)
Sputum culture growth; % (*n*)	
- *Staphylococcus aureus*	34 (12)
- *Pseudomonas aeruginosa*	26 (10)
- *Haemophilus influenzae*	14 (5)
- *Burkholderia cepacia*	6 (2)
- Negative culture	6 (2)

[a]IQR = Interquartile range
[b]Pseudomonas aeruginosa (PA) colonization according to Leeds criteria: Never infected, Free of infection (no PA growth during the previous 12 months), Intermittent infection (PA growth in 50% or less of cultures), or Chronic infection (PA growth in > 50% of cultures)

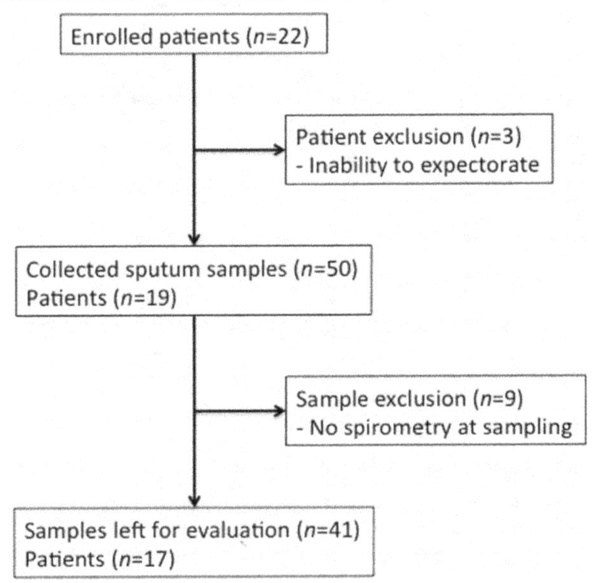

Fig. 1 Flowchart of patients and sputum samples in the cohort

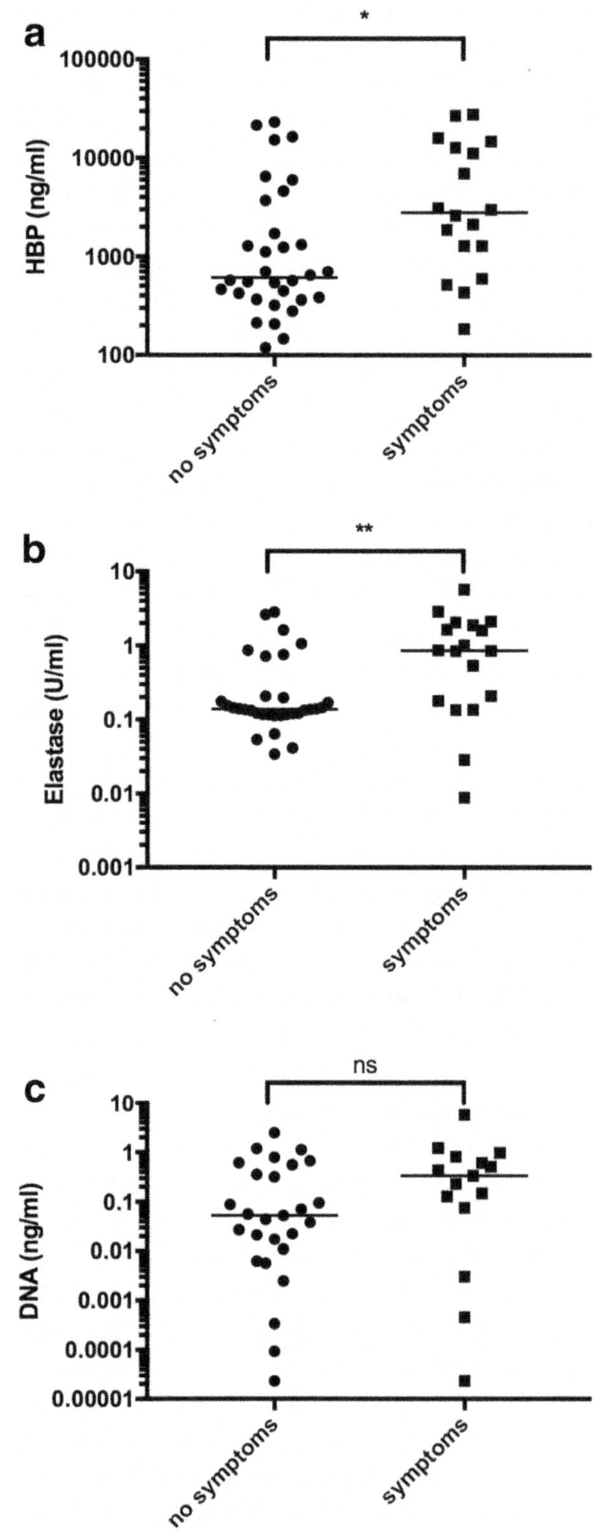

Fig. 2 Sputum levels of HBP (**a**), elastase (**b**), and bacterial load (**c**) in patients with and without symptoms from the respiratory tract. * = $p < 0.05$. ** = $p < 0.005$. Ns = not significant

and bacterial DNA as continuous variables. Using GEE analyses, the odds ratios (ORs) for the prediction of respiratory symptoms were 1.4829 (95% CI 1.02766–2.140) for log(HBP), 1.705 (95% CI 1.082–2.69) for log(Elastase), and 1.124 (95% CI 0.972–1.30) for log(bacterial load).

Six participants had a sputum sample taken at start of antibiotic therapy, and a follow-up sample taken within one month. Median values decreased after therapy for all markers, but only HBP reached statistical significance (Fig. 3). Neither levels of HBP nor elastase differed between induced and naturally expectorated sputum ($p = 0.09$ for HBP and $p = 0.2$ for elastase).

Next, HBP, elastase and bacterial DNA were correlated to FEV_1%predicted at the time of sampling, and to the change in FEV_1%predicted compared to baseline levels (ΔFEV_1). A mean of the patient's two best FEV_1%predicted values from the previous year was used as baseline, and the change in lung function was expressed in percent. Both HBP and elastase correlated more strongly to ΔFEV_1 than FEV_1%predicted, whereas no convincing correlation was found between total bacterial load in sputum and either FEV_1%predicted or ΔFEV_1 (Fig. 4). To account for repeated measurements from the same patient, the correlations between biomarkers and ΔFEV_1 were validated both in a mixed model with patients as random effects, as well as using GEE. The mixed model with random effects estimated log(HBP) to − 2.5 (− 4.63 – − 0.379, $p = 0.0229$) and a semi-partial R-square of 0.122 (0.005–0.344). The estimate for log(elastase) was − 3.17 (− 5.41– − 0.933, $p = 0.0075$) with a semi-partial R-square of 0.161 (0.016–0.389), and for log(bacterial load) the estimate was 0.11 (− 1.23–1.44, $p = 0.8705$) with a semi-partial R-square of 0.001 (0–0.142). Importantly, GEE gave point estimates for the prediction of a decrease in ΔFEV_1 in agreement with the mixed models, but only HBP remained statistically significant. The estimates from the GEE were − 2.57 ($p = 0.023$) for log(HBP), − 2.96 ($p = 0.086$) for log(Elastase), and − 0.0538 ($p = 0.93$) for log(bacterial load).

No correlation was detected between HBP and bacterial DNA ($r = 0.09$, $p = 0.56$) or between elastase and bacterial DNA ($r = 0.24$, $p = 0.13$), whereas HBP and elastase correlated well ($r = 0.85$, $p < 0.001$). No differences in sputum HBP or elastase were found between the different groups of *Pseudomonas* colonisation according to Leeds criteria (data not shown).

In order to reflect involvement of small airway disease [16], sputum HBP levels were also correlated to FEF25/75 in % of predicted values (FEF%predicted), and to a change in FEF%predicted compared to baseline levels (ΔFEF%). HBP showed a weaker, but not statistically different correlation to both FEF%predicted ($r = -0.27$, $p = 0.09$) compared to FEV_1%predicted ($p = 0.43$), and to ΔFEF% ($r = -0.17$, $p = 0.30$) compared to ΔFEV_1, ($p = 0.09$).

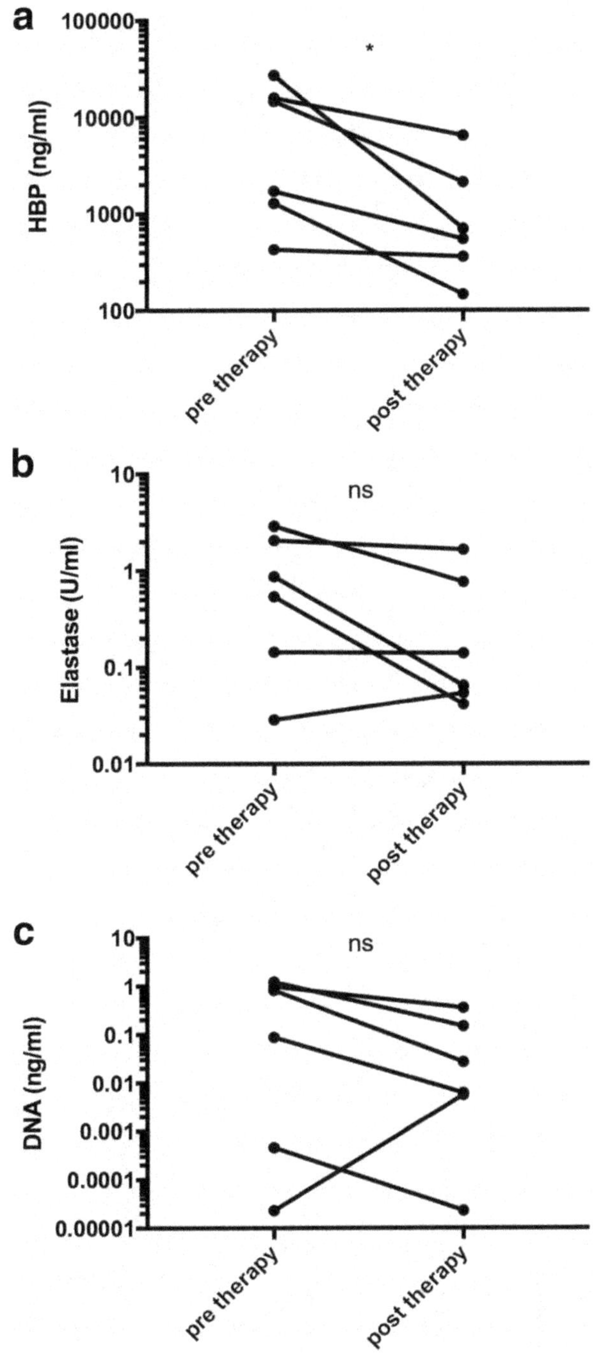

Fig. 3 Levels of HBP (**a**), elastase (**b**), and bacterial load (**c**) before and after antibiotic treatment. * = $p < 0.05$. Ns = not significant

Using 10% decline in ΔFEV_1 compared to baseline as cut-off, both HBP and elastase were significantly increased in the group with a decrease in ΔFEV_1 (Fig. 5). The levels of bacterial DNA were similar in both groups (data not shown). Receiver Operator Characteristics (ROC) analyses for the detection of > 10% decline in ΔFEV_1 are shown in Fig. 6. HBP and elastase performed equally well, with area under the curve (AUC) values of 0.80 (95% CI 0.65–0.94) for HBP and 0.78 (95% CI 0.62–0.93) for elastase. Bacterial DNA presented a lower AUC of 0.54 (95% CI 0.34–0.73) for the detection of a decrease in ΔFEV_1. Based on ROC data, cut-off values for the calculation of sensitivity, specificity and predictive values were identified for HBP, elastase and bacterial DNA. At a cut-off value of 650 ng/ml for HBP, the sensitivity was 81% and the specificity 70% for the detection of > 10% decline in ΔFEV_1. The positive and negative predictive values were 74 and 78%, respectively. Elastase performed similar to HBP, whereas bacterial DNA showed poor sensitivity and specificity (Table 2).

HBP levels in plasma

Eight patients donated a total of 9 plasma samples at the start of *iv* antibiotic treatment during the study period. The median HBP concentration in plasma was 7.0 ng/ml (range 5.1–20.5 ng/ml), which was significantly lower than the HBP concentrations in the corresponding sputum samples (median 1716 ng/ml, range 384–27,051 ng/ml, $p < 0.01$).

Discussion

HBP has received attention over the last years as a promising biomarker of infection in sepsis, urinary tract infections, meningitis, and lately also as a marker of airway infection in broncho-alveolar lavage (BAL) of lung transplant recipients [7–10]. In this prospective study on children with cystic fibrosis, HBP levels in sputum correlated to lung function and to respiratory symptoms, but not to bacterial load. HBP levels in plasma were low and in the same range as reported in healthy individuals [7]. In comparison, levels of HBP in concomitant sputum samples were at least 100-fold and up to 1000-fold higher. The high concentrations of HBP in sputum underline the heavy neutrophil-dominated airway inflammation seen in CF patients, and probably reflect that the lung is the end organ where the neutrophil becomes activated and releases its granular contents.

Expectorated and induced sputum is a non-invasive method to obtain airway samples from CF-patients, as opposed to BAL which is still the gold standard for defining airway inflammation and microbiology in infants and young children [17]. Studies have shown that sputum samples are of equal value as BAL specimens to detect *P. aeruginosa* colonization [18], indicating that sputum biomarkers for the detection of airway inflammation and infection would be a simple and useful tool in clinical practice. However, sputum collection is not as standardized as BAL, which may result in large intra- and inter-individual variations. For example, CF patients often have sputum plugs that cannot be expectorated and thus cause false low levels of inflammatory markers. Moreover, the sampling technique was not identical for all samples in the study, as 17% of samples were

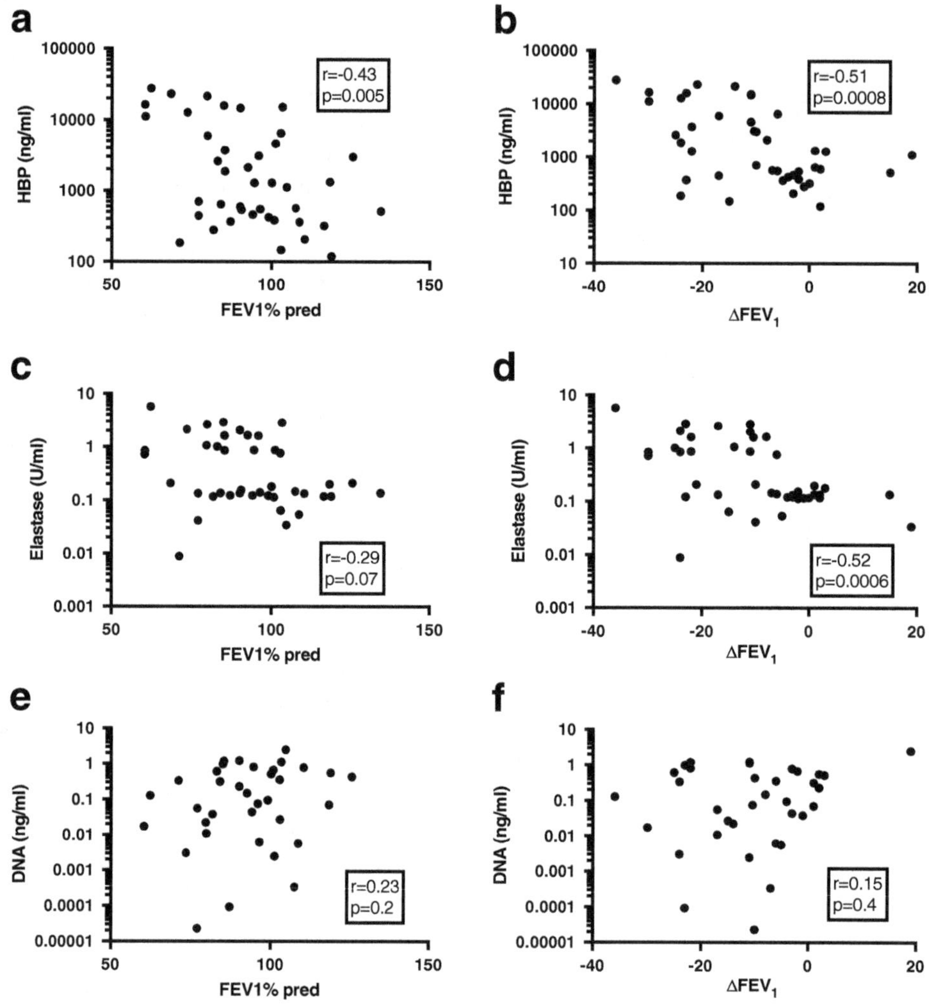

Fig. 4 Correlations between biomarkers and lung function. HBP (**a** and **b**), elastase (**c** and **d**), and bacterial DNA (**e** and **f**) were correlated to FEV_1%predicted or ΔFEV_1. r = nonparametric Spearman rank coefficient

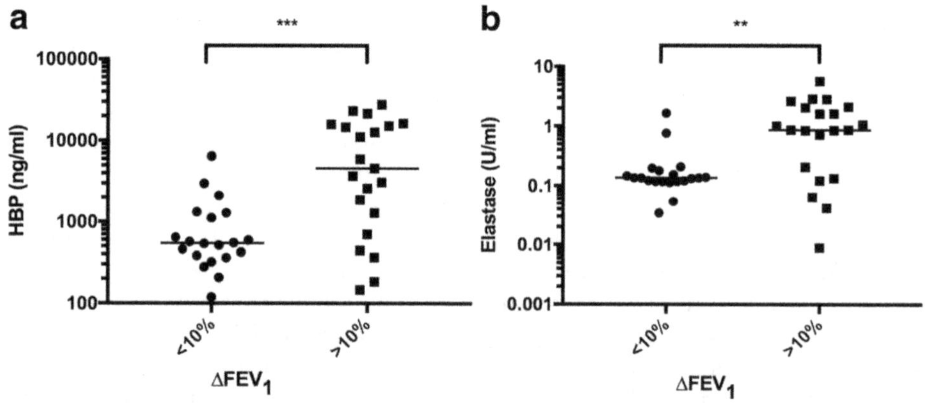

Fig. 5 Sputum levels of HBP (**a**) and elastase (**b**) depending on ΔFEV_1. Sputum samples with more than 10% decline in the patient's ΔFEV_1 were compared to samples with less than 10% decline in lung function. ΔFEV_1 was calculated using the mean of the patient's two best FEV_1%predicted values the previous year as baseline, and comparing to the patient's FEV_1%predicted at the time of sampling, expressed in %. ** = $p < 0.005$. *** = $p < 0.001$

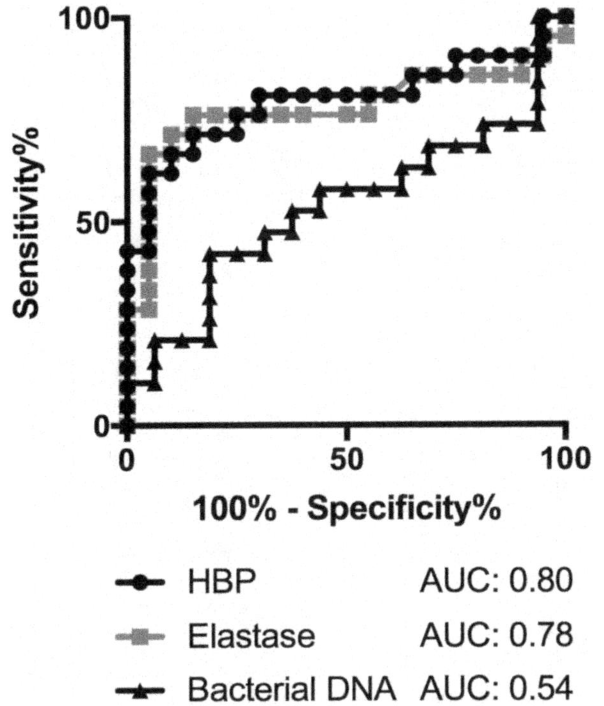

Fig. 6 Receiver-operating characteristics (ROC) curves of HBP, elastase, and bacterial DNA for the detection of > 10% decline in ΔFEV_1

expectorated and 83% were induced with sodium chloride. However, we saw no differences in biomarker levels between induced and non-induced sputum, and it has also been shown by others that there are no differences in microbiology between induced and expectorated sputum [19]. We therefore believe that the sampling technique has a minor impact on the results.

In this study, bacterial DNA tended to increase with pulmonary symptoms but did not reach statistical significance. Nor did bacterial DNA levels correlate to pulmonary function or biomarker levels. Previous work has reported conflicting results. For example, it has been shown that *P. aeruginosa* load correlate to lung function in stable patients, and also decrease after treatment of pulmonary exacerbation [20–22]. On the other hand, a large multicentre study could not attribute any important differences in FEV_1 to bacterial densities [23]. In this study, the cohort was diverse with respect to airway microbiology. We therefore chose to analyse total bacterial load with a universal 16S rDNA primer, as not all participants were colonized with pseudomonas. This PCR-method detects both viable and dead cells, which may be one reason why not more clear results were obtained.

An important shortcoming of the study is the lack of information about sputum neutrophil counts. Instead, we used neutrophil elastase as a marker of the neutrophil burden in our comparisons with HBP. Neutrophil elastase is well studied in sputum from CF patients, and has been reported to decrease after treatment of pulmonary exacerbations [21], to have a longitudinal association with lung function [23], and to be predictive of lung function decline [24]. Both elastase and HBP are neutrophil granule proteins that are released upon cellular activation. It is therefore not surprising that HBP performed equally well to elastase in most, but not all, comparisons made in this study. For example, HBP decreased significantly in sputum after antibiotic treatment, whereas elastase did not. However, only 6 patients had sputum samples taken before and after treatment, which gives the comparison poor power. Moreover, HBP was the only biomarker that remained statistically significant in all comparisons regardless of statistical analysis.

Another difficulty is the definition of airway symptoms in the study. There is no universally accepted definition of pulmonary exacerbations in CF, although Fuchs criteria are commonly used for adults. However, it has been argued that Fuchs criteria are less suited for studies on children, who have a milder lung disease and also milder symptoms of exacerbation [25]. In this study, patients were simply classified based on symptoms from the lower respiratory tract as reported by the patient or staff. Only a few patients experienced exacerbations that required *iv* antibiotic treatment during the study period. Even so, HBP increased significantly in the presence of pulmonary symptoms.

A final limitation is the small number of patients and the fact that participants donated varying numbers of samples to the study. However, even after correction for multiple measurements with mixed models and GEE, we could demonstrate that HBP correlates to ΔFEV_1 and pulmonary symptoms.

Conclusion

Sputum HBP is a promising biomarker for pulmonary inflammation and lung function in children with CF, and could thus be a simple and complementary tool in clinical practice. However, more studies are needed on larger study populations to validate the results.

Table 2 Sensitivity, specificity and predictive values for the detection of > 10% decrease in ΔFEV_1

	Cut-off	Sensitivity (%)	Specificity (%)	PPV (%)	NPV (%)
HBP (ng/ml)	650	81	70	74	78
Elastase (U/ml)	0.15	76	70	73	74
Bacterial load (ng/ml)	0.1	47	44	50	41

PPV positive predictive value, *NPV* negative predictive value

Abbreviations

ΔFEV_1: Change in FEV_1%predicted; BAL: Broncho-alveolar lavage; CF: Cystic Fibrosis; FEV_1%predicted: Forced expiratory volume in one second, % of predicted; HBP: Heparin-binding protein; RT-PCR: Real-Time Polymerase Chain Reaction

Acknowledgements

The authors whish to thank Dr. Adam Linder for helpful discussions, and Maria Mårtensson and all other staff at the Cystic Fibrosis centre, Children's Hospital in Lund, for valuable help with sputum collection.

Funding

This work was funded by the Swedish Heart and Lung foundation, the Alfred Österlund, Magnus Bergvall, and Mats Kleeberg Foundations, Lions research fund in Skåne, The Swedish Heart and Lung Association, and the Swedish Government Funds for Clinical Research (ALF).

Authors' contributions

GH analysed sputum samples and was involved in writing of the manuscript. VP contributed to the concept and design of the study. FK helped with statistical analyses. AE contributed to the concept of the study and writing of the manuscript. LP contributed to the concept and design of the study, analysis and interpretation of samples and patient data, and writing of the manuscript. All authors read and approved the final manuscript.

Consent for publication

Not applicable.

Competing interests

The authors declare that they have no competing interests.

Author details

[1]Department of Clinical Sciences Lund, Division of Infection Medicine, BMC B14, Lund University, Skåne University Hospital, Tornavägen 10, SE-22184 Lund, Sweden. [2]Skåne University Hospital, Clinic of Paediatrics, Lund, Sweden. [3]Department of Clinical Sciences Lund, Respiratory Medicine & Allergology, Lund University, Lund, Sweden.

References

1. Stoltz DA, Meyerholz DK, Welsh MJ. Origins of cystic fibrosis lung disease. N Engl J Med. 2015;372(16):1574–5.
2. Cogen J, Emerson J, Sanders DB, Ren C, Schechter MS, Gibson RL, Morgan W, Rosenfeld M, Group ES. Risk factors for lung function decline in a large cohort of young cystic fibrosis patients. Pediatr Pulmonol. 2015;50(8):763–70.
3. Nkam L, Lambert J, Latouche A, Bellis G, Burgel PR, Hocine MN. A 3-year prognostic score for adults with cystic fibrosis. J Cyst Fibros. 2017;16(6):702-8.
4. Tapper H, Karlsson A, Morgelin M, Flodgaard H, Herwald H. Secretion of heparin-binding protein from human neutrophils is determined by its localization in azurophilic granules and secretory vesicles. Blood. 2002;99(5):1785–93.
5. Linder A, Soehnlein O, Akesson P. Roles of heparin-binding protein in bacterial infections. J Innate Immun. 2010;2(5):431–8.
6. Gautam N, Olofsson AM, Herwald H, Iversen LF, Lundgren-Akerlund E, Hedqvist P, Arfors KE, Flodgaard H, Lindbom L. Heparin-binding protein (HBP/CAP37): a missing link in neutrophil-evoked alteration of vascular permeability. Nat Med. 2001;7(10):1123–7.
7. Linder A, Arnold R, Boyd JH, Zindovic M, Zindovic I, Lange A, Paulsson M, Nyberg P, Russell JA, Pritchard D, et al. Heparin-binding protein measurement improves the prediction of severe infection with organ dysfunction in the emergency department. Crit Care Med. 2015;43(11):2378–86.
8. Linder A, Akesson P, Brink M, Studahl M, Bjorck L, Christensson B. Heparin-binding protein: a diagnostic marker of acute bacterial meningitis. Crit Care Med. 2011;39(4):812–7.
9. Kjolvmark C, Pahlman LI, Akesson P, Linder A. Heparin-binding protein: a diagnostic biomarker of urinary tract infection in adults. Open Forum Infect Dis. 2014;1(1):ofu004.
10. Stjärne, Aspelund A, Hammarström H, Inghammar M, Larsson H, Hansson L, Christensson B, Påhlman LI. Heparin-binding protein, lysozyme and inflammatory cytokines in bronchoalveolar lavage fluid as diagnostic tools for pulmonary infection in lung transplanted patients. Am J Transplant. 2018;18(2):444-52.
11. Zapletal A, Paul T, Samanek M. Significance of contemporary methods of lung function testing for the detection of airway obstruction in children and adolescents (author's transl). Z Erkr Atmungsorgane. 1977;149(3):343–71.
12. Murray PR. Manual of clinical microbiology. Washington: ASM Press; 2007.
13. Wood SN, Pya N, Säfken B. Smoothing parameter and model selection for general smooth models. J Am Stat Assoc. 2016;111(516):1548–63.
14. Yan J, Fine J. Estimating equations for association structures. Statist Med Stat Med. 2004;23(6):859–74.
15. Jaeger BC, Edwards LJ, Das K, Sen PK. An R2 statistic for fixed effects in the generalized linear mixed model. J Appl Stat. 2017;44(6):1086–105.
16. Eckrich J, Zissler UM, Serve F, Leutz P, Smaczny C, Schmitt-Grohe S, Fussbroich D, Schubert R, Zielen S, Eickmeier O. Airway inflammation in mild cystic fibrosis. J Cyst Fibros. 2017;16(1):107–15.
17. Stafler P, Davies JC, Balfour-Lynn IM, Rosenthal M, Bush A. Bronchoscopy in cystic fibrosis infants diagnosed by newborn screening. Pediatr Pulmonol. 2011;46(7):696–700.
18. Jung A, Kleinau I, Schonian G, Bauernfeind A, Chen C, Griese M, Doring G, Gobel U, Wahn U, Paul K. Sequential genotyping of Pseudomonas aeruginosa from upper and lower airways of cystic fibrosis patients. Eur Respir J. 2002;20(6):1457–63.
19. Rogers GB, Skelton S, Serisier DJ, van der Gast CJ, Bruce KD. Determining cystic fibrosis-affected lung microbiology: comparison of spontaneous and serially induced sputum samples by use of terminal restriction fragment length polymorphism profiling. J Clin Microbiol. 2010;48(1):78–86.
20. Deschaght P, Schelstraete P, Van Simaey L, Vanderkercken M, Raman A, Mahieu L, Van Daele S, De Baets F, Vaneechoutte M. Is the improvement of CF patients, hospitalized for pulmonary exacerbation, correlated to a decrease in bacterial load? PLoS One. 2013;8(11):e79010.
21. Ordonez CL, Henig NR, Mayer-Hamblett N, Accurso FJ, Burns JL, Chmiel JF, Daines CL, Gibson RL, McNamara S, Retsch-Bogart GZ, et al. Inflammatory and microbiologic markers in induced sputum after intravenous antibiotics in cystic fibrosis. Am J Respir Crit Care Med. 2003;168(12):1471–5.
22. Reid DW, Latham R, Lamont IL, Camara M, Roddam LF. Molecular analysis of changes in Pseudomonas aeruginosa load during treatment of a pulmonary exacerbation in cystic fibrosis. J Cyst Fibros. 2013;12(6):688–99.
23. Mayer-Hamblett N, Aitken ML, Accurso FJ, Kronmal RA, Konstan MW, Burns JL, Sagel SD, Ramsey BW. Association between pulmonary function and sputum biomarkers in cystic fibrosis. Am J Respir Crit Care Med. 2007;175(8):822–8.
24. Sagel SD, Wagner BD, Anthony MM, Emmett P, Zemanick ET. Sputum biomarkers of inflammation and lung function decline in children with cystic fibrosis. Am J Respir Crit Care Med. 2012;186(9):857–65.
25. Waters V, Ratjen F. Pulmonary exacerbations in children with cystic fibrosis. Ann Am Thorac Soc. 2015;12(Suppl 2):S200–6.

5

Altered deposition of inhaled nanoparticles in subjects with chronic obstructive pulmonary disease

Jonas K F Jakobsson[1], H Laura Aaltonen[2], Hanna Nicklasson[2], Anders Gudmundsson[1], Jenny Rissler[1,3], Per Wollmer[2] and Jakob Löndahl[1*]

Abstract

Background: Respiratory tract deposition of airborne particles is a key link to understand their health impact. Experimental data are limited for vulnerable groups such as individuals with respiratory diseases. The aim of this study is to investigate the differences in lung deposition of nanoparticles in the distal lung for healthy subjects and subjects with respiratory disease.

Methods: Lung deposition of nanoparticles (50 and 100 nm) was measured after a 10 s breath-hold for three groups: healthy never-smoking subjects ($n = 17$), asymptomatic (active and former) smokers ($n = 15$) and subjects with chronic obstructive pulmonary disease ($n = 16$). Measurements were made at 1300 mL and 1800 mL volumetric lung depth. Each subject also underwent conventional lung function tests, including post bronchodilator FEV_1, VC, and diffusing capacity for carbon monoxide, $D_{L,CO}$. Patients with previously diagnosed respiratory disease underwent a CT-scan of the lungs. Particle lung deposition fraction, was compared between the groups and with conventional lung function tests.

Results: We found that the deposition fraction was significantly lower for subjects with emphysema compared to the other subjects ($p = 0.001–0.01$), but no significant differences were found between healthy never-smokers and smokers. Furthermore, the particle deposition correlated with pulmonary function tests, $FEV_{1\%Pred}$ ($p < 0.05$), $FEV_1/VC_{\%Pred}$ ($p < 0.01$) and $D_{L,CO}$ ($p < 0.0005$) when all subjects were included. Furthermore, for subjects with emphysema, deposition fraction correlated strongly with $D_{L,CO}$ (Pearson's $r = 0.80–0.85$, $p < 0.002$) while this correlation was not found within the other groups.

Conclusions: Lower deposition fraction was observed for emphysematous subjects and this can be explained by enlarged distal airspaces in the lungs. As expected, deposition increases for smaller particles and deeper inhalation. The observed results have implications for exposure assessment of air pollution and dosimetry of aerosol-based drug delivery of nanoparticles.

Keywords: Lung deposition, Nanoparticles, Emphysema, Chronic obstructive pulmonary disease, Inhalation exposure, Human, In vivo study

* Correspondence: jakob.londahl@design.lth.se
[1]Division of Ergonomics and Aerosol Technology, Lund University, Lund, Sweden
Full list of author information is available at the end of the article

Background

Factors determining the deposited dose of ambient air pollution include the properties of the inhaled particles as well as individual anatomical and physiological characteristics, such as lung morphology and breathing pattern. The objective of this study was to investigate respiratory tract deposition of nanoparticles in the distal lung in healthy never-smoking subjects, asymptomatic smokers and subjects with diagnosed chronic obstructive pulmonary disease (COPD).

Numerous epidemiological studies show links between airborne pollutants and adverse health effects in terms of both increased morbidity and mortality [1]. By number, ultrafine particles normally dominate in both indoor and outdoor air, and are important for human health, as they are known to be able to penetrate to the deep lungs and deposit there with high efficiency. The material in soluble particles easily translocate into other parts of the body, while insoluble particles are believed to accumulate in the lungs because of low clearance rates in the alveolar region [2]; both prospects may have adverse effects on human health.

Established lung models and previous experimental studies agree that nanoparticles (< 100 nm) to a high degree deposit in the distal lung, with the exception of the very smallest particles below 5–10 nm that deposit higher up in the respiratory tract due to their high diffusion velocity. However, vast intersubject variability have been observed in experimental studies [3–6]. Intersubject variability has also been investigated by modelling [7–9], although there is generally a substantial lack of theoretical calculations for deposition of particles in unhealthy lungs. Experimental data of respiratory tract deposition of nanoparticles is limited to about 50 studies [10], most containing data for small groups (< 10 subjects). Because of differences in methodology and low numbers of subjects, it is not trivial to compare the results between studies or with theoretical models. Especially studies using controlled breathing patterns for larger groups and for subjects with respiratory disease are scarce.

To the best of our knowledge, only five studies have previously reported lung deposition data for nanoparticles in subjects with obstructive lung disease [2, 11–14], and of these only two present data for subjects with explicitly defined emphysema [12, 14]. In a recent publication [14], which included a subset of the material in this study, we have shown that deposition of nanoparticles is reduced in subjects with COPD compared to never-smokers and correlates with the degree of emphysema. This paper extends the observations to a larger number of subjects, two different particle sizes and two different volumetric sample depths. Anderson et al. [11] measured lung deposition for particles in the size range 40–240 nm in obstructive, restrictive and healthy subjects, and reported increased particle deposition efficiency, for subjects with airflow obstruction. Möller et al. [2] also reported increased particle deposition efficiency for obstructive subjects and smokers compared to healthy non-smoking subjects. The measurements were performed with aerosol boluses aimed at the peripheral lung (800 mL volumetric lung depth) and to the more central regions (150 mL volumetric lung depth). Increased deposition efficiency was reported for the peripheral lung, but not for the central airways. Brown et al. [12] showed increased particle deposition for obstructive subjects with bronchitis and decreased particle deposition for emphysematous subjects, compared to healthy subjects. Similar results were also presented by Löndahl et al. [13] who reported decreased particle deposition for COPD subjects for particles < 100 nm and slightly increased lung deposition for larger particles. Thus, depending on phenotype of COPD, the disease can both increase and decrease the deposition of inhaled aerosols.

For particles in the diffusion-dominated range (< 300 nm), the main experimental parameters that govern deposition efficiency are particle size, residence time in the peripheral lung and distance to available surfaces. Previous studies reporting data from experiments using spontaneous [4, 6, 13, 15–17] or controlled [11, 18] natural breathing patterns determine deposited dose of airborne nanoparticles under real life exposure conditions and for different groups, but generally do not provide information on regional deposition.

In this study, we report data for deposition of monodisperse nanoparticles in the peripheral airways (> 1300 mL volumetric sample depth) for three groups of subjects. In order to isolate effects from differences in lung structure, we performed the experiments with a controlled breathing pattern including a breath-hold. We hypothesised that the deposition of nanoparticles will differ between healthy subjects, and subjects with diagnosed respiratory disease. Respiratory disease was assessed with pulmonary function testing and, for subjects with previously diagnosed disease, computed tomography (CT). A detailed analysis of the CT results is provided by Aaltonen et al. in a separate publication [14]. Smoking is known to affect the lungs even for individuals with relatively short smoking history [19, 20] and therefore smokers without symptoms of respiratory disease were included as a separate group.

Methods

Subjects and experimental design

The study was performed on COPD-patients recruited from the department of pulmonary medicine at Skåne University Hospital in Malmö, Sweden, and at a local primary health care clinic, and on two groups of subjects with no symptoms of respiratory disease, whereof one was never-smokers and the other active or former smokers.

All subjects underwent conventional lung function tests, according to current recommendations for diagnosis of respiratory disease [21–23]. Most of the patients (n = 15/16) with previously diagnosed COPD underwent a CT-scan of the lungs, but the other groups were omitted from this part of the study to reduce the exposure to radiation. In addition to conventional lung function tests, all subjects experienced a total of nine measurements of lung deposition of nanoparticles (three replicates at three different measurement conditions) during a total experimental time of approximately 30 min. The deposition measurements were generally performed directly in connection with the clinical lung function tests, or within 6 weeks.

Division of the subjects into the three groups was made based on lung function tests, smoking history and previously diagnosed respiratory disease (Table 1). The healthy never-smoking group (n = 17) was defined as individuals with no previous smoking history and no respiratory disease, normal spirometry (as defined by the Global Initiative for Chronic Obstructive Lung Disease, GOLD [24]), and $D_{L,CO}$. The "asymptomatic smoker" group (n = 15) was defined as present or former smokers, with normal spirometry and $D_{L,CO}$, and no known respiratory disease. In this group the subjects had an average estimated smoking history of 14 pack-years (range 3–41). Two subjects were active smokers and reliable data was missing for 3 subjects. The COPD group (n = 16) consisted of subjects with diagnosed COPD, with airflow obstruction corresponding to spirometric GOLD-stages 1–4 [24]. In the COPD-group, 3 subjects underwent triple therapy, inhaled corticosteroids (ICS), long-acting beta-agonist (LABA) and long-acting muscarinic antagonist (LAMA), while 2 underwent therapy with ICS and LAMA or LABA, 3 subjects had LABA and LAMA therapy. Three individuals reported no inhaled therapy and data was missing for 5 individuals. In this group 4 subjects were never-smokers with alpha-1 antitrypsin deficiency, 10 subjects ex-smokers and 2 subjects active smokers. The COPD subjects that reported smoking history had an average of 37 pack-years (range 0.5–68). Reliable data for estimating pack-years was missing for 4 of these subjects. There were no significant differences on a group level between the subjects with regards to gender, age, weight, height and VC.

Table 1 Subject demographics and lung function

	Healthy Never-Smokers (n = 17)	Asymptomatic Smokers (n = 15)	COPD (n = 16)
Male/Female	9/8	6/9	7/9
Age [y]	64 ± 6	62 ± 3	67 ± 7
Weight [kg]	76 ± 14	76 ± 12	72 ± 13
Height [cm]	173 ± 9	169 ± 9	170 ± 9
FEV_1%pred	110 ± 15	109 ± 13	61 ± 23***
VC %pred	109 ± 20	112 ± 13	107 ± 18
FEV_1/VC %pred	78.6 ± 4.0	78.4 ± 5.6	44.9 ± 14.2***
$D_{L,CO}$ %pred	92.0 ± 10	88.2 ± 13	60.2 ± 22***†
GOLD-stage (1/2/3/4)			3/7/5/1

† Data for $D_{L,CO}$ for one subject in the COPD group is missing
***Significance < 0.001 level
Descriptive demographic data (average ± 1 standard deviation) for the subjects, lung function tests performed post bronchodilation, 1.5 mg terbutaline (Bricanyl Turbuhaler, Astra Zeneca, Mölndal, Sweden)

In total 69 subjects participated, whereof 48 subjects completed the study. Criteria for acceptable quality of particle deposition measurements were measurements with inhalation to > 70% VC, and a complete breathing manoeuvre in less than 17 s. Of the 21 subjects that were omitted, two subjects were not able to exhale the full 1800 mL breath sample, 10 were not able to perform the breathing manoeuvre within the stipulated time, 9 failed to inhale a sufficient volume of test aerosol. It was primarily subjects with more severe COPD that failed to follow the quality criteria, partly due to flow resistance in the inhalation apparatus.

The study was approved by the regional ethical review board of Lund and was performed in accordance with the Declaration of Helsinki. An informed written consent was obtained from all subjects.

Pulmonary function testing

Each subject underwent conventional lung function tests, according to current recommendations for diagnosis of respiratory disease [21–23], including measurement of forced expiratory volume in one second (FEV_1) and vital capacity (VC), as well as diffusing capacity for carbon monoxide ($D_{L,CO}$), (Jaeger MasterScreen PFT, IntraMedic, Sollentuna, Sweden). The lung function tests were performed post bronchodilation (1.5 mg terbutaline (Bricanyl Turbuhaler, Astra Zeneca, Mölndal, Sweden). Lung function variables are, if not explicitly stated otherwise, presented as percentage of predicted values, [21, 25].

Computed tomography

All but one of the patients with previously diagnosed COPD underwent a CT-scan of the lungs. The exclusion of one patient was merely for logistical reasons. A detailed analysis of the CT results, including CT densitometry, is described for a subset of the material in a separate publication [14]. The scans were performed using a multidetector-row CT scanner (Siemens Somatom Definition Flash; Siemens Healthcare, Forchheim, Germany) in suspended full inspiration with a reduced radiation dose, generating an exposure of 120 kV / 15 mAs. The CT scans were visually assessed by a radiologist with 9 years of experience and a radiology resident with 2 years of experience, and classified as having none, mild, moderate or severe emphysema [26].

Particle deposition measurements

The instrumentation used for the particle deposition measurements has been described in detail elsewhere [27]. An overview is shown in Fig. 1. In short, a test aerosol was produced by aerosolizing polystyrene latex nanospheres (PSL) (Polymer Microsphere Suspension, Microgenics Corp, Fremont CA, US) with an electrospray aerosol generator (Model 3480, TSI Inc., Shoreview, MN, US). The produced aerosol was size controlled by a differential mobility analyser (DMA, Model 3071, TSI GmbH, Aachen, Germany) and diluted with particle free air to a concentration of 3000–6000 particles cm^{-3}. The test aerosol was continuously produced and led into a semi-flexible aerosol reservoir with an exhaust in a flow-through design that ensured a steady supply of fresh test aerosol during the measurements. A high-speed computer controlled valve administered the test aerosol or particle-free air to the subjects through a mouthpiece connected to a pneumotachograph flow meter (as used in MasterScreen PFT, Viasys GmbH - Erich Jaeger, Hoechberg, Germany). The high speed valve was also connected to a sample collector, enabling sampling from well-defined exhaled volumes corresponding to specific volumetric lung depths. The particle concentration was monitored in the aerosol reservoir, and in the exhaled samples by a condensation particle counter (CPC, Model a20, Airmodus Ltd., Helsinki, Finland). The instrument was constructed according to the design criteria described by Löndahl et al. [10] and particle losses were characterized and compensated for [27].

The deposition measurements (Fig. 2) started with a period when the subject breathed particle free air to wash out resident ambient air particles and to get accustomed to the instrument. After a minimum period of 30 s, the subject performed a total exhalation to residual volume (RV), followed by a deep inhalation to total lung capacity (TLC). When the inhalation started, the altered flow direction detected by the pneumotachograph automatically triggered the high speed valve to switch, so that the subject inhaled the test aerosol. When the subject reached TLC all valves were shut, and the subject held his breath for a determined time period (10 s). Thereafter the valve opened towards the sample collector and the subject exhaled a predetermined volume, before the valve was turned and the rest of the breath was discarded to exhaust. Measurements were carried out with spherical 50 nm particles (mobility equivalent diameter) and from exhaled samples corresponding to air with a sample front at 1300 mL and 1800 mL volumetric lung depth, and with 100 nm particles from

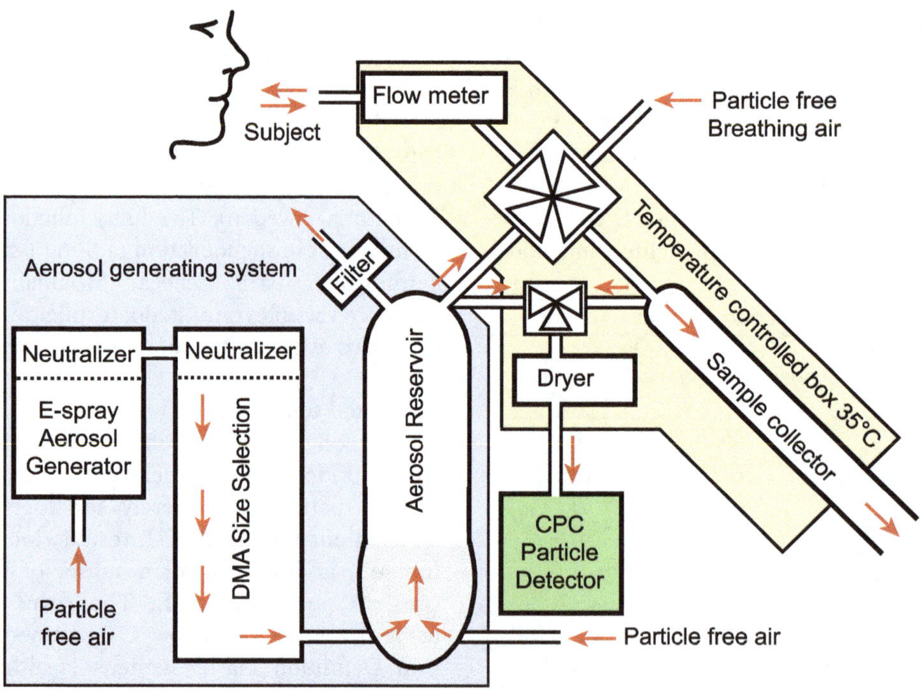

Fig. 1 The aerosol deposition measurement system. The aerosol deposition measurement system can be divided into three sub-systems. Aerosol generation system (blue): the test aerosol is generated by an electrospray aerosol, followed by size-selection and dilution with particle free air. Inhalation system (red): a four-way, high-speed, computer-controlled valve directs particle free air or test aerosol to the subject, monitors the breathing pattern and collects exhaled samples from a well-defined volumetric sample depth. The system is enclosed in a temperature controlled box held at 35°c. Particle detection system (green): the particle number concentration in the test aerosol and in exhaled samples are measured with a condensation particle counter

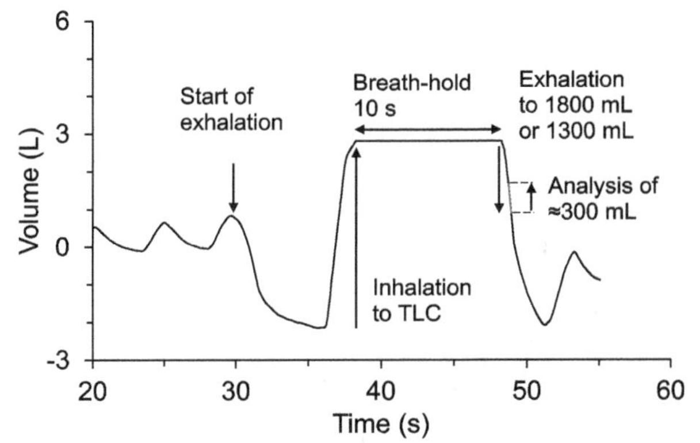

Fig. 2 The breathing pattern. The breathing protocol, illustrated by breathing data for a standard measurement, recorded at 100 Hz. The protocol starts with a period of tidal breathing of particle free air. The breathing manoeuvre is initiated with exhalation to RV followed by an inhalation of the test aerosol to TLC, a breath-hold of 10 s and then relaxed exhalation. A sample is collected from the exhaled air after a controlled volume has passed the sample collector. The particle number concentration is monitored continuously in the test aerosol until the inhalation, and then determined in the exhaled sample immediately after exhalation. The aerosol residence time in the lungs is calculated from the recorded breathing pattern

1800 mL volumetric lung depth. The breathing pattern is shown in Fig. 2.

The particle deposition fraction (DF) is defined as the fraction of the exhaled particle concentration related to the inhaled particle concentration, and is corrected for particle losses in the instrument according to the relation:

$$DF = 1 - \frac{C}{C_0 R_i(t_i)}$$

Here C is the particle number concentration in the exhaled sample and C_0 is the particle number concentration in the inhaled test aerosol. R_i is the instrument recovery, which describes particle losses in the instrument as a function of residence time during measurements, t_i. The relation for R_i is semi-empirical and derived from theory for particle diffusion in confined spaces combined with data for simulated breathing manoeuvres with a physical model, as described in detail elsewhere [27]. The measured DF was reported as the mean value of three measurements. The standard deviation for the measurements was typically 0.001, 0.007 and 0.02 for 50 nm particles/1300 mL, 50 nm particles/1800 mL and 100 nm/1800 mL sample depth respectively.

For the breathing pattern used, the respiratory flow-rates during inhalation and exhalation has previously been shown to have minimal influence on the measurements [27], as long as the total residence time in the lungs does not change. Thus the subjects could inhale and exhale at uncontrolled breathing flow-rates. The residence time in the lungs was defined as the time between midpoint times of inhalation and the exhaled sample in similarity with standard for measurement of $D_{L,CO}$ [22].

Analysis

Although all subjects used similar breath-hold times, there were variations in the total residence time of the particles in the lungs due to differences in exhaled flow rate. To decrease variations in measured DF that were only due to these differences in breathing pattern, we time normalized data to 13 s total residence time. The time normalization was based on the previously observed relationship between DF and breath-hold time for 50 nm and 100 nm particles in healthy subjects [27], which was also found in the present group. We used a linear approximation of the exponential diffusion deposition equation [28] to avoid overestimates of the time correction. Even though the correction may be less valid for severely diseased subjects, this normalization was considered necessary to avoid bias due to the prolonged aerosol residence time in the lungs caused by slower exhalation by the COPD subjects. In the previous study by Anderson et al. [11], a deviation in breathing pattern among the COPD subjects biased the data and made valid conclusions more difficult. The linear approximation was also implemented with the aim to be a conservative approach. The effect of the time normalization on the DF was on average a decrease of 0.015 ± 0.010 for 50 nm particles and 1300 mL sample depth, 0.012 ± 0.008 for 50 nm particles and 1800 mL sample depth, and 0.030 ± 0.020 for 100 nm particles and 1800 mL volumetric sample depth. Statistical analysis was made with IBM SPSS Statistics 23 (Release 23.0.0.0, 2015). Non-parametric statistics, (Kruskal-Wallis test followed by Mann-Whitney) was used for group comparisons, and Pearson's chi square analysis was performed to check for gender differences between groups. The correlation analysis was calculated with Pearson's product moments. The significances considered were those at the 0.05 or higher levels. For group comparisons between three groups, Bonferroni correction was applied, thus the significance level was adjusted to 0.05/3 = 0.016.

Results

The average demographics and measured lung function for the included subjects are shown in Table 1. Using the Kruskal-Wallis test, it was shown that there were no significant differences on a group level between the subjects with regards to age, weight, height and VC. Pearson's chi square analysis revealed no significant gender differences between the groups.

The average deposition fractions, DF, at different sample volumes and particle sizes are shown in Fig. 3

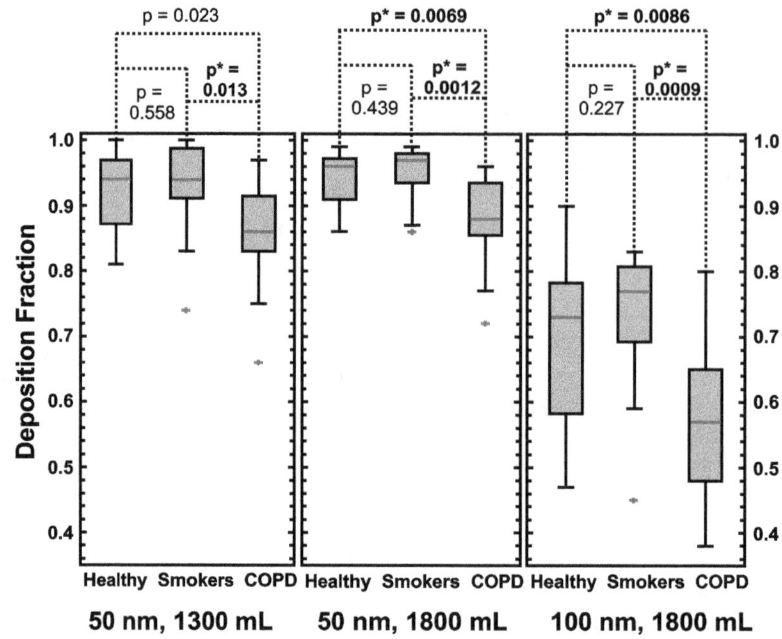

Fig. 3 Boxplot of particle deposition for the three groups. Particle deposition fraction, DF, in the peripheral lungs for the three groups, measured for 50 nm particles and from 1300 mL volumetric sample depth (left panel), 50 nm particles and 1800 mL sample depth (middle panel) and 100 nm particles and 1800 mL sample depth (right panel). The red line indicates the median, the box 25th and 75th percentiles and the whiskers minimum and maximum values (two outliers displayed as a red marks). The *p*-values (Mann-Witney asymptotic significance, 2-tailed) are given in the figure. Significant differences between the groups are indicated with *. The 5% significance level for rejecting the null hypothesis is adjusted to 0.016 (Bonferroni correction)

and the mean values for each group are provided in Table 2.

The DF was significantly higher for the healthy never-smoking subjects and the asymptomatic smokers, than for the subjects diagnosed with COPD. There were no significant differences in DF between the healthy never-smokers and asymptomatic smokers and no significant gender differences. Neither did DF correlate with age.

Figure 4 shows the correlation between the DF measured for each individual for different particle sizes and volumetric sample depths. DF varied in a consistent way for the subjects – with some subjects having a low DF for all measurements and others a high. Especially in the COPD group there was a larger intra-subject variability in DF (coefficient of variance 8–21% for the COPD group compared to 5–16% on average for the healthy groups), and this group also included subjects with a considerably low DF.

Table 2 Particle deposition fractions

	DF 50 nm 1300 mL	DF 50 nm 1800 mL	DF 100 nm 1300 mL
Healthy Never-Smokers (*n* = 17)	0.92 ± 0.06	0.94 ± 0.05	0.69 ± 0.12
Asymptomatic Smokers (*n* = 15)	0.93 ± 0.08	0.95 ± 0.04	0.73 ± 0.11
COPD (*n* = 16)	0.86 ± 0.08*	0.88 ± 0.07*	0.57 ± 0.12*
All Subjects (*n* = 48)	0.90 ± 0.08	0.92 ± 0.06	0.66 ± 0.14

* Significance < 0.016 level. Particle deposition fraction, DF, for the different groups (average DF ± 1 standard deviation). Significant differences compared to the healthy reference group marked by *, (Bonferroni adjusted significance level 0.016)

The measured DF was found to correlate with $FEV_{1\%pred}$ and $FEV_1/VC_{\%pred}$ when all (n = 48) subjects were included in the analysis. This is most likely an effect of group differences (Table 3). There was no significant correlation between DF and sex, age, weight, height or VC for any of the groups or when all subjects were analysed together. For healthy never-smokers a negative correlation was found between DF and $FEV_{1\%pred}$. The correlation was weak for 50 nm particles, at 1300 mL and 1800 mL respectively (Pearson's $r = -0.489$, $p = 0.047$ and Pearson's $r = -0.491$, $p = 0.045$), but much stronger for 100 nm particles at 1800 mL sample depth (Pearson's $r = -0.728$, $p = 0.001$). No significant correlation was found between the spirometry parameters and DF for the COPD group or for the asymptomatic smokers.

Significant correlation between DF and $D_{L,CO\ \%pred}$ was found for the COPD group. Especially when studying the subjects with < 90% $D_{L,CO\ \%pred}$, (Fig. 5). Computed tomography data was available for all but one of these subjects, and a visual grading [26] of the group confirmed that the subjects with > 90% $D_{L,CO\ \%pred}$ had no or minor

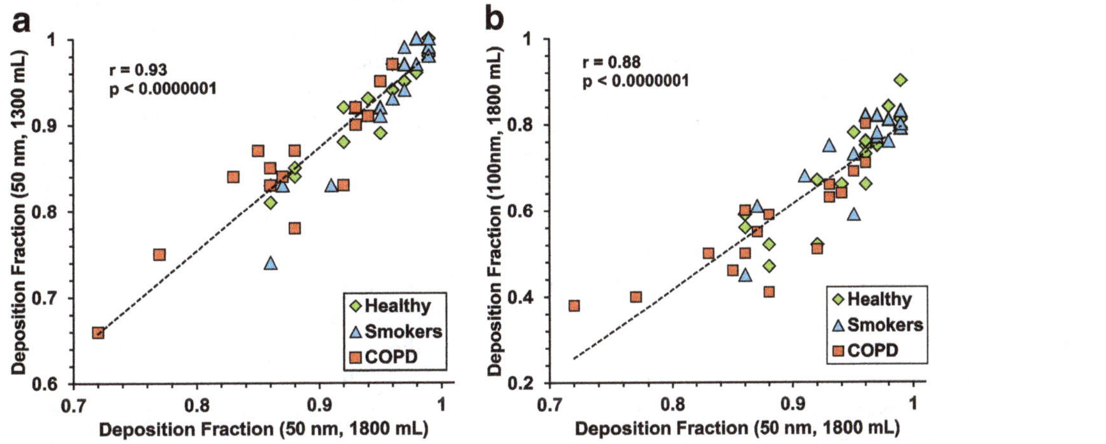

Fig. 4 (**a**, **b**). Correlations for volumetric sample depth and particle size. The relation between lung particle deposition measured at different sample depths and for different particle sizes. In **a** (left panel), for 50 nm particles at sample depths 1300 ml and 1800 ml, and in **b** (right panel), for 50 nm and 100 nm particles at sample depth 1800 ml. Pearson's correlation coefficient and *p*-values are indicated in the figure. Healthy = green, smokers = blue, COPD = red

emphysema, while the other subjects generally had moderate to severe emphysema. An analysis of the CT results, including CT densitometry, is described in a separate publication [14]. The correlations for all subjects are summarized in Table 3 and the correlation between $D_{L,CO}$ and DF for 50 nm particles (1300 mL, 1800 mL sample depth) and 100 nm (1800 mL sample depth) for the COPD group with < 90% $D_{L,CO\ \%pred}$ is shown in Fig. 5. There was no correlation between DF and $D_{L,CO}$ for the healthy subjects.

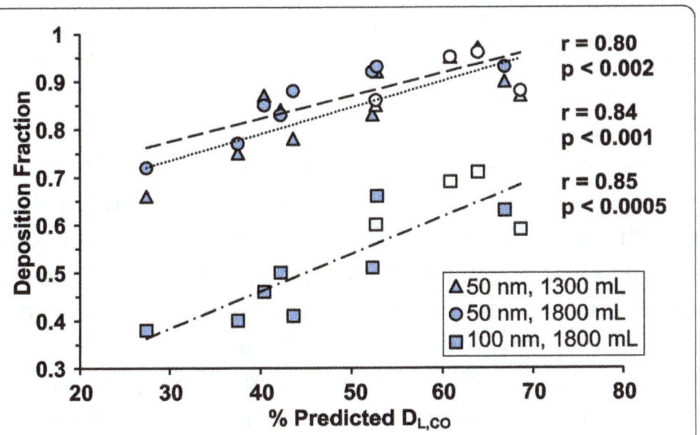

Fig. 5 Correlation between particle DF and $D_{L,CO}$ for COPD subjects. Correlation between $D_{L,CO}$ and particle deposition for emphysematous subjects (*n* = 12). The included subjects were confirmed to have emphysema by visual CT evaluation and graded to have mild (*n* = 2), moderate (*n* = 2) and severe (*n* = 8) emphysema. The visual grading is indicated by colour intensity (white = mild, light blue = moderate, dark blue = severe). Four subjects were omitted from the analysis based on a $D_{L,CO}$ > 95% of predicted, or missing data. Of these one had no emphysema and one was graded as having mild emphysema but 97% of predicted $D_{L,CO}$, CT data was missing for one subject and $D_{L,CO}$ was missing for one subject

Discussion

This study presents measurements of deposition of nanoparticles in the distal lungs, for healthy never-smoking subjects, asymptomatic (active or former) smokers and subjects with diagnosed COPD. Measurements were performed using a controlled breathing pattern including a breath hold. There was a significant difference in particle deposition between COPD patients and the other subjects, but no significant differences between the healthy never-smokers and asymptomatic smokers. Significant correlation was also found between DF and $D_{L,CO\%pred}$ for

Table 3 Correlation between deposition fractions and lung function

		DF 50 nm 1300 mL	DF 50 nm 1800 mL	DF 100 nm 1800 mL
$FEV_{1\%pred}$	Pearson's r	0.317*	0.391**	0.357**
	p-value	0.028	0.0060	0.013
$FEV_1/VC_{\%pred}$	Pearson's r	0.452**	0.530***	0.574***
	p-value	0.0013	0.00011	0.000020
$DL_{CO\ \%pred}$ †	Pearson's r	0.494***	0.571***	0.518***
	p-value	0.00049	0.000034	0.00023

† *n* = 46, $D_{L,CO}$ data for two subjects is missing
*Significance < 0.05 level
**Significance < 0.01 level
***Significance < 0.001 level
Pearson's correlation coefficients, r, and p-values for the associations between particle deposition and clinical lung function tests for all subjects (n = 48)

patients with confirmed emphysema, but not for the other subjects.

The method used in this study is specifically designed to examine particle deposition in the alveolar region of the lung during a breath-hold. Although the controlled breathing pattern deviates from normal tidal breathing, and therefore does not reflect a typical everyday exposure scenario, it enables investigation of specific relations between lung morphology and particle deposition mechanisms. We used monodisperse nanoparticles, known to deposit mainly by diffusion in the distal lung, with small influence of the larger conducting airways, [28]. Time normalization was applied to minimize differences in breathing pattern, and measurements were performed at full lung inflation. As a consequence, most of the observed particle deposition is expected to occur by diffusion during the breath-hold, with the lung at a fixed state of inflation. It is therefore likely that the variation of particle deposition in this study primarily reflects individual variation of lung morphology in the peripheral lung.

Mainly two features of lung morphology can be assumed to affect lung deposition in diseased lungs: narrowing of the bronchioles (bronchiolitis), causing increased deposition, and enlargement of distal airspaces (emphysema) with the opposite effect [29]. Generally it can be supposed that COPD subjects have varying proportions of both bronchiolitis and emphysema, and that the asymptomatic smokers primarily have some irritation and narrowing of the bronchioles [19, 20, 30].

The observed decrease in DF for the COPD subjects in this study is most probably caused by the presence of pulmonary emphysema, a conclusion that is supported by the correlation between DF and $D_{L,CO}$ for the COPD group. However, other lung features that could provide an alternative explanation should be further investigated. Local alterations to the lung morphology, such as chokes, collapsing airways or poorly ventilated airspaces (i.e. bullae) most probably also have some effect on particle deposition. However, these conditions would more likely increase than decrease particle deposition, and thus do not explain the observed findings. It is also important to note that even though we found a significantly lower DF for subjects with COPD in this study, the total particle burden may be increased for this group during natural tidal breathing, as individuals with COPD generally have increased minute ventilation and thus process more air than healthy individuals [13, 31].

Previous studies of lung deposition of nanoparticles (< 100 nm) are scarce and the reported data show much divergence. This can be attributed to differences in methodology as well as differences between individual subjects [5]. Several studies of the deposition of nanoparticles have been performed with natural or spontaneous breathing patterns [4, 12, 13, 15–17, 32–38]. Generally, the studies report lower particle deposition than found in the present study, as expected since most of these previous studies are performed at lower degrees of lung inflation and shorter residence times of aerosol in the lung. Studies with controlled breathing patterns [2, 11, 12, 39–43], usually defined by controlled volumes and flow rates, result in particle deposition being measured at different degrees of lung inflation and from different anatomical regions of the lung. Several studies report increased DF both for smokers [2, 17] and for subjects with airflow obstruction [16, 37]. This is contrary to our results. However, most of the studies measure particle deposition at shallower volumetric lung depths, leading to a stronger influence of the deposition in the conducting airways (such as turbulent diffusion at local anatomical alterations) rather than in the alveolar region of the lung targeted by this study.

Several mechanisms for the increased DF of nanoparticles in obstructed subjects have been proposed by Anderson et al. [11]. The obstructed subjects in their study (n = 5) were characterized as having mainly chronic bronchitis or asthma. Among the suggested mechanisms, it was shown that failure to comply with the predetermined breathing pattern, resulting in longer residence times for the patients, did not fully explain the observed differences in deposition, and they suggest that abnormal expiratory collapse of airways and narrowing of airway calibre combined with excessive airway secretion is a more likely mechanism.

Using a similar breathing protocol and particle size (92–103 nm) as the present study, Möller et al. [2], found significant differences in DF between healthy subjects (n = 9), asymptomatic smokers (n = 10) and COPD patients (n = 7), with increased DF for smokers and COPD patients. The particle deposition was measured after bolus administration of aerosol to 800 and 150 mL volumetric lung depth. Differences were only found at 800 mL. The authors concluded that the observed increased DF was caused by narrowing of the distal airways, bronchiolitis, and that at the more shallow bolus, (reaching mainly central airways), the relative changes in airway diameter for obstructive subjects were not expected to have a strong influence on diffusional particle deposition.

To our knowledge, the only study reporting data for confirmed emphysematous subjects (with exception for the measurements performed within this project [14]), Brown et al. [12], agrees with our results [14]. In that study lower DF is reported for subjects with emphysema (n = 3) than for healthy subjects (n = 9), and higher DF for subjects with bronchitis (n = 7) than for healthy subjects. Another study by Löndahl et al. [13], using continuous breathing of polydisperse diesel exhaust particles has also showed lowered DF in subjects with COPD in the size range < 100 nm, similar to the results in this study, but increased DF for larger particles, that have a higher probability to deposit by inertial impaction and sedimentation in the conducting airways.

More data on DF in the peripheral lungs are available for larger aerosol particles, than for nanoparticles. Techniques have been developed to use airborne particles to infer information about the lung, using controlled breathing patterns similar to the present study, but with particles close to 1 μm in size [44, 45]. In similarity with our results, these studies also found a decreased DF in the distal lung for subjects with emphysema [46–50]. Particles around 1 μm inhaled at low flow rates are assumed to deposit mainly by sedimentation, and models have been developed to use these techniques to derive effective airway diameters (EADs) from particle deposition measurements [51–53]. The most well-explored of these techniques are the different versions of the aerosol-derived airway morphometry technique (ADAM) [45] and the bolus dispersion technique [44]. ADAM has been proposed as a diagnostic method with specificity for pulmonary emphysema [45] although the technique has not been established in clinical practice.

The conclusion that the decreased DF observed in the COPD group in this study is an effect of enlarged distal airspaces is also consistent with the correlations between lung function tests and DF. The influence of particle deposition in the upper airways have been minimized by the choice of particle size, volumetric sample depth and the inclusion of a breath hold. Correlations were found both with spirometric parameters and $D_{L,CO}$ when all subjects (n = 48) were included in the analysis, but not within all of the separate groups. Interestingly, correlation with $D_{L,CO}$ was only found within the COPD group, and a negative correlation to spirometry was only found in the healthy never-smoking group. The reason for the negative correlation between FEV_1 and particle deposition found for the healthy never-smoking subjects is not clear, but may be an effect of flow rate-dependent particle losses during the dynamic part of the breathing manoeuvre. The effect may be present for the other groups, but distorted by less uniform changes to the conducting airways and therefore not detected in this study. The found correlations agree with the results presented by Brown et al. [12], who report significant correlation between both $D_{L,CO}$ and particle deposition for the emphysematous subjects but not for the non-emphysematous subjects, who instead had a weak ($p = 0.045$) correlation between particle deposition and spirometry.

The DF was consistently higher for 1800 mL than for 1300 mL volumetric sample depth in all groups, but the effect of volume is small compared to the influence of particle size. The observed relation between DF and volume was not merely an effect of different residence times in the lungs and in agreement with previous studies [2, 11], which attribute the increased DF to the increasingly narrowing dimensions in the tracheobronchial tree. The lower DF for 100 nm particles, compared to 50 nm particles, is consistent with the theory of Brownian diffusion and previous studies [4, 11, 15, 16, 43, 54].

$D_{L,CO}$ is known to correlate with degree of emphysema, and thus the correlation between $D_{L,CO}$ and DF suggests that the lower DF in the diseased group is not primarily caused by airflow obstruction, but rather by the extent of emphysema. Visual grading of the available CT-data for the obstructed subjects confirmed that those with $D_{L,CO} < 90\%$ of the predicted values had varying degrees of emphysema. This is also consistent with the full data set. As most subjects from the healthy groups are expected to have no or neglible emphysema, no correlation was expected for the healthy subjects. Correlations between particle deposition and CT-densitometry [14] also support this interpretation. Similar relations between particle deposition and lung function tests have also been observed for larger particles [46, 55, 56].

Although the number of subjects with COPD, to the best of our knowledge, exceeds previous comparable studies [10], the group is limited and more data is needed to support the conclusions. No clear differences were detected between healthy never-smokers and asymptomatic smokers. This could likely be explained by the classification of smokers (any reported tobacco use qualified the subject as a "smoker") that resulted in a diverse group with a wide range of smoking history. A more targeted recruitment of a group of "heavy smokers" may have generated clearer results. Another limitation that should be investigated further is the ability to perform measurements on diseased subjects. Several subjects were excluded from the study for not meeting the quality criteria of the particle deposition measurement. It was also observed that the intra-subject variability was elevated for the COPD group. The variability may reflect individual lung abnormalities, but may also be related to the ability of COPD subjects to comply with the measurement protocol. A re-design of the breathing manoeuvre with a shorter breath-hold and smaller exhaled volumes may be considered for future studies.

The results presented in this study suggest that measurement of lung deposition of nanoparticles could be utilized to detect and quantify respiratory disease, potentially giving medically relevant information about diffusion distances in the lungs similar to magnetic resonance imaging (MRI) with hyperpolarized noble gas [57, 58]. Such a technique, named AiDA, has recently been suggested by Löndahl et al. [29]. By measuring particle deposition for different breath-holding times and determining the particle half-life time in the lungs, it is possible to determine effective airspace radii in the distal lung. In two recent proof-of-concept studies the technique was compared to MRI [57] and CT [14]. In the MRI study the authors found that AiDA-derived airspace radii correlated with lung tissue density. In the CT study it was found that particle deposition correlated with CT densitometry for emphysematous subjects. These findings are in agreement with the results of this study.

Conclusions

This study presents measurements of nanoparticle deposition in the distal lung for healthy subjects and subjects with COPD during a breath-hold. DF was significantly lower for subjects with COPD compared to the healthy group, which can be explained by enlarged distal airspaces caused by emphysema. The conclusion was further strengthened by a strong correlation between DF and emphysema, as assessed by $D_{L,CO\%pred}$, within the COPD group. The results show that lung morphology has a significant influence on the deposition of nanoparticles in humans, and should be considered when estimating the lung burden of airborne particles, when identifying especially vulnerable groups and in dosimetry of aerosol based drug delivery.

Abbreviations

ADAM: Aerosol-derived Airway Morphometry; AiDA: Airspace Dimension Assessment by nanoparticles; bCPC: (Butanol) Condensation particle counter; COPD: Chronic obstructive pulmonary disease; CT: Computed tomography; DF: Deposition fraction; $D_{L,CO}$: Diffusing capacity for carbon monoxide; DMA: Differential mobility analyser; FEV_1: Forced expiratory flow during one second; GOLD: Global Initiative on Obstructive Disease; ICS: Inhaled corticosteroid; LABA: long-acting beta-agonist; LAMA: long-acting muscarinic antagonist; PSL: Polystyrene Latex; RV: Residual volume; TLC: Total lung capacity; VC: Vital capacity

Acknowledgements

The authors would like to acknowledge Eeva Piitulainen, dept. of Respiratory Medicine and Allergology, Lund University, Sweden, for recruiting volunteers to the study and Sandra Diaz, dept. of Translational Medicine, Lund University, Sweden, for aiding in designing the CT protocol used and reviewing the CT images.

Funding

The following organizations are gratefully acknowledged for financial support: The Swedish Research Council, the Crafoord foundation, the Swedish Governmental Agency for Innovation Systems (VINNOVA), the ERA-NET project EuroNanoMed2, the Swedish Research Council for Health, Working Life and Welfare (FORTE) and the Swedish Heart and Lung Foundation.

Authors' contributions

JKFJ, JL, HLA and PW designed the study. All authors reviewed and had input to the protocol. HLA recruited the patients. JKFJ and HN performed the particle deposition measurements. HLA reviewed the CT images. All authors took part in the data analysis and data interpretation. JKFJ wrote the first version of the manuscript. All authors had input to the manuscript and approved the final version.

Consent for publication

Not applicable.

Competing interests

Jakob Löndahl and Per Wollmer have a patent pending for the lung deposition measurement technology, Airspace Dimension Assessment with nanoparticles (AiDA). Jonas Jakobsson, H Laura Aaltonen, Hanna Nicklasson, Anders Gudmundsson and Jenny Rissler declare no competing interests.

Author details

[1]Division of Ergonomics and Aerosol Technology, Lund University, Lund, Sweden. [2]Department of Translational Medicine, Lund University, Malmö, Sweden. [3]Chemistry, Materials and Surfaces, SP Technical Research Institute of Sweden, Lund, Sweden.

References

1. Heal MR, Kumar P, Harrison RM. Particles, air quality, policy and health. Chem Soc Rev. 2012;41(19):6606–30.
2. Möller W, Felten K, Sommerer K, Scheuch G, Meyer G, Meyer P, Haussinger K, Kreyling WG. Deposition, retention, and translocation of ultrafine particles from the central airways and lung periphery. Am J Respir Crit Care Med. 2008;177(4):426–32.
3. Tarroni G, Melandri C, Prodi V, De Zaiacomo T, Formignani M, Bassi P. An indication on the biological variability of aerosol total deposition in humans. Am Ind Hyg Assoc J. 1980;41(11):826–31.
4. Löndahl J, Massling A, Pagels J, Swietlicki E, Vaclavik E, Loft S. Size-resolved respiratory-tract deposition of fine and ultrafine hydrophobic and hygroscopic aerosol particles during rest and exercise. Inhal Toxicol. 2007; 19(2):109–16.
5. Heyder J, Gebhart J, Stahlhofen W, Stuck B. Biological variability of particle deposition in the human respiratory-tract during controlled and spontaneous mouth-breathing. Ann Occup Hyg. 1982;26(1–4):137–47.
6. Rissler J, Gudmundsson A, Nicklasson H, Swietlicki E, Wollmer P, Londahl J. Deposition efficiency of inhaled particles (15-5000 nm) related to breathing pattern and lung function: an experimental study in healthy children and adults. Part Fibre Toxicol. 2017;14:10.
7. Hofmann W, Bergmann R, Ménache MG. The effect of intersubject variability in airway morphology on intersubject variations in particle deposition. J Aerosol Sci. 1998;29(SUPPL.2):S943–4.
8. Hofmann W, Asgharian B, Winkler-Heila R. Modeling intersubject variability of particle deposition in human lungs. J Aerosol Sci. 2002;33(2):219–35.
9. Hussain M, Renate WH, Werner H. Effect of intersubject variability of extrathoracic morphometry, lung airways dimensions and respiratory parameters on particle deposition. Journal of Thoracic Disease. 2011; 3(3):156–70.
10. Löndahl J, Möller W, Pagels JH, Kreyling WG, Swietlicki E, Schmid O. Measurement techniques for respiratory tract deposition of airborne nanoparticles: a critical review. J Aerosol Med Pulm Drug Deliv. 2014;27(4): 229–54.
11. Anderson PJ, Wilson JD, Hiller FC. Respiratory-tract deposition of ultrafine particles in subjects with obstructive or restrictive lung-disease. Chest. 1990; 97(5):1115–20.
12. Brown JS, Zeman KL, Bennett WD. Ultrafine particle deposition and clearance in the healthy and obstructed lung. Am J Resp Crit Care. 2002; 166(9):1240–7.
13. Löndahl J, Swietlicki E, Rissler J, Bengtsson A, Boman C, Blomberg A, Sandstrom T. Experimental determination of the respiratory tract deposition of diesel combustion particles in patients with chronic obstructive pulmonary disease. Part Fibre Toxicol. 2012;9:30.
14. Aaltonen HL, Jakobsson JK, Diaz S, Zackrisson S, Piitulainen E, Londahl J, Wollmer P: Deposition of inhaled nanoparticles is reduced in subjects with COPD and correlates with the extent of emphysema: proof of concept for a novel diagnostic technique. Clin Physiol Funct Imaging 2018; doi:https://doi.org/10.1111/cpf.12517.
15. Daigle CC, Chalupa DC, Gibb FR, Morrow PE, Oberdorster G, Utell MJ, Frampton MW. Ultrafine particle deposition in humans during rest and exercise. Inhal Toxicol. 2003;15(6):539–52.

16. Chalupa DC, Morrow PE, Oberdorster G, Utell MJ, Frampton MW. Ultrafine particle deposition in subjects with asthma. Environ Health Perspect. 2004; 112(8):879–82.
17. Morawska L, Barron W, Hitchins J. Experimental deposition of environmental tobacco smoke submicrometer particulate matter in the human respiratory tract. Am Ind Hyg Assoc J. 1999;60(3):334–9.
18. Wilson FJ Jr, Hiller FC, Wilson JD, Bone RC. Quantitative deposition of ultrafine stable particles in the human respiratory tract. J Appl Physiol (1985). 1985;58(1):223–9.
19. Niewoehner DE, Kleinerman J, Rice DB. Pathologic changes in the peripheral Airways of Young Cigarette Smokers. N Engl J Med. 1974;291(15):755–8.
20. Woodruff PG, Barr RG, Bleecker E, Christenson SA, Couper D, Curtis JL, Gouskova NA, Hansel NN, Hoffman EA, Kanner RE, et al. Clinical significance of symptoms in smokers with preserved pulmonary function. N Engl J Med. 2016;374(19):1811–21.
21. Quanjer PH, Tammeling GJ, Cotes JE, Pedersen OF, Peslin R, Yernault JC. Lung volumes and forced ventilatory flows. Work Group on Standardization of Respiratory Function Tests. European Community for Coal and Steel. Official position of the European Respiratory Society. Rev Mal Respir. 1994; 11(Suppl 3):5–40.
22. Macintyre N, Crapo RO, Viegi G, Johnson DC, van der Grinten CP, Brusasco V, Burgos F, Casaburi R, Coates A, Enright P, et al. Standardisation of the single-breath determination of carbon monoxide uptake in the lung. Eur Respir J. 2005;26(4):720–35.
23. Celli BR, MacNee W, Force AET. Standards for the diagnosis and treatment of patients with COPD: a summary of the ATS/ERS position paper. Eur Respir J. 2004;23(6):932–46.
24. Gomez FP, Rodriguez-Roisin R. Global initiative for chronic obstructive lung disease (GOLD) guidelines for chronic obstructive pulmonary disease. Curr Opin Pulm Med. 2002;8(2):81–6.
25. Miller MR, Hankinson J, Brusasco V, Burgos F, Casaburi R, Coates A, Crapo R, Enright P, van der Grinten CP, Gustafsson P, et al. Standardisation of spirometry. Eur Respir J. 2005;26(2):319–38.
26. Bankier AA, De Maertelaer V, Keyzer C, Gevenois PA. Pulmonary emphysema: subjective visual grading versus objective quantification with macroscopic morphometry and thin-section CT densitometry 1. Radiology. 1999;211(3):851–8.
27. Jakobsson JKF, Hedlund J, Kumlin J, Wollmer P, Löndahl J. A new method for measuring lung deposition efficiency of airborne nanoparticles in a single breath. Sci Rep. 2016;6:36147.
28. ICRP. Human respiratory tract model for radiological protection. A report of a task Group of the International Commission on radiological protection. Ann ICRP. 1994;24(1–3):1–482.
29. Löndahl J, Jakobsson JKF, Broday DM, Aaltonen HL, Wollmer P. Do nanoparticles provide a new opportunity for diagnosis of distal airspace disease? Int J Nanomedicine. 2017;12:41–51.
30. Wright JL, Lawson LM, Pare PD, Wiggs BJ, Kennedy S, Hogg JC. Morphology of peripheral airways in current smokers and ex-smokers. Am Rev Respir Dis. 1983;127(4):474–7.
31. Tobin MJ, Chadha TS, Jenouri G, Birch SJ, Gazeroglu HB, Sackner MA. Breathing patterns. 2. Diseased subjects. Chest. 1983;84(3):286–94.
32. Morrow PE, Mehrhof E, Casarett LJ, Morken DA. An experimental study of aerosol deposition in human subjects. AMA Arch Ind Health. 1958; 18(4):292–8.
33. Wiebert P, Sanchez-Crespo A, Falk R, Philipson K, Lundin A, Larsson S, Moller W, Kreyling WG, Svartengren M. No significant translocation of inhaled 35-nm carbon particles to the circulation in humans. Inhal Toxicol. 2006;18(10):741–7.
34. Wiebert P, Sanchez-Crespo A, Seitz J, Falk R, Philipson K, Kreyling WG, Moller W, Sommerer K, Larsson S, Svartengren M. Negligible clearance of ultrafine particles retained in healthy and affected human lungs. Eur Respir J. 2006; 28(2):286–90.
35. Invernizzi G, Ruprecht A, De Marco C, Paredi P, Boffi R. Residual tobacco smoke: measurement of its washout time in the lung and of its contribution to environmental tobacco smoke. Tob Control. 2007;16(1):29–33.
36. Löndahl J, Pagels J, Boman C, Swietlicki E, Massling A, Rissler J, Blomberg A, Bohgard M, Sandstrom T. Deposition of biomass combustion aerosol particles in the human respiratory tract. Inhal Toxicol. 2008;20(10):923–33.
37. Olvera HA, Perez D, Clague JW, Cheng YS, Li WW, Amaya MA, Burchiel SW, Berwick M, Pingitore NE: The effect of ventilation, age, and asthmatic condition on ultrafine particle deposition in children. Pulmonary Medicine 2012. https://doi.org/10.1155/2012/736290.
38. Rissler J, Swietlicki E, Bengtsson A, Boman C, Pagels J, Sandstrom T, Blomberg A, Londahl J. Experimental determination of deposition of diesel exhaust particles in the human respiratory tract. J Aerosol Sci. 2012;48:18–33.
39. Blanchard JD, Willeke K. Total deposition of ultrafine sodium chloride particles in human lungs. J Appl Physiol Respir Environ Exerc Physiol. 1984; 57(6):1850–6.
40. Schiller CF, Gebhart J, Heyder J, Rudolf G, Stahlhofen W. Deposition of monodisperse insoluble aerosol particles in the 0.005 to 0.2 µm size range within the human respiratory tract. Annals of Occupational Hygiene. 1988; 32(inhaled particles VI):41–9.
41. Kim CS, Jaques PA. Respiratory dose of inhaled ultrafine particles in healthy adults. Philos T Roy Soc A. 2000;358(1775):2693–705.
42. Jaques PA, Kim CS. Measurement of total lung deposition of inhaled ultrafine particles in healthy men and women. Inhal Toxicol. 2000;12(8):715–31.
43. Kim CS, Jaques PA. Analysis of total respiratory deposition of inhaled ultrafine particles in adult subjects at various breathing patterns. Aerosol Sci Technol. 2004;38(6):525–40.
44. Blanchard JD. Aerosol bolus dispersion and aerosol-derived airway morphometry: Assessment of lung pathology and response to therapy .1. J Aerosol Med. 1996;9(2):183–205.
45. Blanchard JD. Aerosol bolus dispersion and aerosol-derived airway morphometry: Assessment of lung pathology and response to therapy .2. J Aerosol Med. 1996;9(4):453–76.
46. Lehnigk B, Schleiss M, Bluhme P, Jörres R, Brand P, Heyder J, Magnussen M. Aerosol-derived effective air space diameter (EAD) in different types of emphysema as characterized by computer tomography compared to healthy subjects. J Aerosol Med. 1995;8:126. (Abstract)
47. Brand P, Kohlhaufl M, Meyer T, Selzer T, Heyder J, Haussinger K. Aerosol-derived airway morphometry and aerosol bolus dispersion in patients with lung fibrosis and lung emphysema. Chest. 1999;116(2):543–8.
48. Kohlhaufl M, Brand P, Rock C, Radons T, Scheuch C, Meyer T, Schulz H, Pfeifer KJ, Haussinger K, Heyder J. Noninvasive diagnosis of emphysema - aerosol morphometry and aerosol bolus dispersion in comparison to HRCT. Am J Resp Crit Care. 1999;160(3):913–8.
49. Brand P, Letzel S, Buchta M, Scheuch G, Windorfer K, Hilla W, Smith HJ, Kraus T. Can aerosol-derived airway morphometry detect early, asymptomatical lung emphysema? J Aerosol Med. 2003;16(2):143–51.
50. Lehnigk B, Schleiss M, Brand P, Heyder J, Magnussen H, Jorres RA. Aerosol-derived airway morphometry (ADAM) in patients with lung emphysema diagnosed by computed tomography--reproducibility, diagnostic information and modelling. Eur J Med Res. 2007;12(2):74–83.
51. Heyder J. Gravitational deposition of aerosol particles within a system of randomly oriented tubes. J Aerosol Sci. 1975;6(2):133–7.
52. Heyder J. Assessment of airway geometry with inert aerosols. J Aerosol Sci. 1989;2(2):89–97.
53. Rosenthal FS. Aerosol recovery following breath-holding derived from the distribution of chord-lengths in pulmonary tissue. J Aerosol Sci. 1989;20(2): 267–77.
54. Brown JH, Cook KM, Ney FG, Hatch T. Influence of particle size upon the retention of particulate matter in the human lung. Am J Public Health Nations Health. 1950;40(4):450–80.
55. Blanchard JD, Heyder J, Odonnell CR, Brain JD. Comparison of aerosol-derived small airway caliber estimates with lung-function tests. Am Rev Respir Dis. 1986;133(4):A29.
56. Beinert T, Brand P, Behr J, Vogelmeier C, Heyder J. Peripheral airspace dimensions in patients with COPD. Chest. 1995;108(4):998–1003.
57. Aaltonen HL, Kindvall S, Jakobsson JKF, Löndahl J, Olsson LE, Diaz S, Zackrisson S, Wollmer P. Airspace dimension assessment with nanoparticles reflects lung density as quantified by MRI. Int J Nanomedicine. 2018;13:2989–95.
58. Yablonskiy DA, Sukstanskii AL, Leawoods JC, Gierada DS, Bretthorst GL, Lefrak SS, Cooper JD, Conradi MS. Quantitative in vivo assessment of lung microstructure at the alveolar level with hyperpolarized 3He diffusion MRI. Proc Natl Acad Sci. 2002;99(5):3111–6.

6

Unilateral diaphragm paralysis: a dysfunction restricted not just to one hemidiaphragm

Mayra Caleffi-Pereira[1], Renata Pletsch-Assunção[1], Letícia Zumpano Cardenas[1], Pauliane Vieira Santana[1], Jeferson George Ferreira[1], Vinícius Carlos Iamonti[1], Pedro Caruso[1], Angelo Fernandez[2], Carlos Roberto Ribeiro de Carvalho[1] and André Luís Pereira Albuquerque[1,3*]

Abstract

Background: Most patients with unilateral diaphragm paralysis (UDP) have unexplained dyspnea, exercise limitations, and reduction in inspiratory muscle capacity. We aimed to evaluate the generation of pressure in each hemidiaphragm separately and its contribution to overall inspiratory strength.

Methods: Twenty-seven patients, 9 in right paralysis group (RP) and 18 in left paralysis group (LP), with forced vital capacity (FVC) < 80% pred, and 20 healthy controls (CG), with forced expiratory volume in 1 s (FEV_1) > 80% pred and FVC > 80% pred, were evaluated for lung function, maximal inspiratory (MIP) and expiratory (MEP) pressure measurements, diaphragm ultrasound, and transdiaphragmatic pressure during magnetic phrenic nerve stimulation (Pdi_{TW}).

Results: RP and LP had significant inspiratory muscle weakness compared to controls, detected by MIP (− 57.4 ± 16.9 for RP; − 67.1 ± 28.5 for LP and − 103.1 ± 30.4 cmH_2O for CG) and also by Pdi_{TW} (5.7 ± 4 for RP; 4.8 ± 2.3 for LP and 15.3 ± 5.7 cmH_2O for CG). The Pdi_{TW} was reduced even when the non-paralyzed hemidiaphragm was stimulated, mainly due to the low contribution of gastric pressure (around 30%), regardless of whether the paralysis was in the right or left hemidiaphragm. On the other hand, in CG, esophagic and gastric pressures had similar contribution to the overall Pdi (around 50%). Comparing both paralyzed and non-paralyzed hemidiaphragms, the mobility during quiet and deep breathing, and thickness at functional residual capacity (FRC) and total lung capacity (TLC), were significantly reduced in paralyzed hemidiaphragm. In addition, thickness fraction was extremely diminished when contrasted with the non-paralyzed hemidiaphragm.

Conclusions: In symptomatic patients with UDP, global inspiratory strength is reduced not only due to weakness in the paralyzed hemidiaphragm but also to impairment in the pressure generated by the non-paralyzed hemidiaphragm.

Keywords: Diaphragm paralysis, Diaphragm strength, Diaphragm dysfunction, Electromagnetic phrenic nerve stimulation

* Correspondence: drean.albuquerque@gmail.com
[1]Pulmonary Division, Heart Institute (Incor), Hospital das Clínicas da Faculdade de Medicina da Universidade de São Paulo, Av. Dr. Enéas Carvalho Aguiar, n°44. Cerqueira Cesar., São Paulo 05403-900, Brazil
[3]Sírio-Libanês Teaching and Research Institute, São Paulo, Brazil
Full list of author information is available at the end of the article

Background

Dysfunction of the diaphragm is an important, underdiagnosed cause of breathlessness. Most patients with bilateral involvement already experience dyspnea on mild effort or even at rest, mainly while in the supine position. In unilateral diaphragm weakness, the presentation can be asymptomatic or with dyspnea on exercise, frequently discovered incidentally [1, 2]. The association of comorbidities, such as cardiopulmonary diseases or obesity, frequently increases the clinical symptoms, but the mechanisms involved in the genesis of dyspnea still have not been elucidated regarding unilateral involvement.

During normal inspiration, the contraction of the diaphragm draws a caudal movement as a whole. In other words, both right and left sides work harmoniously generating positive pressure in the abdominal compartment and negative pressure in the pleural space. In unilateral diaphragm paralysis (UDP), it is believed that the non-paralyzed hemidiaphragm increases in strength to compensate for the dysfunction of the paralyzed hemidiaphragm; therefore, most of these patients are able to maintain appropriate ventilatory conditions at rest and during mild exercise [3]. However, this is not true for all patients, because many of them have unexplained dyspnea, exercise limitations, and a reduction in inspiratory muscle capacity [1, 4]. Taking into account the fact that the paralyzed hemidiaphragm usually has a pendulum movement into the thorax (paradoxical movement) [1, 2], it has the potential to impair the pressure generated during inspiration even in the non-paralyzed hemidiaphragm.

We hypothesized that UDP also impairs the function of the non-paralyzed hemidiaphragm, mainly influenced by the low abdominal pressure. The aim of the present study was to evaluate the generation of pressure in each hemidiaphragm separately and their contribution to the overall transdiaphragmatic pressure (Pdi) in healthy subjects and patients with UDP.

Methods

Subjects

This was a cross-sectional study involving 27 patients with UDP (9 with right paralysis [RP] and 18 with left paralysis [LP]), who were consecutively recruited from a tertiary university hospital. All diagnoses were confirmed by the respiratory physician, using complementary imaging studies with ultrasound (USG), chest computed tomography, or radiography. The inclusion criteria were the restrictive pattern (FVC < 80% pred) and body mass index (BMI) between 20 and 30 kg/m^2. Patients with lung diseases and neuromuscular disorders were excluded. A control group (CG) was included composed of 20 healthy, age-matched subjects with normal lung function (FEV_1 > 80% pred and FVC > 80% pred) who were physically inactive (exercise activity less than twice a week). The study was approved by the local Ethics Committee (CapPesq) (protocol number: 0835/11), and all subjects provided written informed consent.

Study protocol

The individuals were evaluated with the following measurements at rest: lung function tests, maximal inspiratory (MIP) and expiratory (MEP) pressures, esophageal and gastric pressures during electromagnetic phrenic nerve stimulation with Twitches, and diaphragm motion and thickness with ultrasound. All the measurements were completed during a single visit.

Measurements

Lung function tests

All measurements were performed according to American Thoracic Society/European Respiratory Society (ATS/ERS) guidelines [5–7]. Spirometry was performed using a calibrated pneumotachograph (Medical Graphics Corporation - MGC, St. Paul, MN, USA), whereas lung volumes and carbon monoxide diffusion capacity (DL_{CO}) were obtained on a body plethysmograph (Elite Dx, Elite Series™ – MGC). The following variables were obtained: forced vital capacity (FVC), expiratory forced volume in the first second (FEV_1), total lung capacity (TLC), residual volume (RV), and DL_{CO}. The control group underwent only forced spirometry to measure FEV_1 and FVC.

Dyspnea

The degree of dyspnea was assessed using the Medical Research Council Breathlessness Scale [8].

Maximal inspiratory (MIP) and expiratory (MEP) pressures

MIP and MEP were measured using a digital manovacuometer (MicroRPM®, CareFusion, Yorba Linda, CA, USA). In the sitting position with a nose clip, subjects were asked to exhale to RV and then perform a maximal inspiratory effort for at least 3 s for MIP measurement; for MEP measurement, they were asked to inhale to TLC followed by a maximal expiratory effort for at least 3 s. The maneuvers were repeated 3 to 5 times, and the highest pressures were selected for analysis [9].

The predicted values for lung function and ventilatory pressures were derived from the Brazilian population [10–12].

Transdiaphragmatic pressure (Pdi)

To measure Pdi, 2 air-filled balloon catheters (Adult Esophageal Balloon Catheter Set, CooperSurgical, Trumbull, CT, USA) were used. One was positioned into the distal esophagus and filled with 1 mL of air, ensuring the correct position by correlating esophageal pressure (Pes) with mouth pressure (Pmo) by using the occlusion technique [13]. To access gastric pressure (Pga), the distal balloon was introduced 65 cm from the nares and positioned in the stomach, filled with 1.5 mL of air. Both catheters were connected to pressure transducers (TruStability® Standard Accuracy Silicon Ceramic, Honeywell, Morris Plains, NJ, USA), which were calibrated before each test with a graded water column at 3 different levels (0, 10, and 20 cmH_2O). Both Pes and Pga were measured continuously, and Pdi was calculated automatically (Pdi = Pga − Pes) during the entire acquisition.

To measure non-volitional Pdi we performed magnetic phrenic nerve stimulation (Twitch) (MagProCompact®, MagVenture-Denmark), with two 45-mm figure-of-eight coils (MC-B35, MagPro, MagVenture), to create a field focused on the phrenic nerve [14]. With the patient in a sitting position, arms relaxed, with a nose clip and a mouthpiece, the coils were placed on the posterior edge of the sternocleidomastoid muscle at the level of the cricoid cartilage [15]. The individuals were instructed to exhale to the functional residual capacity (FRC), the mouthpiece was occluded, and a maximal stimulus was applied 5 times, with 30-s intervals between them. At the time of magnetic stimulation, the Pes and Pmo were mandatory to be in plateau after expiration to ensure the Twitch was applied from the FRC. This protocol was performed in 3 phrenic magnetic stimulations: bilateral (two 45-mm coil synchronized), unilateral right, and unilateral left. The highest transdiaphragmatic pressure during magnetic phrenic nerve stimulation (Pdi_{Tw}) value among at least 3 reproducible maneuvers (< 10% of difference) in each position was considered for analyses.

AqDados 7.0 software (Lynx technology, Brazil) was used for data acquisition and the AqAnalysis 7.0 (Lynx technology, Brazil) for data analysis.

Diaphragm ultrasound

Ultrasound imaging of the diaphragm was performed using a portable ultrasound system (Nanomaxx; Sonosite, Bothell, WA, USA) while subjects were in a semi-recumbent position. For the evaluation of diaphragmatic mobility, we installed a 2–5 MHz convex transducer. For the right hemidiaphragm, the probe was placed over the right anterior subcostal region between the midclavicular and anterior axillary lines. The transducer was directed medially cephalad, and dorsally, so that the ultrasound beam reached perpendicularly the posterior third of the right hemidiaphragm. The 2-dimensional (2D) mode was initially used to visualize and obtain the best approach, with the liver serving as an acoustic window to the right, and to select the exploration line. Then, the M-mode was used to display and measure the amplitude of the cranio-caudal diaphragmatic excursion during quiet breathing and deep breathing. For the left measurement, the probe was placed on subcostal or low intercostal regions between the anterior and mid axillary lines to obtain the best image of the left hemidiaphragm dome. The same respiratory maneuvers were performed to measure the left hemidiaphragm excursion [16, 17]. The ultrasound images acquired were measured on scans off-line using ImageJ software (available at: http://rsb.info.nih.gov/ij/docs/index.html). We recorded the averaged value of 3 consecutive measurements. The mobility of the diaphragm during a sniff test was performed to exclude paradoxical movement.

Right and left diaphragm thickness was measured in B-mode with a 6–13 MHz linear transducer placed over the zone of apposition (ZA) of the diaphragm to the rib cage, between the anterior and medial axillary lines. In the ZA, the diaphragm is observed as a structure made of 3 distinct layers: a nonechogenic central layer bordered by 2 echogenic layers, the peritoneum, and the diaphragmatic pleurae. The thickness was measured from the middle of the pleural line to the middle of the peritoneal line [18, 19]. We measured the thickness of the diaphragm during quiet spontaneous breathing at FRC, and at breath holding after a maximal inspiratory effort at TLC. Again, the averaged value of 3 consecutive measurements was recorded for each. We also calculated the thickening fraction (TF, proportional thickening of the diaphragm from FRC to TLC), an index of diaphragmatic thickening as defined by the following equation: $TF = ([Th_{TLC} - Th_{FRC}] \ / \ Th_{FRC}) \times 100$, where Th_{FRC} is thickness of the diaphragm measured at the end of a quiet expiration (at FRC), and Th_{TLC} is the maximum thickness of the diaphragm measured at the end of deep breathing (at TLC).

Statistical analysis

Statistical analysis was performed using SPSS 21.0 software (IBM SPSS Statistics®, US). The Shapiro-Wilk test was used to verify the normality of data distribution. The data are presented as mean ± standard deviation and percentage. To compare anthropometric data, lung function, and respiratory strength among the 3 groups (CG, RP, and LP), we used 1-way ANOVA with the Tukey posthoc test. The *t* test for independent samples was used to compare lung capacities (TLC, RV, and DLCO) between RP and LP, and also to compare the mobility and thickness between paralyzed hemidiaphragm and non-paralyzed hemidiaphragm. The significance level was set to 5% ($p < 0.05$).

Results

The most frequent causes of diaphragm paralysis (DP) were trauma and idiopathic reasons. Among the comorbidities, systemic arterial hypertension was prevalent in almost half of patients, with former smokers being 30%

(Table 1). None of the subjects had airflow obstruction (all had $FEV_1/FVC >$ the lower limit of normal and RV preserved) or lung parenchyma involvement (emphysema or air trapping areas) on lung function and chest CT, respectively.

No difference was found related to sex, age, and BMI among the groups (Table 2). Patients with UDP had lower FEV_1 and FVC than controls, irrespective of the hemidiaphragm involved. Furthermore, patients were characterized by reduced lung volumes (FVC and TLC), with a normal or mild reduction in DL_{CO}, and irrespective of which hemidiaphragm was involved, they had dyspnea with mild and moderate exercise (MRC score) (Table 2).

Table 3 shows muscle strength measurements. Considering inspiratory and expiratory strength measures, patients with UDP had significant respiratory muscle weakness detected by volitional tests. No statistical difference existed in transdiaphragmatic pressure during sniff (Pdi_{sniff}) between RP and LP groups compared with controls.

During bilateral Twitch, the controls had Pes, Pga, and Pdi approximately 2 to 3 times higher than RP and LP. In controls, Pdi produced by unilateral stimulation was similar for both right (7.4 cmH_2O) and left (8.9 cmH_2O) hemidiaphragms, suggesting that each hemidiaphragm contributed equally to total Pdi during bilateral stimulation (15.3 cmH2O). In patients, unilateral Pdi was reduced not only during paralyzed-hemidiaphragm stimu lation but also during non-paralyzed hemidiaphragm stimulation in both RP group (3 cmH_2O for right twitch and 4.1 cmH_2O for left twitch) and LP group (2.1 cmH_2O for left twitch and 2.9 cmH_2O for right twitch), contributing to their decreased total Pdi during bilateral stimulation (5.7 cmH_2O for RP and 4.8 cmH_2O for LP) compared with controls. (Fig. 1).

Pes and Pga have nearly equal contributions to Pdi in CG for all Twitch conditions. In patients with UDP, however, the contribution of Pga (around 30% of total Pdi) was significantly reduced compared to controls, regardless of the side of involvement (RP or LP), and the Pes was the main component for total Pdi (around 70% of total Pdi) (Fig. 2).

The paralyzed hemidiaphragm had major impairments related to mobility and thickness compared with the non-paralyzed hemidiaphragm. The mobility, defined as total diaphragm displacement during inspiration, was

Table 1 Causes of diaphragmatic paralysis, associated comorbidities, and smoking history

	n (%)
Causes of DP	
Idiopathic	8 (29.6)
Trauma	10 (37.0)
Cardiac surgery	6 (22.2)
Thoracic surgery	3 (11.1)
Comorbidities	
Arterial hypertension	12 (44.4)
Valvopathy	4 (14.8)
Acute myocardial infarction	2 (7.4)
Active smoker	–
Former smoker	8 (29.6)
Pack/years	19.6

Data expressed as n (%). *DP* diaphragmatic paralysis

Table 2 Anthropometric data, lung function, and dyspnea of CG, RP, and LP

	CG ($n = 20$)	RP ($n = 9$)	LP ($n = 18$)
Anthropometric data			
Male, n (%)	10 (50)	3 (33.3)	12 (66.7)
Age, years	50 ± 6.5	57 ± 11	55 ± 11.4
BMI, kg/m^2	27.9 ± 2.1	29.4 ± 4.6	27.9 ± 3.0
Lung Function			
FEV_1, L	2.9 ± 0.5	1.5 ± 0.6*	2.0 ± 0.7*
% predicted	91.9 ± 8.5	52.9 ± 15.3*	60.9 ± 14.1*
FVC, L	3.5 ± 0.7	1.9 ± 0.6*	2.6 ± 0.8*
% predicted	91.6 ± 8.1	56.0 ± 13.2*	64.4 ± 13.7*
FEV_1/ FVC	82.2 ± 4.9	77.0 ± 9.0*	75.8 ± 6.6*
TLC, L	–	3.9 ± 0.9	4.6 ± 1.0
% predicted		76.9 ± 11.8	78.8 ± 12.1
RV, L	–	2.1 ± 0.8	1.9 ± 0.5
% predicted		119.2 ± 46.7	94.9 ± 20.9
DL_{CO}	–	16.2 ± 9.9	23.3 ± 7.6
% predicted		61.9 ± 27.1	82.9 ± 24.3
MRC	–	2 ± 0.7	1.5 ± 0.7

Data expressed as mean ± standard deviation and n (%) for sex. *CG* control group, *RP* right paralysis group, *LP* left paralysis group, *BMI* body mass index, FEV_1 forced expiratory volume in 1 s, *FVC* forced vital capacity, *TLC* total lung capacity, *RV* residual volume, *L* liters, DL_{CO} carbon monoxide diffusing capacity, *MRC* Medical Research Council Breathlessness Scale. *$p < 0.05$ compared with control

Table 3 Respiratory muscle strength data of CG, RP, and LP

	CG ($n = 20$)	RP ($n = 9$)	LP ($n = 18$)
Respiratory muscle strength			
MIP, cmH_2O	−103.1 ± 30.4	−57.4 ± 16.9*	−67.1 ± 28.5*
% predicted	99.5 ± 20.9	59.9 ± 13.4*	63.4 ± 21.2*
MEP, cmH_2O	120.9 ± 41.6	78.8 ± 24.8*	95.8 ± 43.8*
% predicted	115.5 ± 35.6	85.1 ± 24.8*	85.8 ± 32.3*
SNIP, cmH_2O	95.9 ± 20.0	53.9 ± 16.7*	62.0 ± 17.5*
% predicted	88.5 ± 28.0	56.0 ± 15.2*	60.0 ± 13.7*
Pdi_{Sniff}, cmH_2O	70.3 ± 25.5	51.7 ± 10.9	53.4 ± 21.6

Data expressed as mean ± standard deviation. *CG* control group, *Pdi* transdiaphragmatic pressure, *RP* right paralysis group, *LP* left paralysis group, *MIP* maximal inspiratory pressure, *MEP* maximal expiratory pressure, *SNIP* sniff nasal inspiratory pressure. *$p < 0.05$ compared with control

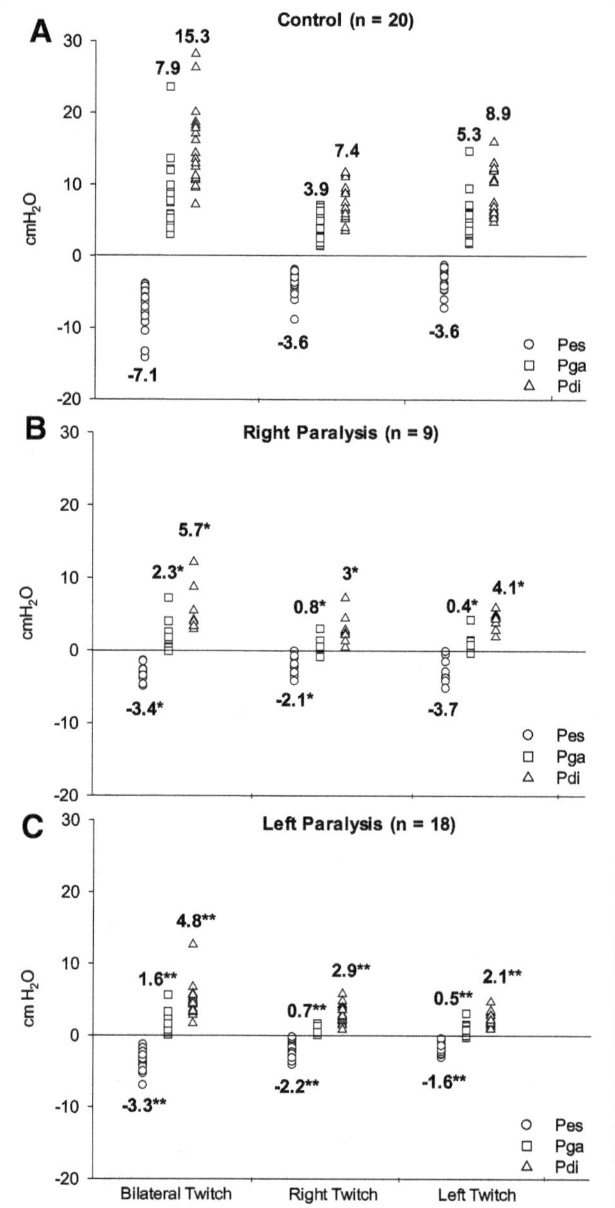

Fig. 1 Pes, Pga, and Pdi during bilateral, right, and left Twitch. **a** Control; **b** Right paralysis; **c** Left paralysis. Pes: esophageal pressure; Pga: gastric pressure; Pdi: transdiaphragmatic pressure. $*p < 0.05$ Right Paralysis vs Control; $**p < 0.05$ Left Paralysis vs Control. Bold numbers mean the mean value (cmH_2O)

significantly reduced not only during quiet breathing but also during deep breathing. The thickness was also reduced at FRC and TLC, and the thickness fraction was extremely diminished when contrasted with the non-paralyzed hemidiaphragm. Moreover, the ratio between transdiaphragmatic pressure during unilateral stimuli and thickness at TLC ($PdiTw_U/Thick_{TLC}$) is significantly higher in paralyzed hemidiaphragm than non-paralyzed hemidiaphragm (Fig. 3). Paradoxical movement of the paralyzed hemidiaphragm during sniff was found in 11 (38%) patients. It was not possible to evaluate sniff in 4 patients, because the left hemidiaphragm was not properly accessible in the USG window.

Discussion

This study describes the contribution of each hemidiaphragm to the inspiratory pressure generated in patients with UDP during Twitch and compared with healthy individuals. Of note, the reduced inspiratory pressure is not restricted to the side with paralysis. Regardless of whether it is right or left paralysis, the maximal inspiratory pressures generated by paralyzed and non-paralyzed hemidiaphragms were lower, with a significantly diminished unilateral Pdi_{TW} compared with healthy controls. The drop in inspiratory pressure was mainly attributed to a significant reduction in gastric pressure.

Our patients already reported a higher level of dyspnea (increased MRC) and had lower lung volumes than controls, but with similar BMI and no significant comorbidities that could influence this increased breathlessness. The inspiratory strength was reduced regardless of the side of hemidiaphragm involvement (MIP 59.9% of predicted in RP and 63.4% of predicted in LP), which was confirmed by the other volitional tests. A previous study [4] of UDP found similar values for MIP, around 60% of predicted. Lisboa et al. [20] reported that MIP values are below normal in these patients. Of note, Laroche et al. [4] also considered UDP to be the cause of exercise intolerance and dyspnea, because their patients had no relevant clinical comorbidity that would cause these symptoms.

It is well established that lung volume influences the inspiratory strength and diaphragmatic paralysis is related to a restrictive pattern, which is characterized by reduced FVC [2]. However, correcting the Pdi during bilateral twitch by FVC, patients with UDP persisted with reduced values (2.5 ± 1.7 vs 4.6 ± 2.2 cmH_2O / L, $p = 0.001$) reinforcing that the low Pdi values are related mainly to diaphragm weakness and not due the lower lung volume. The normalization of Pdi during bilateral twitch by FRC would be also another option, however the FRC was not measured in control group.

Magnetic phrenic nerve stimulation has been described as a useful tool to evaluate diaphragmatic dysfunction [14, 15, 21–23]. However, just one study evaluated the two hemidiaphragms separately, involving 11 patients with recent UDP (symptoms started within 12 months of a normal chest radiograph), and no controls were available to use for comparison [4]. In contrast to our results, the Pdi_{Tw} was reduced in the paralyzed hemidiaphragm but preserved in the non-paralyzed hemidiaphragm. It is important to highlight that some patients with UDP have the possibility of improving the phrenic function in a short

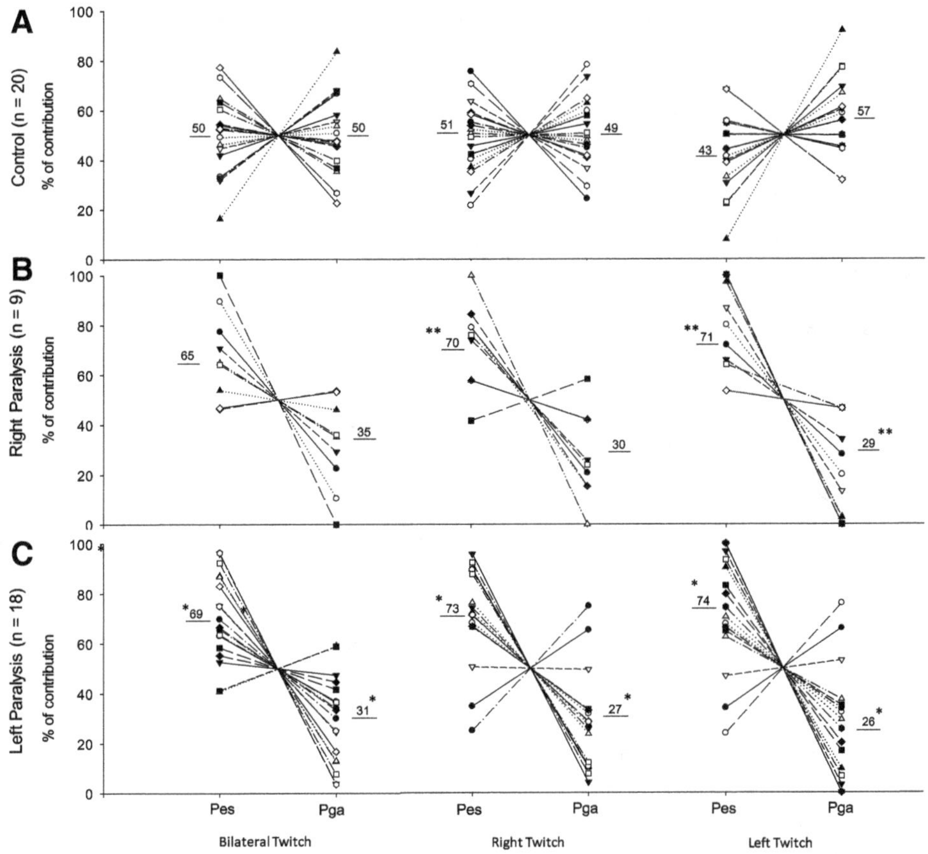

Fig. 2 Pes and Pga contributions to Pdi during bilateral, right, and left Twitch. **a** Control; **b** Right paralysis; **c** Left paralysis. Pes: esophageal pressure; Pga: gastric pressure. **$p < 0.05$ Right Paralysis vs Control; *$p < 0.05$ Left Paralysis vs Control. Underlined numbers mean the mean value (%)

period [1, 24]. On the other hand, after 12 months the chance of recovery decreases. Because over half of our patients were evaluated more than 12 months after onset or radiograph alteration, we ascribe the difference between the results to the shorter time of disease in the patients evaluated by Laroche et al. [4]. Probably, the shorter time of disease resulted in a more preserved hemidiaphragm, because even 2 patients had normal phrenic nerve conduction times [4]. Thus, the paralyzed hemidiaphragm possibly was not so flaccid and, as a result, contributed to the greater pressures in the non-paralyzed hemidia phragm.

Our most important finding was that Pga is the main factor that influences the decrease in Pdi_{TW} in UDP, and it also affects the generation of pressure by the non-paralyzed hemidiaphragm. Mills et al. [14] evaluated that the pattern of pressure changes during Twitch and also found a decline in Pga, justifying that it was due to the diaphragm being sucked up into the chest on inspiration, thus reducing abdominal pressure. However, this study involved only 5 patients who had bilateral diaphragmatic paralysis.

Gibson [25] reported that each hemidiaphragm could apparently operate independently, because "the tension on one side was not well transmitted to the other." Our USG evaluation confirmed the normal mobility and thickness of the non-paralyzed hemidiaphragm during normal and deep breathing, in which we cannot rule out some influence of accessory inspiratory muscle. However, this independence and the preservation of the non-paralyzed hemidiaphragm were not confirmed by our results during isolated phrenic magnetic stimulation. We believe that Pdi_{TW} and mainly the Pga of the non-paralyzed hemidiaphragm were reduced because the paralyzed hemidiaphragm was not secured and was sucked up into the chest, as described by Mills et al. [14]. Consequently, the non-paralyzed hemidiaphragm could not generate positive pressure in the abdominal compartment and even the pleural pressure was less negative. However, studies are required to confirm this assumption. Because the 2 diaphragmatic crura are joined by a fibrous median arcuate ligament [2], we cannot rule out possible interference of the paralyzed hemidiaphragm decreasing the tension and, therefore,

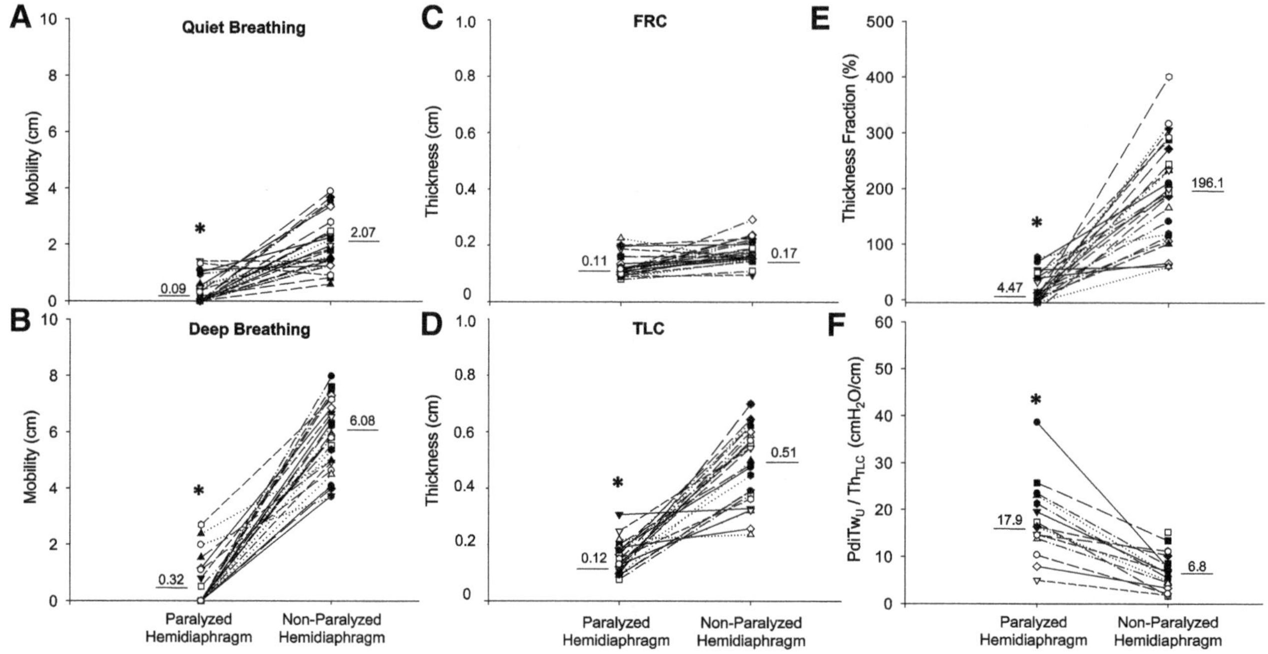

Fig. 3 Ultrasound data of the paralyzed and normal hemidiaphragms. Mobility during quiet breathing (**a**) and deep breathing (**b**); Thickness during FRC (**c**) and TLC (**d**); Thickness Fraction (**e**) and $PdiTW_U$ / Th_{TLC} ratio (**f**). FRC: forced residual capacity; TLC: total lung capacity; $PdiTW_U$ / Th_{TLC}: ratio between transdiaphragmatic pressure during unilateral stimuli and thickness during TLC. *$p < 0.001$ paralyzed hemidiaphragm vs non-paralyzed hemidiaphragm. Underlined numbers mean the mean value

impairing the generation of pressure by the non-paralyzed hemidiaphragm during Twitch stimulation. Finally, adjusting the Pdi to the respective diaphragm atrophy ($Thickness_{TLC}$), we found an inspiratory weakness even more evident in UDP patients.

Bellemare et al. [21] reported that bilateral Pdi is greater than the sum between right plus left Pdi during unilateral stimulus in 6 healthy individuals, but stimulation by the phrenic nerve was electrical and with a different frequency (5-35 Hz). Our results showed similar Pdi during bilateral Twitch compared with the sum of the right and left stimulus, and it was consistently found in all healthy controls. It is probable that the high-frequency phrenic stimulation impacted the results preventing high values in bilateral Pdi. Finally, even in this study [21], the authors suggested there is an upward displacement of the abdominal contents on the normal hemidiaphragm, stretching it.

The diaphragm plication effects reinforce the importance of having a stable hemidiaphragm to allow positive pressure in the abdominal compartment. Surgery plication has the goal of avoiding the dysfunctional movement of the hemidiaphragm during inspiration, with no interference in the force generation by the paralyzed hemidiaphragm. Despite this, studies of diaphragm plication have shown an increase from 10 to 30% in lung function, reduction in dyspnea [26], and an increase in maximal transdiaphragmatic pressure ($Pdi_{Máx}$) [27].

There are relevant findings of respiratory mechanics in diaphragm paralysis induced in dogs [28, 29]. De Troyer et al. [28] using radiographic evaluation found that the electrical stimulation of preserved hemidiaphragm reduces the caudal displacement of the central portion of the preserved contralateral hemidiaphragm. Scillia et al. [29] found a caudal displacement of the paralyzed hemidiaphragm during electrical stimulation of the non-paralyzed hemidiaphragm. However, this caudal movement was observed in dogs with induced injury in the parasternal intercostal muscles besides a pneumothorax, factors that interfere significantly with pressure generation in the pleural space. In this way, there is no negative pressure secondary to the inspiratory accessory muscle recruitment, which in fact sucks the paralyzed hemidiaphragm in a cranial direction.

This study has some limitations. First, the patients had predominantly left hemidiaphragm paralysis, which was found in another study as well [4]. Nevertheless, we have not found any difference in pressures or USG variables between left and right hemidiaphragm involvement. Second, we postulate that the reduced inspiratory strength by the normal hemidiaphragm is related to the cranial movement of the involved muscle; however, this was not confirmed by imaging techniques, and future studies are required to confirm this assumption. Third, although the coils were positioned to create a field more focused on the phrenic nerve, we cannot confirm that the accessory and rib cage muscles were not activated during the stimuli. However, cervical magnetic stimulation would be responsible merely for stiffening the rib cage, and the diaphragm would be allowed to contract against a stable rib cage, acting efficiently [14]. Finally, magnetic phrenic nerve stimulation is considered a useful tool to evaluate more specifically diaphragmatic dysfunction for many studies [14, 15, 21–23].

Conclusion

The results of the current study show that in symptomatic patients with UDP global inspiratory strength is reduced not only due to the weakness in the paralyzed hemidiaphragm but also to the impairment in the generation of pressure by the non-paralyzed hemidiaphragm. This comes from the flaccidness of the affected side, which does preclude the generation of positive pressure in the abdominal compartment during diaphragm contraction. Studies of diaphragm plication over these physiological mechanisms are highly relevant for gaining a better understanding of the process.

Abbreviations

BMI: Body mass index; CG: Control group; DL_{CO}: Carbon monoxide diffusion capacity; FEV1: Expiratory forced volume in the first second; FRC: Functional residual capacity; FVC: Forced vital capacity; LP: Left paralysis; MEP: Maximal expiratory pressure; MIP: Maximal inspiratory pressure;
Pdi: Transdiaphragmatic pressure; Pes: Esophageal pressure; Pga: Gastric pressure; Pmo: Mouth pressure; RP: Right paralysis; RV: Residual volume; TLC: Total lung capacity; Twitch: Phrenic nerve stimulation; UDP: Unilateral diaphragm paralysis; USG: Ultrasound

Acknowledgments

The authors thank all participating investigators of the Respiratory Muscles Group (Heart Institute – Incor) from the Hospital das Clínicas da Faculdade de Medicina da Universidade de São Paulo for their contribution to the collected data, Ann Conti Morcos (Medical Writer/Editor) for her contribution to language editing, and São Paulo Research Foundation (Fapesp) for supporting this research.

Funding

This study was supported by São Paulo Research Foundation [Fapesp]. Protocol number: 2011/20979-6. Mayra Callefi-Pereira receives a PhD-bursary from Conselho Nacional de Desenvolvimento Científico e Tecnológico [CNPq], Process number 142298/2016-6.

Authors' contributions

MCP, ALPA, PC, CRRC, and AF contributed to the study conception and design. MCP, LZC, RP, JGF, VCI, and AA contributed to data acquisition. MCP, LZC, and PVS contributed to data analysis. MCP and ALPA contributed to manuscript drafting. All authors contributed to the final manuscript approval.

Consent for publication

Not applicable.

Competing interests

The authors declare that they have no competing interests.

Author details

[1]Pulmonary Division, Heart Institute (Incor), Hospital das Clínicas da Faculdade de Medicina da Universidade de São Paulo, Av. Dr. Enéas Carvalho Aguiar, n°44. Cerqueira Cesar., São Paulo 05403-900, Brazil. [2]Thoracic Surgery Division, Heart Institute (Incor), Hospital das Clínicas da Faculdade de Medicina da Universidade de São Paulo, São Paulo, Brazil. [3]Sírio-Libanês Teaching and Research Institute, São Paulo, Brazil.

References

1. McCool FD, Tzelepis GE. Dysfunction of the diaphragm. N Engl J Med. 2012;366:932–42.
2. Nason LK, Walker CM, McNeeley MF, Burivong W, Fligner CL, Godwin JD. Imaging of the diaphragm: anatomy and function. Radiographics. 2012;32:E51–70.
3. Verin E, Marie JP, Tardif C, Denis P. Spontaneous recovery of diaphragmatic strength in unilateral diaphragmatic paralysis. Respir Med. 2006;100:1944–51.
4. Laroche CM, Mier AK, Moxham J, Green M. Diaphragm strength in patients with recent hemidiaphragm paralysis. Thorax. 1988;43:170–4.
5. Macintyre N, Crapo RO, Viegi G, Johnson DC, van der Grinten CP, Brusasco V, Burgos F, Casaburi R, Coates A, Enright P, et al. Standardisation of the single-breath determination of carbon monoxide uptake in the lung. Eur Respir J. 2005;26:720–35.
6. Miller MR, Hankinson J, Brusasco V, Burgos F, Casaburi R, Coates A, Crapo R, Enright P, van der Grinten CP, Gustafsson P, et al. Standardisation of spirometry. Eur Respir J. 2005;26:319–38.
7. Wanger J, Clausen JL, Coates A, Pedersen OF, Brusasco V, Burgos F, Casaburi R, Crapo R, Enright P, van der Grinten CP, et al. Standardisation of the measurement of lung volumes. Eur Respir J. 2005;26:511–22.
8. Mahler DA, Wells CK. Evaluation of clinical methods for rating dyspnea. Chest. 1988;93:580–6.
9. Caruso P, Albuquerque AL, Santana PV, Cardenas LZ, Ferreira JG, Prina E, Trevizan PF, Pereira MC, Iamonti V, Pletsch R, et al. Diagnostic methods to assess inspiratory and expiratory muscle strength. J Bras Pneumol. 2015;41:110–23.
10. Neder JA, Andreoni S, Castelo-Filho A, Nery LE. Reference values for lung function tests. I. Static volumes. Braz J Med Biol Res. 1999;32:703–17.
11. Neder JA, Andreoni S, Peres C, Nery LE. Reference values for lung function tests. III. Carbon monoxide diffusing capacity (transfer factor). Braz J Med Biol Res. 1999;32:729–37.
12. Pereira CA, Sato T, Rodrigues SC. New reference values for forced spirometry in white adults in Brazil. J Bras Pneumol. 2007;33:397–406.
13. Baydur A, Behrakis PK, Zin WA, Jaeger M, Milic-Emili J. A simple method for assessing the validity of the esophageal balloon technique. Am Rev Respir Dis. 1982;126:788–91.
14. Mills GH, Kyroussis D, Hamnegard CH, Wragg S, Polkey MI, Moxham J, Green M. Cervical magnetic stimulation of the phrenic nerves in bilateral diaphragm paralysis. Am J Respir Crit Care Med. 1997;155:1565–9.
15. Man WD, Moxham J, Polkey MI. Magnetic stimulation for the measurement of respiratory and skeletal muscle function. Eur Respir J. 2004;24:846–60.
16. Boussuges A, Gole Y, Blanc P. Diaphragmatic motion studied by m-mode ultrasonography: methods, reproducibility, and normal values. Chest. 2009;135:391–400.
17. Testa A, Soldati G, Giannuzzi R, Berardi S, Portale G, Gentiloni Silveri N. Ultrasound M-mode assessment of diaphragmatic kinetics by anterior transverse scanning in healthy subjects. Ultrasound Med Biol. 2011;37:44–52.
18. Boon AJ, Harper CJ, Ghahfarokhi LS, Strommen JA, Watson JC, Sorenson EJ. Two-dimensional ultrasound imaging of the diaphragm: quantitative values in normal subjects. Muscle Nerve. 2013;47:884–9.
19. Ueki J, De Bruin PF, Pride NB. In vivo assessment of diaphragm contraction by ultrasound in normal subjects. Thorax. 1995;50:1157–61.
20. Lisboa C, Pare PD, Pertuze J, Contreras G, Moreno R, Guillemi S, Cruz E. Inspiratory muscle function in unilateral diaphragmatic paralysis. Am Rev Respir Dis. 1986;134:488–92.

21. Bellemare F, Bigland-Ritchie B, Woods JJ. Contractile properties of the human diaphragm in vivo. J Appl Physiol (1985). 1986;61:1153–61.
22. Hamnegard CH, Wragg SD, Mills GH, Kyroussis D, Polkey MI, Bake B, Moxham J, Green M. Clinical assessment of diaphragm strength by cervical magnetic stimulation of the phrenic nerves. Thorax. 1996;51:1239–42.
23. Zoumot Z, Jordan S, Hopkinson NS, Polkey MI. Twitch transdiaphragmatic pressure morphology can distinguish diaphragm paralysis from a diaphragm defect. Am J Respir Crit Care Med. 2013;188:e3.
24. Gayan-Ramirez G, Gosselin N, Troosters T, Bruyninckx F, Gosselink R, Decramer M. Functional recovery of diaphragm paralysis: a long-term follow-up study. Respir Med. 2008;102:690–8.
25. Gibson GJ. Diaphragmatic paresis: pathophysiology, clinical features, and investigation. Thorax. 1989;44:960–70.
26. Groth SS, Andrade RS. Diaphragm plication for eventration or paralysis: a review of the literature. Ann Thorac Surg. 2010;89:S2146–50.
27. Ciccolella DE, Daly BD, Celli BR. Improved diaphragmatic function after surgical plication for unilateral diaphragmatic paralysis. Am Rev Respir Dis. 1992;146:797–9.
28. De Troyer A, Cappello M, Meurant N, Scillia P. Synergism between the canine left and right hemidiaphragms. J Appl Physiol (1985). 2003;94:1757–65.
29. Scillia P, Cappello M, De Troyer A. Determinants of diaphragm motion in unilateral diaphragmatic paralysis. J Appl Physiol (1985). 2004;96:96–100.

7

Pulmonary nocardiosis mimicking small cell lung cancer in ectopic ACTH syndrome associated with transformation of olfactory neuroblastoma

Keigo Kobayashi[1], Takanori Asakura[1], Makoto Ishii[1*], Soichiro Ueda[1], Hidehiro Irie[1], Hiroyuki Ozawa[2], Kohei Saitoh[3], Isao Kurihara[3], Hiroshi Itoh[3] and Tomoko Betsuyaku[1]

Abstract

Background: Pulmonary nocardiosis frequently develops as an opportunistic infection in cell-mediated immunosuppressive patients, and sometimes requires differentiation from pulmonary malignancy. Ectopic adrenocorticotropic hormone (ACTH) syndrome (EAS) is a neoplastic disorder which leads to impaired cell-mediated immunity, and is commonly associated with small cell lung cancer (SCLC). Because pulmonary infection and causative malignancy can appear as pulmonary lesions with EAS, differentiation of these diseases remains a critical issue for physicians.

Case presentation: A 52-year-old woman with progressive lower limb paralysis and general fatigue was referred to us. She had been diagnosed with olfactory neuroblastoma (ONB) and treated with surgery and radiation therapy 10 years before the referral and had required stereotactic radiosurgery and chemotherapy 4 years later for a relapse of the ONB. On referral, she presented with Cushing's syndrome with elevated cortisol and ACTH levels. Potassium supplement improved her symptoms; however, a month later, she was urgently hospitalized due to acute pleuritic chest pain on inspiration. Chest computed tomography revealed left lower lobular consolidations and a contralateral nodule in the right middle lobe. The clinical history and laboratory work-up suggested that her Cushing's syndrome had most likely arisen from EAS. Additionally, the lungs were suspected as the ACTH source due to high levels of progastrin-releasing peptide and progressive pulmonary consolidation with a contralateral nodule, suggesting SCLC. However, histological examination from bronchoscopy revealed no evidence of malignancy, and *Nocardia cyriacigeorgica* was isolated from bronchoalveolar lavage fluid. Sulfamethoxazole/trimethoprim improved her pulmonary lesions. Somatostatin receptor scintigraphy revealed strong tracer uptake in the ONB lesions, indicating that the origin of the EAS was the olfactory tumor. However, histological examination of ONB specimens resected 10 years earlier showed no intracytoplasmic immunopositivity for ACTH.

Conclusions: We highlight a rare case of pulmonary nocardiosis, which was associated with EAS mimicking SCLC, and was related to ONB transformation. Nocardiosis has to be considered even though anamnestic, clinical, and radiological aspects suggest the presence of metastasis. Additionally, physicians should carefully monitor patients with ONB for the development of Cushing's symptoms because the tumor can transform into an ACTH-producing form, even after long-term follow-up.

Keywords: Ectopic adrenocorticotropic hormone syndrome, Olfactory neuroblastoma, Pulmonary nocardiosis, Small cell lung cancer, Transformation

* Correspondence: ishii@keio.jp
[1]Division of Pulmonary Medicine, Department of Medicine, Keio University School of Medicine, 35 Shinanomachi, Shinjuku, Tokyo 160-8582, Japan
Full list of author information is available at the end of the article

Background

Pulmonary nocardiosis is an uncommon gram-positive bacterial lung infection caused by aerobic actinomycetes of the genus *Nocardia*, which can be found in environmental sources such as soil, decomposing vegetation, other organic matter, and fresh and salt water [1]. It develops mainly as an opportunistic infection in patients with cell-mediated immunosuppressive conditions, including various malignancies and human immunodeficiency virus (HIV) infection, and those receiving long-term systemic steroids or immunosuppressive agents [1, 2]. In addition to nonspecific symptoms, pulmonary nocardiosis can present as various radiographic abnormalities. The most common findings include focal or multifocal consolidations and nodules, as well as cavitary lesions [1, 3]. It can be very difficult to clinically and radiographically differentiate pulmonary nocardiosis from other infections, such as fungal or mycobacterial infections, and malignancy [1, 4].

Ectopic adrenocorticotropic hormone (ACTH) syndrome (EAS) is a well-known paraneoplastic disorder, and accounts for about 10% of cases of all types of Cushing's syndrome, and leads to impaired cell-mediated immunity by markedly raising cortisol levels [5]. The most prevalent tumors associated with EAS include small cell lung cancer (SCLC), neuroendocrine tumors, pheochromocytomas, and medullary carcinoma of the thyroid; it is said that the SCLC association is observed in over 50% of EAS patients [6]. Olfactory neuroblastoma (ONB), an indolent progressive tumor accounting for 3% of all intranasal tumors [7], can also cause EAS on rare occasions [8, 9].

Patients with EAS have a high prevalence of unusual pulmonary infections caused by opportunistic pathogens, including *Cryptococcus*, *Aspergillus*, *Pneumocystis*, and *Nocardia* [5, 10], which mimics lung malignancy as previously mentioned. Therefore, in patients with EAS of unknown origin, both pulmonary infection and causative malignancy of EAS can present as pulmonary lesions. Additionally, hypercortisolism in EAS may mask symptoms and signs of infection, leading to a delay in the diagnosis, which contributes to the high mortality rate [11]. Thus, differentiation of the pulmonary lesions with EAS remains a clinical issue for physicians.

Here, we report on a patient with ONB who was diagnosed with EAS of unknown origin and developed pulmonary lesions, which required differentiation from SCLC. We confirmed that the pulmonary lesions were caused by *Nocardia cyriacigeorgica* in EAS with ONB, which may have transformed to produce ACTH during the 10-year follow-up, as indicated by somatostatin receptor scintigraphy.

Case presentation

A 52-year-old woman was referred to our hospital due to progressive lower limb paralysis and general fatigue. She had been diagnosed with ONB 10 years before the referral and had undergone skull base surgery and postoperative radiation therapy against ONB. Four years after her initial diagnosis, chemotherapy with paclitaxel, carboplatin, and cetuximab was administered after completion of CyberKnife (Accuray Inc., Sunnyvale, CA) treatment against a relapsed pterygopalatine fossa tumor. Although the tumor had gradually worsened after the treatment, the patient had been followed up without treatment because of its slow rate of growth. On referral, she had a Cushingoid appearance: moon face, central obesity, and thin skin with purpura. Laboratory examination revealed hypokalemia (2.4 mEq/L) and metabolic alkalosis. Elevated cortisol level (59.6 μg/dl, range 3.5–18.4), elevated ACTH level (469 pg/ml, range 7.2–63.3), and raised pro-gastrin releasing peptide level (ProGRP; 2110 pg/ml, range 0–81) were also detected. Chest and abdominal computed tomography (CT) revealed no abnormality except for a new pulmonary nodule in the left lower lobe (Fig. 1a). Head and neck magnetic resonance imaging (MRI) scans showed that there were no remarkable findings in the pituitary gland, and the ONB had slightly increased in size in the right nasal cavity and the right ethmoid sinus over 3 years. Thus, the history and laboratory data appeared to be consistent with EAS, however, an obvious source was not apparent. Potassium supplement improved her symptoms, and she was planned to be admitted for further work-up and management for EAS, at a later date.

One month after the referral, she was urgently hospitalized due to acute pleuritic chest pain on inspiration. She had no high fever (36.2 °C) or any other symptoms indicating respiratory infection. Chest CT revealed left lower lobular consolidations with pleural effusion and a new pulmonary nodule in the right middle lobe (Fig. 1b). Laboratory results revealed elevated levels of C-reactive protein (CRP: 12.77 mEq/L, range 0.00–0.35) and β-D-glucan (77.8 pg/ml, range 0–11), but were negative for *Aspergillus* antigen, *Aspergillus* precipitating antibody, and *Cryptococcus* antigen test. Her HIV screening was negative. Blood and sputum culture showed no remarkable findings. As evidence for Cushing's syndrome, a raised cortisol level (72.3 μg/dl at 6 a.m., range 3.5–18.4) and ACTH level (466 pg/ml, 7.2–63.3) were also detected. The cortisol level was not suppressed by a low-dose dexamethasone suppression test (LDDST: 1 mg dexamethasone per day for 48 h): plasma cortisol level was 59.3 μg/dl and 24 h urine cortisol level was 439 μg/day after the LDDST. The history and laboratory work-up suggested that her Cushing's syndrome was more likely arising from EAS. The lungs were suspected as the source of ACTH due to the high level of ProGRP and progressive pulmonary

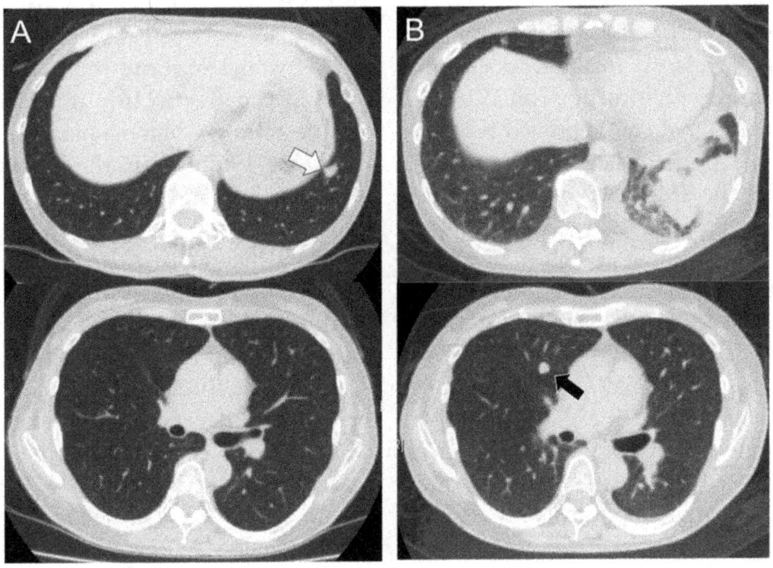

Fig. 1 **a** Chest computed tomography (CT) performed 1 month before admission showed a pulmonary nodule in the left lower lobe (white arrow). **b** Chest CT on admission showed consolidations in the same lobe, and a new pulmonary nodule in the right middle lobe (black arrow)

consolidation with a contralateral nodule, suggesting SCLC.

Although treatment with piperacillin-tazobactam (18 g/day) for pneumonia improved her pleuritic chest pain after 5 days, the pulmonary consolidation did not resolve. Hence, we proceeded with bronchoscopy to differentiate SCLC from pulmonary infections. Histological examination of the transbronchial biopsy specimen and cytology of the bronchoalveolar lavage fluid (BALF) showed no evidence of malignancy or fungi. Two weeks later, the BALF culture was positive for *Nocardia spp.*, identified as *Nocardia cyriacigeorgica* by 16S ribosomal RNA gene sequencing. Table 1 shows the minimum inhibitory concentration of the indicated antibiotics against *N. cyriacigeorgica*. We used the

Table 1 Antimicrobial Suscepibilities of an Isolated Strain of *N.cyriacigeorgica*

Agents	MIC (μg/ml)	Susceptible	Intermediate	Resistant
Amikacin	1	≤8	–	≥16
Amoxicillin / Clavulanate	> 32/16	≤8/4	16/8	≥32/16
Ceftriaxone	8	≤8	16–32	≥64
Ciprofloxacin	> 4	≤1	2	≥4
Imipenem	2	≤4	8	≥16
Linezolid	2	≤8	–	–
Minocycline	2	≤1	2–4	≥8
Sulfamethoxazole / Trimethoprim	19/1	≤38/2	–	≥76/4
Tobramycin	< 0.5	≤4	8	≥16
Cefotaxime	16	≤8	16–32	≥64
Cefepime	16	≤8	16	≥32
Doxycycline	2	≤1	2–4	≥8
Gentamicin	1	≤4	8	≥16
Ampicillin	> 8			
Clarithromycin	> 8	≤2	4	≥8
Erythromycin	> 2			

This table shows the minimum inhibitory concentration (MIC) of the indicated antibiotics against *N. cyriacigeorgica*. The specific susceptible breakpoint of Sulfamethoxazole / Trimethoprim (SMX/TMP) for Nocardia species was ≤2/38 and the specific resistance breakpoint was ≥4/76. The MICs of SMX/TMP for *N. cyriacigeorgica* were 1/19. Thus, the *N. cyriacigeorgica* was regarded as sensitive to SMX/TMP

Mueller-Hinton agar to culture *N. cyriacigeorgica* at 37 °C for 72 h. Susceptibility testing was performed according to Clinical and Laboratory Standards Institute document M24-A [12]. Oral sulfamethoxazole/trimethoprim 1920 mg (SMX 1600 mg/day, TMP 320 mg/day) improved her pulmonary lesions, as well as decreased the β-D-glucan level (Fig. 2). It was decided that the SMX/TMP would be continued for more than 1 year because she was an immunocompromised host [13]. Treatment with metyrapone (2.25 g/day) and mitotane (0.5 g/day) improved her plasma ACTH and cortisol levels. Scintigraphy performed using Octreoscan (Mallinckrodt, St Louis, MO) as an additional investigation for the origin of the EAS, revealed strong tracer uptake consistent with the ONB (Fig. 3); however, there was no uptake in the lung. Moreover, histological specimens of the ONB resected 10 years earlier showed no evidence of intracytoplasmic immunopositivity of ACTH. Therefore, this ONB may have transformed to produce ACTH over the 10-year clinical course.

Discussion and conclusions

In the present case report, we highlight a rare case of pulmonary nocardiosis, which was associated with EAS mimicking SCLC, and was related to transformation of an ONB. Although there is still no clear cutoff value to distinguish between EAS and Cushing's disease, plasma ACTH values of more than 200 pg/ml were reported in most EAS patients [14]. In this patient, matched clinical manifestations, higher plasma ACTH values, no remarkable findings in the hypothalamus and pituitary gland on brain MRI, and the confirmation with uptake consistent with the ONB in Octreoscan strongly supported a diagnosis of EAS, even though bilateral inferior petrosal sinus sampling, which is one of the confirmatory tests, was not performed because of its invasiveness and frequency of false-positives in ONB [15].

There are three important issues that made it difficult to differentiate pulmonary nocardiosis from SCLC in this case. First, the left pulmonary nodule was found in the first CT scan along with a high serum ProGRP level. Second, the chest CT on admission revealed a new pulmonary nodule in the right middle lobe, mimicking pulmonary metastasis. Third, the patient had no Cushingoid appearance over a 10-year period from the initial diagnosis of ONB, and the histological examination of resected specimens revealed no intracytoplasmic immunopositivity of ACTH.

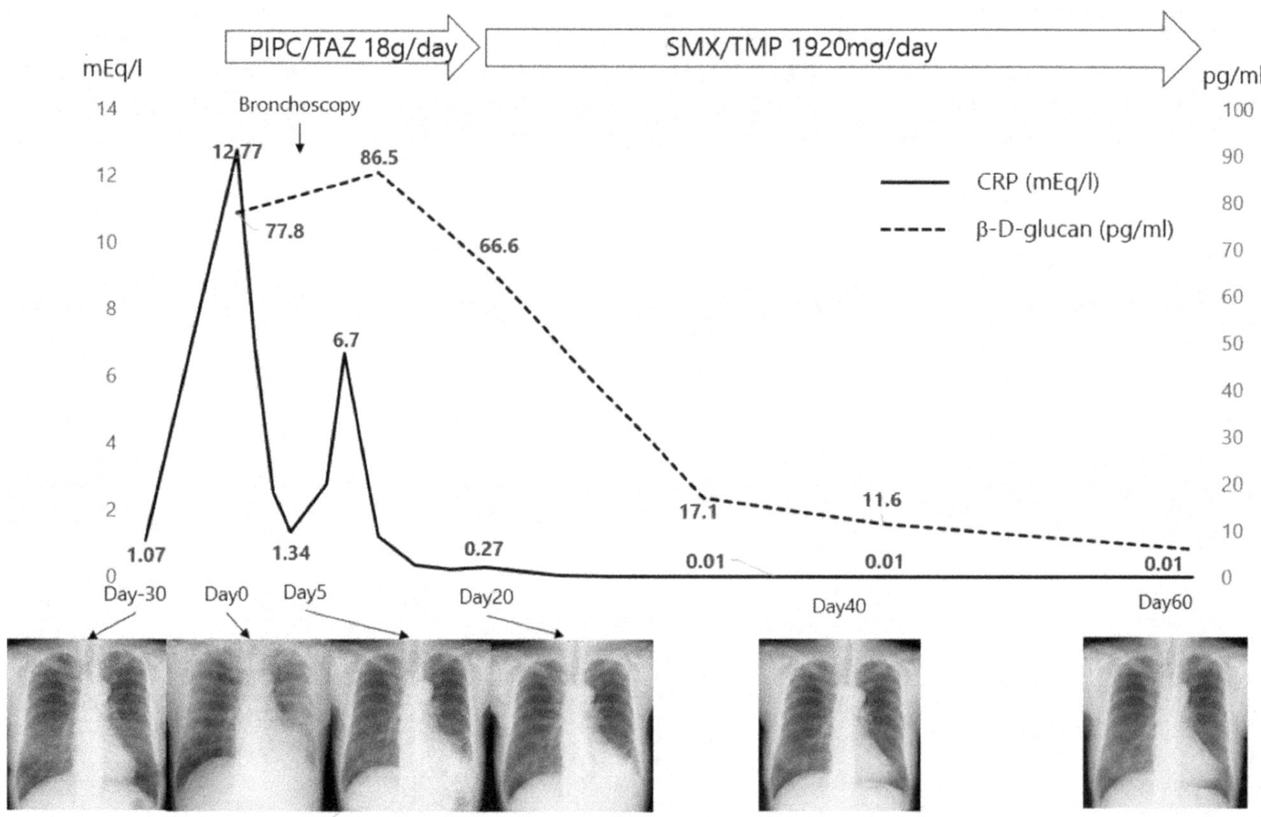

Fig. 2 Clinical course of our case including the changes of serum CRP (solid line) and β-D-glucan (dotted line) levels is shown. Dates of the referral and admission are presented as day − 30 and day 0, respectively. Bronchoscopy was performed at day 5. PIPC/TAZ; piperacillin/tazobactum, SMX/TMP; sulfamethoxazole/trimethoprim, CRP; c-reactive protein

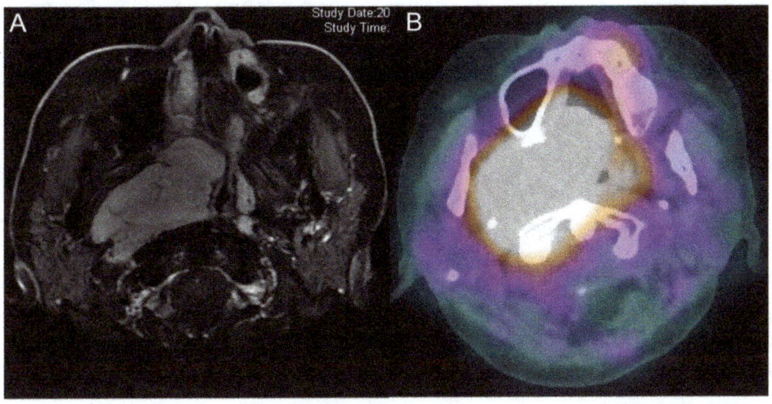

Fig. 3 a T1-weighted contrast-enhanced magnetic resonance imaging of an axial image showed an enhancing mass in the right nasal cavity and ethmoid sinus. **b** Somatostatin receptor scintigraphy (Octreoscan) showed strong tracer uptake consistent with the tumor

Nocardia infection can mimic lung cancer in various situations: some reports revealed that cerebral or cutaneous nocardiosis mimics metastases of the lung [16]; pulmonary nocardiosis also mimics both primary and metastatic lung cancer because the *Nocardia* can gain access into the lung by direct inoculation or by hematogenous spread from the primary site [17]. Although a rapidly progressive radiological shadow (around 1 month) generally indicates an infective etiology rather than malignancy, SCLC could also cause rapid progression with poor prognosis. In our case, progressive pulmonary consolidation from a nodule and a new contralateral nodule during the follow-up suggested primary and metastatic lesions, respectively. Additionally, the presence of EAS and a high serum ProGRP level, one of the diagnostic markers for neuroendocrine tumors, such as SCLC, thyroid medullary carcinoma, and pancreatic endocrine tumor [6], made the diagnosis difficult.

Our patient also had a high level of β-D-glucan, which is a polysaccharide glucose polymer present in a broad range of commonly encountered fungal agents, including *Candida spp.*, *Aspergillus spp.*, and *Pneumocistis jirovecii.* Furthermore, a recent study reported a case of *Nocardia* infection with elevated serum β-D-glucan levels due to its possible cross-reactivity [18]. β-D-glucan may have been useful in the diagnosis of pulmonary infections in our situation; however, we could not exclude the possibility that these infections were complications of SCLC.

Our patient had Cushing's syndrome due to EAS 10 years after the onset of the ONB, which may be as a result of the transformation that was confirmed by immunohistochemistry and Octreoscan. A recent study reviewed 18 cases of EAS with ONB: Cushing's syndrome developed simultaneously with ONB diagnosis or its recurrence in nine cases; Cushing's syndrome after diagnosis with ONB in five; and the location of the ACTH-secreting tumor was occult in four. The median times from ONB diagnosis to EAS development was 18 months [15], which is much shorter than in our case. In terms of confirming the source of ACTH production, Octreoscan is useful to diagnose ACTH-secreting tumors that have somatostatin receptors, which are expressed in 80% of EAS tumors [19]. Regarding immunohistochemical staining for ACTH, some tumors in Cushing's syndrome have been shown to be negative due to their secretion of corticotropin-releasing hormone rather than ACTH [8]. Although investigation of the ACTH source was limited until the referral, we believe that the ONB underwent a transformation to start producing ACTH because Cushing's syndrome was not evident until the referral, 10 years after the onset of the ONB.

In conclusion, we described a case of pulmonary nocardiosis mimicking SCLC in EAS, and associated with transformation of an ONB. In patients with EAS, physicians should consider both SCLC and pulmonary infection, including pulmonary nocardiosis, as differential diagnoses of pulmonary lesions. Additionally, physicians should carefully monitor patients with ONB for the development of Cushing's symptoms because the tumor can transform to produce ACTH, even after a long-term follow-up.

Abbreviations

ACTH: Adrenocorticotropic hormone; BALF: Bronchoalveolar lavage fluid; CRP: C-reactive protein; CT: Computed tomography; EAS: Ectopic adrenocorticotropic hormone syndrome; LDDST: Low-dose dexamethasone suppression test; MRI: Magnetic resonance imaging; ONB: Olfactory neuroblastoma; ProGRP: Pro-gastrin releasing peptide; SCLC: Small cell lung cancer; SMX/TMP: Sulfamethoxazole/trimethoprim

Authors' contributions

KK, TA, HI1, and MI drafted the manuscript and were responsible for the clinical care of the patient. SU, HO, KS, IK, HI2, and TB supervised the manuscript revision. All authors read and approved the final manuscript.

Consent for publication
Written informed consent was obtained from the patient for publication of this case report.

Competing interests
The authors declare that they have no competing interests.

Author details
[1]Division of Pulmonary Medicine, Department of Medicine, Keio University School of Medicine, 35 Shinanomachi, Shinjuku, Tokyo 160-8582, Japan. [2]Department of Otorhinolaryngology, Head and Neck Surgery, Keio University School of Medicine, 35 Shinanomachi, Shinjuku, Tokyo, 160-8582, Japan. [3]Division of Endocrinology, Metabolism and Nephrology, Department of Medicine, Keio University School of Medicine, 35 Shinanomachi, Shinjuku, Tokyo, 160-8582, Japan.

References
1. Wilson JW. Nocardiosis: updates and clinical overview. Mayo Clin Proc. 2012; 87(4):403–7.
2. Martinez Tomas R, Menendez Villanueva R, Reyes Calzada S, Santos Durantez M, Valles Tarazona JM, Modesto Alapont M, Gobernado Serrano M. Pulmonary nocardiosis: risk factors and outcomes. Respirology. 2007;12(3): 394–400.
3. Tsujimoto N, Saraya T, Kikuchi K, Takata S, Kurihara Y, Hiraoka S, Makino H, Yonetani S, Araki K, Ishii H, et al. High-resolution CT findings of patients with pulmonary nocardiosis. J Thorac Dis. 2012;4(6):577–82.
4. Yagi K, Ishii M, Namkoong H, Asami T, Fujiwara H, Nishimura T, Saito F, Kimizuka Y, Asakura T, Suzuki S, et al. Pulmonary nocardiosis caused by Nocardia cyriacigeorgica in patients with Mycobacterium avium complex lung disease: two case reports. BMC Infect Dis. 2014;14:684.
5. Ilias I, Torpy DJ, Pacak K, Mullen N, Wesley RA, Nieman LK. Cushing's syndrome due to ectopic corticotropin secretion: twenty years' experience at the national institutes of health. J Clin Endocrinol Metab. 2005;90(8): 4955–62.
6. Alexandraki KI, Grossman AB. The ectopic ACTH syndrome. Rev Endocr Metab Disord. 2010;11(2):117–26.
7. Wormald R, Lennon P, O'Dwyer TP. Ectopic olfactory neuroblastoma: report of four cases and a review of the literature. Eur Arch Otorhinolaryngol. 2011; 268(4):555–60.
8. Koo BK, An JH, Jeon KH, Choi SH, Cho YM, Jang HC, Chung JH, Lee CH, Lim S. Two cases of ectopic adrenocorticotropic hormone syndrome with olfactory neuroblastoma and literature review. Endocr J. 2008;55(3):469–75.
9. Doi M, Sugiyama T, Izumiyama H, Yoshimoto T, Hirata Y. Clinical features and management of ectopic ACTH syndrome at a single institute in Japan. Endocr J. 2010;57(12):1061–9.
10. Sarlis NJ, Chanock SJ, Nieman LK. Cortisolemic indices predict severe infections in Cushing syndrome due to ectopic production of adrenocorticotropin. J Clin Endocrinol Metab. 2000;85(1):42–7.
11. Graham BS, Tucker WS Jr. Opportunistic infections in endogenous Cushing's syndrome. Ann Intern Med. 1984;101(3):334–8.
12. Susceptibility Testing of Mycobacteria, Nocardia, and Other Aerobic Actinomycetes; Approved Standard. 2011, Clinical and Laboratory Standards Institute, Wayne, PA. https://jmedicalcasereports.biomedcentral.com/articles/10.1186/1752-1947-7-103.
13. Lerner PI. Nocardiosis. Clin Infect Dis. 1996;22(6):891–903. quiz 904-895
14. Wajchenberg BL, Mendonca B, Liberman B, Adelaide M, Pereira A, Kirschner MA. Ectopic ACTH syndrome. J Steroid Biochem Mol Biol. 1995;53(1–6):139–51.
15. Kunc M, Gabrych A, Czapiewski P, Sworczak K. Paraneoplastic syndromes in olfactory neuroblastoma. Contemp Oncol. 2015;19(1):6–16.
16. Nenoff P, Kellermann S, Borte G, Horn LC, Ponisch W, Winkler J, Haustein UF. Pulmonary nocardiosis with cutaneous involvement mimicking a metastasizing lung carcinoma in a patient with chronic myelogenous leukaemia. Eur J Dermatol. 2000;10(1):47–51.
17. Outhred AC, Watts MR, Chen SC, Sorrell TC. Nocardia infections of the face and neck. Curr Infect Dis Rep. 2011;13(2):132–40.
18. Sawai T, Nakao T, Yamaguchi S, Yoshioka S, Matsuo N, Suyama N, Yanagihara K, Mukae H. Detection of high serum levels of β-D-glucan in disseminated nocardial infection: a case report. BMC Infect Dis. 2017;17:272.
19. Uwaifo GI, Koch CA, Hirshberg B, Chen CC, Hartzband P, Nieman LK, Pacak K. Is there a therapeutic role for octreotide in patients with ectopic Cushing's syndrome? J Endocrinol Investig. 2003;26(8):710–7.

8

Regional heterogeneity in response of airway epithelial cells to cigarette smoke

Hario Baskoro[1], Tadashi Sato[1*], Keiko Karasutani[1], Yohei Suzuki[1], Aki Mitsui[1], Naoko Arano[1], Fariz Nurwidya[1,2], Motoyasu Kato[1], Fumiyuki Takahashi[1], Yuzo Kodama[1], Kuniaki Seyama[1] and Kazuhisa Takahashi[1]

Abstract

Background: Cigarette smoke (CS) exposure causes an abnormal inflammatory response, which can result in chronic obstructive pulmonary disease (COPD). Previous studies show that this disorder predominantly occurs in peripheral or small-airway areas, whereas the same condition has not been identified in the larger airways during the course of COPD. However, the different biochemical and genetic alterations occurring in response to CS exposure among airway epithelial cells from different sites in the lungs have not been fully investigated.

Methods: Human small airway epithelial cells (SAECs) and normal human bronchial epithelial cells (NHBEs) were exposed to CS extract (CSE), and microarray analysis was used to determine gene- and protein-expression profiles and identify alterations following CSE exposure in both cell types. An in vivo smoking experiment was also performed to confirm differential responses to CS between sites in the lung.

Results: Microarray analysis of SAECs and NHBEs following 24 h of CSE exposure showed that inflammatory related pathways and terms, including the tumor necrosis factor-signaling pathway, were overrepresented, especially in SAECs. Clustering analysis highlighted *prostaglandin-endoperoxide synthase-2* [also known as cyclooxygenase (COX)-2] as a gene specifically upregulated in SAECs, with COX-2 mRNA and protein expression significantly elevated by CSE exposure in SAECs (3.1- and 3.1-fold, respectively), but not in NHBEs. Furthermore, time-course analysis of COX-2 expression revealed earlier increases in SAECs compared with NHBEs following CS exposure. Short-term exposure of mouse lungs to CS was found to predominantly induce COX-2 expression in the small airway.

Conclusions: The small airway is more susceptible to CSE than the large airway and could be the initial site of development of CS-related respiratory diseases, such as COPD.

Keywords: Cigarette smoke, Airway epithelial cells, Small airway, Inflammation, Cyclooxygenase-2, Chronic obstructive pulmonary disease

Background

Cigarette smoke (CS) produces oxidant and reactive oxygen species in the lungs [1] and the unfavorable impacts of CS represent a primary cause of respiratory diseases, such as chronic obstructive pulmonary disease (COPD) and a leading contributor to preventable morbidity and mortality [2]. Preventing CS-related diseases can be best achieved by avoiding smoking initiation [3]; however, when the smoking habit has already started, smoking cessation considerably decreases numerous adverse health effects [4]. Intervention by smoking cessation during the early stages of COPD can decrease the rate of lung-function loss [5]. Moreover, CS-induced oxidant burden can irreversibly change endogenous antioxidant protection in airways. CS-derived oxidants injure airway epithelial cells by affecting lipid-membrane, carbohydrate, protein, and DNA structures and lead to the persistent inflammation evident in COPD development [6].

In addition to its status as a leading cause of mortality worldwide, COPD is also the only major cause of death that continues to increase annually [2]. Two main features of COPD include progressive limitation of expiratory airflow, which is not completely reversible, and an abnormal inflammatory response in the lungs [7]. Hogg et al. [8]

* Correspondence: satotada@juntendo.ac.jp
[1]Department of Respiratory Medicine, Juntendo University Graduate School of Medicine, 3-1-3 Hongo, Bunkyo-ku, Tokyo 113-8431, Japan
Full list of author information is available at the end of the article

suggested that the initial locus of inflammation in COPD is the small airways represented by membranous (diameter, < 2 mm), terminal and respiratory bronchioles. In smokers, the small airways show structural abnormalities, with or without COPD. The relationship between inflammatory mucus exudates from airway lumen and COPD severity was investigated by analyzing lung tissue from patients with all clinical stages of COPD [9], revealing that small-airway obstruction associated with COPD is related to thickening of the airway wall as a consequence of the remodelling process marked by mucociliary clearanc e-component malfunction and tissue repair related to innate-immune mechanisms, finally resulting in acculumation of lumen inflammatory exudates [9, 10]. A more recent study from the same group, based on multidetector computed tomography obtained from patients at various stages of COPD, showed that narrowing and loss of small conducting airways occurs before the emphysematous changes associated with COPD [11]. However, the genetic and biochemical alterations involved in responses to CS exposure by airway epithelial cells from different sites in the lungs have not been fully investigated.

In this study, we investigated the response to CS in two commercially available human airway epithelial cell lines [small airway epithelial cells (SAECs) and normal human bronchial epithelial cells (NHBEs)]. SAECs were isolated from the distal portion of a healthy lung in the 1-mm bronchiole area, and NHBEs were derived from the epithelial lining of airways above the bifurcation of the lung (according to documentation from Lonza, Basel, Switzerland). We explored the genetic differences between SAECs and NHBEs during the initial phase of CS-exposure using microarray analysis and performed in vivo smoking experiments using a mouse model to confirm that cells from different lung sites respond differently to CS exposure.

Methods

Preparation of CS extract

CS extract (CSE) was prepared using commercially marketed Peace unfiltered cigarettes (29 mg of tar and 2.5 mg of nicotine per cigarette; Japan Tobacco, Tokyo, Japan). The smoke from one cigarette was bubbled through 15 mL of sterilized purified water, and this solution passed through a 0.22-µm pore filter (Pall Corporation, Port Washington, NY, USA), to generate 100% CSE. Pilot cell-growth experiments showed that concentrations of ≤2.5% CSE were not cytotoxic; therefore, cultured cells were exposed to 2.5% CSE.

Cell culture

SAECs and NHBEs were purchased from Lonza. Three batches of each cell type, each originally isolated from three different healthy never-smoker donors, were used. SAECs were cultured with small airway epithelial cell growth medium (Lonza), and NHBEs were cultured with bronchial epithelial cell growth medium (Lonza), according to the manufacturer's instructions (SAECs and NHBEs were seeded at 2500 and 3500 cells/cm^2, respectively, in 25 cm^2 plastic flasks). Both cell types were used at passages three to six and assayed at the same passages for direct comparisons. After reaching approximately 80% confluence, cells were treated with or without 2.5% CSE until assayed.

RNA extraction and real-time quantitative polymerase chain reaction (qPCR)

Total RNA was extracted using miRNeasy mini kits (Qiagen, Hilden, Germany). For cDNA synthesis, total RNA was transcribed using ReverTra Ace qPCR RT master mix with gDNA remover (Toyobo, Osaka, Japan). Real-time qPCR for *cyclooxygenase* (*COX*)*-2* mRNA detection was performed using Thunderbird SYBR qPCR mix (Toyobo), an ABI 7500 Fast real-time PCR instrument (Applied Biosystems, Foster City, CA, USA), and *COX-2*-specific primers [(5′ → 3′) Fw: CTGGCGCTCAGCCATACAG; Rv: CCGGGTACAATCGCACTTATACT; Thermo Fisher Scientific, Waltham, MA, USA] according to manufacturer instructions. The expression of β-actin was measured using specific primers [(5′ → 3′) Fw: CTCTTCCAGCCTTC CTTCCT; Rv: AGCACTGTGTTGGCGTACAG; Thermo Fisher Scientific] as an internal control.

Microarray analysis

Two different batches of SAECs and NHBEs were used for microarray analysis. RNA samples (2 µg) were labeled using the low input Quick Amp labeling kit (Agilent Technologies, Waldbronn, Germany). Labeled RNA was hybridized to an oligonucleotide microarray (Whole Human Genome 4× 44 K; Agilent Technologies) at 60 °C for 17 h. After washing with reagents from the gene expression wash buffer kit (Agilent Technologies) and drying, slides were scanned with an Agilent microarray scanner and analyzed using Feature Extraction software (v9.5.1; Agilent Technologies). Normalization was performed using global normalization methods. Data from the microarray analysis have been deposited in the Gene Expression Omnibus database (accession ID: GSE107200). Differentially expressed genes were defined based on unpaired *t*-test p values < 0.01 and fold change ≥2. Gene-set enrichment analysis (GSEA) of differentially expressed genes was conducted using the DAVID functional annotation tool (https://david.ncifcrf.gov/home.jsp). Gene sets from the Kyoto Encyclopedia of Genes and Genomes (KEGG; http://www.genome.jp/kegg/) and the Gene Ontology (GO) biological process database (http://www.geneontology.org/) were used. Pathways and ontology terms with a $p <$ 0.05 were considered significant.

The Benjamini-Hochberg procedure was used in the analysis to control the false discovery rate.

Western blot analysis

Whole-cell lysates were prepared, and the total protein content of each measured using a BCA kit (Thermo Fisher Scientific). Protein aliquots (10 μg) were separated by electrophoresis on 10% sodium dodecyl sulfate polyacrylamide gels. After transferring the proteins to Immobilion-P membranes (Merck Millipore Corporation, Darmstadt, Germany), membranes were blocked with 5% skim milk in Tris-buffered saline with Tween-20 and allowed to react with an anti-COX-2 (1:400; Santa Cruz Biotechnology, Dallas, TX, USA) and anti-β-actin (1:10,000; Wako, Tokyo, Japan) monoclonal antibodies at 4 °C overnight. Membranes were then incubated with the appropriate horseradish-peroxidase-conjugated secondary antibody (1:20,000; Sigma-Aldrich, St. Louis, MO, USA), followed by detection with the Clarity western enhanced chemiluminescence substrate (Bio-Rad Laboratories, Hercules, CA, USA). Western blot signals were captured using an ImageQuant LAS-4000 mini fluorescence imager (GE Healthcare, Pittsburgh, PA, USA) and quantified using Multi Gauge image analysis software (Fujifilm Corporation, Tokyo, Japan).

In vivo exposure to CS and preparation of lung sections

C57BL/6 J male mice (3 months old; $n = 6$) were purchased from Oriental Yeast Co., Ltd. (Tokyo, Japan) and used for the smoking experiment. The procedures for animal experimentation were approved by the Animal Care and Use Committee of Juntendo University School of Medicine (Tokyo, Japan). Mice were maintained in a limited-access barrier facility and housed in a humidity (55% ± 10%) and temperature (24 °C ± 2 °C) controlled room under 12-h light/dark cycles. Mice were fed with standard commercial chow (CRF-1; Oriental Yeast) and provided water ad libitum. Mice were exposed to CS using Peace unfiltered cigarettes and a tobacco smoke-inhalation experimental system for small animals (Model SIS-CS; Shibata Scientific Technology, Tokyo, Japan) [12–15]. The experimental settings were as follows: 15 mL stroke volume, six puffs per minute, and 3.5% CS diluted with compressed air (the mass concentration of total particulate matter; 1430 ± 100 mg/m^3). Mice were exposed to either diluted CS or fresh air (as a control, $n = 3$ each) for 30 min/day over 5 days.

Mice were sacrificed at day 5 and their lungs subsequently processed as described previously [13–15]. Briefly, mice were anesthetized and then sacrificed by exsanguination of the left atrium with perfusion of phosphate-buffered saline (PBS) through the main pulmonary artery. Lungs were inflated and fixed by intratracheal instillation of 10% buffered formalin (pH 7.4; Wako) at a constant pressure of 25 cm H_2O for 48 h. Frontal plane sections of the lungs were taken at the depth of the hilum, followed by further sectioning of each block into two equal-sized pieces, and from the frontal plane, and embedded in paraffin.

Immunohistochemistry

Paraffin-embedded lung sections (4 μm) were deparaffinized in xylene and rehydrated in ethanol. Heat-induced epitope retrieval (10 min at 125 °C) was performed in citrate buffer (pH 6.0; LSI Medience Corporation, Tokyo, Japan). After blocking with 2% bovine serum albumin in PBS, tissue sections were incubated at 4 °C overnight with anti-COX-2 antibody (1:300; BD Biosciences, San Jose, CA, USA). Tissue sections were then incubated with biotin-labeled anti-mouse IgG antibody (1:300; Agilent Technologies) and labeled with avidin (1:50; Vector Laboratories, Burlingame, CA, USA) for 40 min at between 25 °C and 28 °C. Signals were detected using hydrogen peroxide and 3,3-diaminobenzidine tetrahydrochloride. Tissue sections were counterstained with hematoxylin and dehydrated in xylene. The ratio of positively immuno-stained nuclei to the total count of nuclei present in a field at 400× magnification was determined in 10 different lung areas per mouse.

Statistical analysis

Data are expressed as the mean ± standard error of the mean (SEM) and were analyzed using GraphPad Prism 6 (GraphPad Software, San Diego, CA, USA). Analysis of variance was performed using a non-parametric Kruskal–Wallis test. When applicable, the Mann–Whitney *U* test was used for comparisons between groups. Differences were considered significant at $p < 0.05$.

Results

Gene-expression profiles altered by CSE exposure in SAECs and NHBEs

As shown in the scatter plots, exposure to CSE for 24 h altered the expression of several probes in NHBEs and SAECs (Fig. 1a and b). In NHBEs, 83 probes were upregulated (≥ 2-fold) by CSE exposure, while in SAECs 116 probes were upregulated (Fig. 1c). Among upregulated probes, 72 were upregulated only in SAECs (46% of the total upregulated probes), whereas 39 were upregulated only in NHBEs (25%). Ninety-four and 78 probes were downregulated (≤ 2-fold) by CSE exposure in NHBEs and SAECs, respectively, with 71 probes (48% of the total downregulated probes) downregulated in NHBEs alone and 55 (37%) downregulated in SAECs alone (Fig. 1d). Differentially expressed probes are listed in Additional file 1: Tables S1–S6.

To elucidate the biological significance of altered gene-expression profiles in NHBEs and SAECs, we performed GSEA based on two different gene sets chosen using KEGG and GO biological-process analyses. As

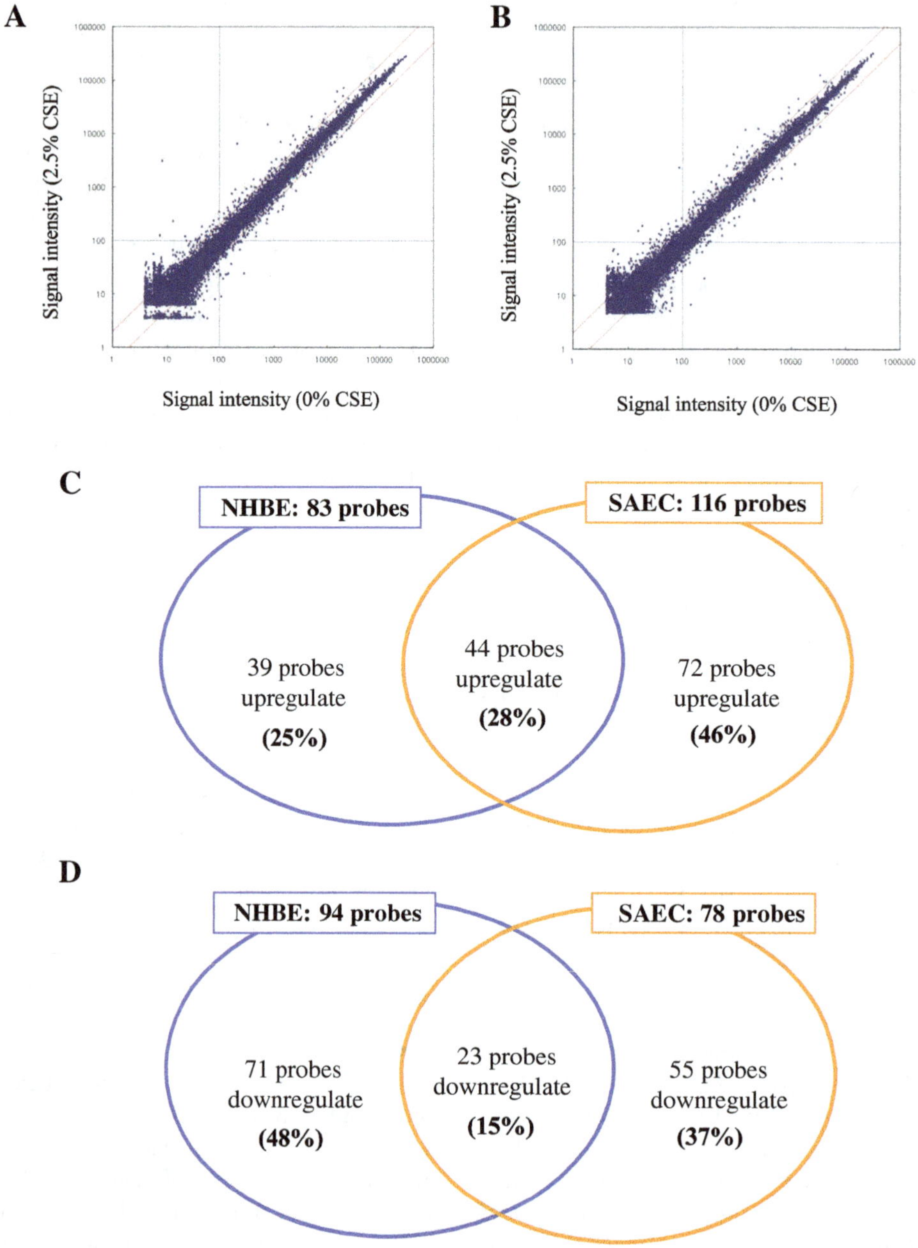

Fig. 1 Gene-expression profiles after exposure to CSE in SAECs and NHBEs. Two different batches of SAECs and NHBEs were used. Cells were exposed to 2.5% CSE for 24 h or not (controls). Scatter plot of (**a**) NHBEs and (**b**) SAECs. The vertical axis represents the relative signal intensity in CSE-exposed cells, and the horizontal axis represents the control (without CSE exposure). Both axes show log scales. **c** Venn diagram of probes showing significant upregulation in SAECs and NHBEs after CSE exposure. **d** Venn diagram of probes showing significant downregulation in SAECs and NHBEs after CSE exposure. CSE, cigarette smoke extract; SAECs, small airway epithelial cells; NHBEs, normal human bronchial epithelial cells.

shown in Table 1, KEGG analysis showed that 10 pathways, including the tumor necrosis factor (TNF)- and nuclear factor (NF)-κB-signaling pathways, were significantly and specifically overrepresented in SAECs subjected to CSE exposure. Additionally, GO analysis revealed that 29 GO terms, mostly related to inflammation, were significantly enriched in SAECs (Table 2). In contrast, no pathways or terms were identified by analysis of enrichment of genes downregulated in either CSE-exposed SAECs or NHBEs. In contrast, two pathways, including the JAK-STAT signaling pathway and arachidonic acid metabolism, and five GO terms related to oxidative stress metabolism, were significantly overrepresented in NHBEs subjected to CSE exposure (Tables 3, 4).

Table 1 Overrepresented pathways in SAECs based on KEGG analysis

Pathway	*p*	Genes
Rheumatoid arthritis	< 0.001	*CCL20, MMP1, IL1B, TLR2, FOS, IL8*
TNF-signaling pathway	0.001	*CCL20, PTGS2, IL1B, MAP3K8, FOS, TRAF1*
Toll-like receptor-signaling pathway	0.001	*SPP1, IL1B, MAP3K8, TLR2, FOS, IL8*
Leishmaniasis	0.001	*NCF1, PTGS2, IL1B, TLR2, FOS*
Malaria	0.004	*CSF3, IL1B, TLR2, IL8*
Amoebiasis	0.005	*IL1B, IL1R2, TLR2, IL8, SERPINB2*
NF-κB-signaling pathway	0.020	*PTGS2, IL1B, TRAF1, IL8*
MAPK-signaling pathway	0.026	*NR4A1, PLA2G4A, IL1B, IL1R2, MAP3K8, FOS*
Chagas disease (American trypanosomiasis)	0.032	*IL1B, TLR2, FOS, IL8*

SAECs small airway epithelial cells, *KEGG* Kyoto Encyclopedia of Genes and Genomes

Next, we focused on the TNF-signaling pathway and performed hierarchical clustering analysis of the 82 identified genes included in this pathway. As shown in Fig. 2, CSE exposure significantly upregulated genes in a specific cluster in SAECs compared with NHBEs, and the cluster included several inflammation-related genes, including *TNF-receptor-associated factor-1* and *prostaglandin-endoperoxide synthase-2* (*PTGS2*).

COX-2 expression is altered by CSE exposure in SAECs and NHBEs

Hierarchical clustering analysis revealed that *PTGS2* is highly upregulated after CSE exposure, especially in SAECs. *PTGS2* encodes a key enzyme (COX-2) involved in prostaglandin (PG) biosynthesis. COX-2 is not expressed under normal conditions in most cells; however, elevated levels are observed during inflammation. Furthermore, our previous studies identified a relationship between COX-2 and the abnormal inflammatory response in COPD [16, 17]. Therefore, we evaluated COX-2 mRNA and protein expression following exposure to CSE. After 24 h of exposure, COX-2 mRNA and protein levels were both significantly elevated in SAECs (3.1- and 3.1-fold compared with no CSE treatment, respectively), but not in NHBEs (1.2- and 1.4-fold, respectively) (Fig. 3a and b). To explore the mechanism of COX-2 overproduction in SAECs, we performed time-course analysis of COX-2 expression in response to CSE exposure in NHBEs and SAECs. Our results showed that *COX-2* mRNA levels began to increase 1 h earlier in SAECs than in NHBEs, and that COX-2 production was significantly higher in SAECs than in NHBEs (Fig. 3c). Time-course results for COX-2 protein expression were similar to those obtained for *COX-2* mRNA expression (Fig. 3d).

COX-2 expression in the lungs of CS-exposed mice

To investigate the initial effect of CS exposure on COX-2 expression in vivo, we performed a short-duration in vivo smoking experiment using C57BL/6 J mice. Immunohistochemical analysis revealed that, after 5 days of exposure to CS, COX-2 expression increased compared with that in air-exposed mice, with more immuno-stained cells observed in small airways than in large airways (Fig. 4a–d). After 5 days of CS exposure, COX-2-positive cells were significantly increased in the small airways of mouse lungs, but not in the large airways (4.6-fold vs. 1.2-fold; Fig. 4e).

Discussion

This study demonstrated that small and large airways differed in their initial responses to CS exposure. Microarray analysis revealed that small airways showed higher susceptibility to CS compared with large airways and displayed enhanced expression of genes associated with inflammatio n-related pathways, including TNF-signaling. Among TNF-pathway related genes, *PTGS2*, also known as *COX-2*, showed the greatest difference in expression levels, with higher CSE-induced increases in both mRNA and protein expression in SAECs compared with NHBEs. In vivo short-duration smoking experiments also showed that initial COX-2 expression occurred in lung small-airways. This is the first study clarifying initial genetic and biochemical alterations associated with inflammatory responses to CS exposure in the small and large airways.

CS is the most typical source of exogenous oxidants [18], and oxidants derived from CS can injure airway epithelial cells, leading to persistent inflammation. Oxidative stress and persistent inflammation combine to result in increases in airway free radicals and amplification of the expression of proinflammatory genes that contribute to the release of inflammatory proteins, thereby promoting inflammatory cell infiltration [6]. The present study demonstrated that the expression of proinflammatory genes, and initiation of signaling associated with their related pathways, were more greatly enhanced in SAECs relative to NHBEs following a comparatively short period of CSE exposure. Further, we identified initial induction of *COX-2* expression in the small airway of CS-exposed mice. These results suggest that SAECs represent the initial targets of CS and play an important role in the development of CS-mediated inflammation, which might contribute to CS-related respiratory diseases, such as COPD.

Accumulating evidence suggests that the small airway is the initial locus of inflammation in COPD and plays a critical role in disease development [19]. Based on clinical findings, even patients with mild COPD already show some pathological abnormalities in the small-airway area,

Table 2 Overrepresented terms in SAECs by GO enrichment analysis

GO term	*p*	Genes
Inflammatory response	< 0.001	*CCL20, SPP1, PTGS2, IL1F9, IL1B, BMP2, TLR2, FOS, ELF3, CYP4F11, IL24, IL8*
Response to vitamin D	< 0.001	*SPP1, PLA2G4A, PTGS2, IL1B*
Response to hypoxia	< 0.001	*SOD2, MUC1, IL1B, CYP1A1, BMP2, ALDH3A1, TLR2*
Positive regulation of fever generation	0.001	*PLA2G4A, PTGS2, IL1B*
Wound healing	0.001	*EREG, CCL20, IL1B, IL24, SERPINB2*
Response to lipopolysaccharide	0.002	*SOD2, PLA2G4A, CCRN4L, PTGS2, CYP1A1, FOS*
Ovulation	0.002	*EREG, PTGS2, IL1B*
Aging	0.003	*NQO1, PLA2G4A, IL1B, CYP1A1, ALDH3A1, FOS*
Cellular response to organic cyclic compound	0.004	*IL1B, CYP1A1, BMP2, CYP1B1*
Positive regulation of apoptotic process	0.004	*ALDH1A3, NR4A1, PLA2G4A, PTGS2, IL1B, BMP2*
Decidualization	0.005	*SPP1, PLA2G4A, PTGS2*
Positive regulation of NF-κB import into nucleus	0.005	*PTGS2, IL1B, TLR2*
Epithelial cell differentiation	0.005	*DHRS9, MUC1, AKR1C1, ELF3*
Arachidonic acid metabolic process	0.007	*CYP4F12, PLA2G4A, CYP1B1*
Positive regulation of vascular endothelial growth factor production	0.007	*PTGS2, IL1B, CYP1B1*
Response to immobilization stress	0.007	*SOD2, CYP1A1, FOS*
Transcription from RNA polymerase II promoter	0.012	*OVOL1, NFYC, ATF3, CCRN4L, PIR, FOSB, FOS, ELF3*
Negative regulation of cell cycle	0.013	*NR4A1, PTGS2, BMP2*
Apoptotic process	0.019	*NCF1, NR4A1, IL1B, MAP3K8, TLR2, TRAF1, MAL, IL24*
Positive regulation of transcription from RNA polymerase II promoter	0.019	*NFYC, NR4A1, ATF3, FOSB, MYO6, CSF3, IL1B, BMP2, TLR2, FOS, ELF3*
Embryo implantation	0.019	*SPP1, PTGS2, IL1B*
Positive regulation of nitric oxide biosynthetic	0.019	*SOD2, PTGS2, IL1B*
Cellular response to lipopolysaccharide	0.023	*CCL20, CSF3, IL24, IL8*
Response to progesterone	0.024	*FOSB, TLR2, FOS*
Skeletal muscle cell differentiation	0.024	*NR4A1, ATF3, FOS*
Response to cAMP	0.027	*FOSB, ALDH3A1, FOS*
Cell-cell signaling	0.033	*EREG, CCL20, IL1F9, IL1B, BMP2*
Positive regulation of gene expression	0.034	*PRDM1, ID1, IL1B, BMP2, TLR2*
Neutrophil chemotaxis	0.040	*CCL20, IL1B, IL8*

SAECs small airway epithelial cells, *GO* gene ontology

including active inflammation and obstruction [9]. Based on the results of multidetector computed-tomography, McDonough et al. [11] reported that small-airway injury precedes the development of centrilobular emphysema, and another study of pathology in smokers who

Table 3 Overrepresented pathways in NHBEs based on KEGG analysis

Pathway	*p*	Genes
JAK-STAT signaling pathway	0.029	*CCND1, IL13RA2, LIF, CSF3*
Arachidonic acid metabolism	0.033	*PLA2G3, AKR1C3, GPX2*

NHBEs normal human bronchial epithelial cells, *KEGG* Kyoto Encyclopedia of Genes and Genomes

Table 4 Overrepresented terms in NHBEs by GO enrichment analysis

GO term	*p*	Genes
Doxorubicin metabolic process	< 0.001	*AKR1C3, AKR1B10, AKR1C1*
Daunorubicin metabolic process	< 0.001	*AKR1C3, AKR1B10, AKR1C1*
Retinoid metabolic process	0.001	*AKR1C3, LRP8, AKR1B10, AKR1C1*
Positive regulation of peptidyl-tyrosine	0.003	*CD4, LIF, LRP8, CSF3*
Response to nutrient	0.038	*NQO1, AKR1C3, ALDH3A1*

NHBEs normal human bronchial epithelial cells, *GO* gene ontology

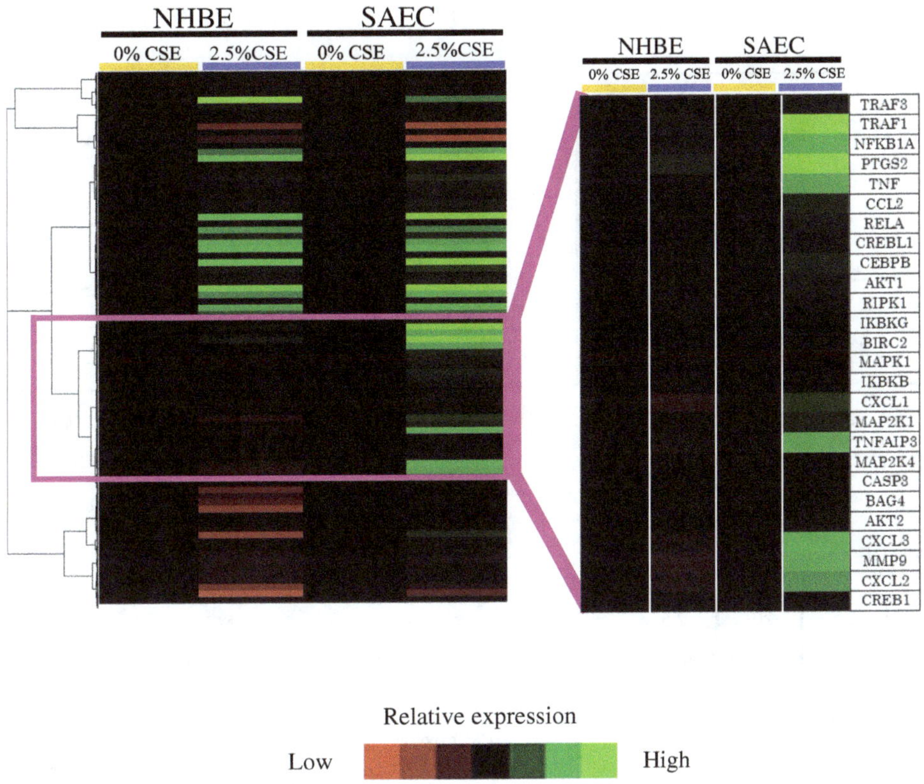

Fig. 2 Hierarchical clustering analysis of the TNF-signaling pathway. SAECs and NHBEs were exposed to 2.5% CSE for 24 h or not (controls). Two different batches of SAECs and NHBEs were used. The specific cluster containing genes upregulated by CSE exposure predominantly in SAECs is highlighted (right). High relative expression is indicated in green, and low relative expression is indicated in red. CSE, cigarette smoke extract; SAECs, small airway epithelial cells; NHBEs, normal human bronchial epithelial cells.

underwent surgical resection showed that the number of neutrophils and mast cells infiltrating the small airway was higher than that in the large airway [20]. In terms of genetic analysis, Mercer et al. [21] performed microarray analyses using CSE-exposed SAECs and showed differential regulation of 425 genes involved in various biological processes, including immune function, signal transduction, apoptosis, the cell cycle, cell proliferation, and anti-oxidation. The results of the present study were consistent with the findings of Mercer et al. [21], and further demonstrate that CSE exposure affects gene groups related to diverse biological processes in SAECs, including the inflammatory response, wound healing, aging, apoptosis, cell differentiation, and neutrophil chemotaxis (Table 2). Importantly, these findings extend previous results by demonstrating that SAECs exhibit greater alterations in gene regulation and a higher susceptibility to CSE exposure than NHBEs.

A recent study by Yang et al. demonstrated that smoking induced *distal-to-proximal repatterning* of the adult human small airway epithelium, which is a pathologic feature of COPD [22] . The authors showed that the proximal airway epithelium is enriched for molecular features related to oxidative stress, xenobiotic metabolism, and nicotine degradation, suggesting that the proximal airway epithelium can more robustly tolerate oxidants and toxins compared with the small airway epithelium. In the current study, the GSEA in NHBEs indicated that a smaller number of pathways and GO terms were overrepresented following CSE exposure compared to SAECs (Tables 3, 4); however, *GPX-2* [glutathione peroxidase] was one of the enriched genes in the arachidonic acid metabolism pathway, according to KEGG analysis (Table 3). Furthermore, GO enrichment analysis showed that several *AKR* [aldo-keto reductase] family members, which encode enzymes that detoxify oxidative stress-induced carbonyl proteins, were enriched (Table 4). These findings are consistent with those of Yang et al. [22], showing that *GPX-2* is a proximal airway epithelial signature gene. Interestingly, Yang et al. [22] also showed that the expression of proximal signature genes was increased in the small airway epithelium of healthy smokers and COPD patients compared with nonsmokers. They named this phenomenon, which may be relevant to the pathogenesis of small airway disorder in COPD, *distal-to-proximal repatterning*. Here, we investigated the initial response towards CS-exposure to determine whether the small-airway is the initial site of the CS-induced lung damage; however, investigations

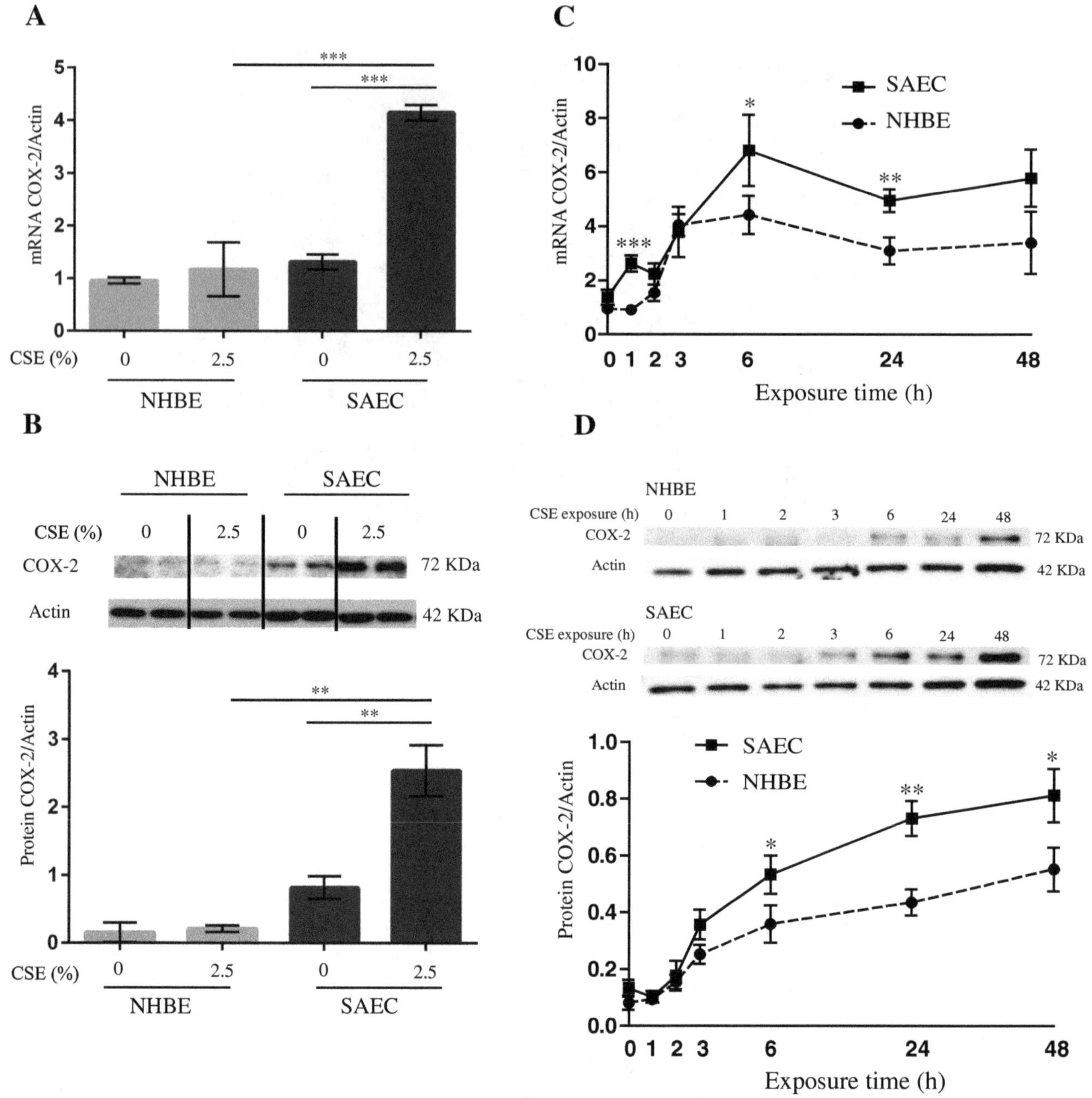

Fig. 3 Effects of CSE exposure on COX-2 expression in SAECs and NHBEs. **a** COX-2 mRNA and (**b**) protein expression, with β-actin used as an internal and loading control, respectively. Band size is indicated on the right. Cells were exposed to 2.5% CSE for 24 h or not (controls). **c** Time-course of *COX-2* mRNA expression in SAECs and NHBEs following 2.5% CSE exposure. β-Actin was used as an internal control. **d** Time course of COX-2 protein expression in SAECs and NHBEs following 2.5% CSE exposure. β-Actin was used as a loading control. Band size is indicated on the right. Values are shown as the mean ± SEM. *$p < 0.05$; **$p < 0.01$; *** $p < 0.001$ compared with NHBEs in (**c**) and (**d**). Three batches each of SAECs and NHBEs were evaluated on three separate occasions in all experiments. CSE, cigarette smoke extract; SAECs, small airway epithelial cells; NHBEs, normal human bronchial epithelial cells; COX-2, cyclooxygenase-2

during longer periods of CSE exposure will likely be fruitful beyond the current study.

Here, we focused on COX-2 as an important factor that initiates an inflammatory response to CSE exposure in the lung. COX-2 is a key mediator of inflammation that catalyzes the transformation of arachidonic acid to thromboxanes and PGs, such as prostaglandin E_2 (PGE_2) [23]. COX-2 is also believed to be associated with COPD pathogenesis [24]. A previous animal study showed that treatment with a COX-2 inhibitor attenuated PGE_2 synthesis and protected against the development of CS-induced pulmonary emphysema [25]. Our previous

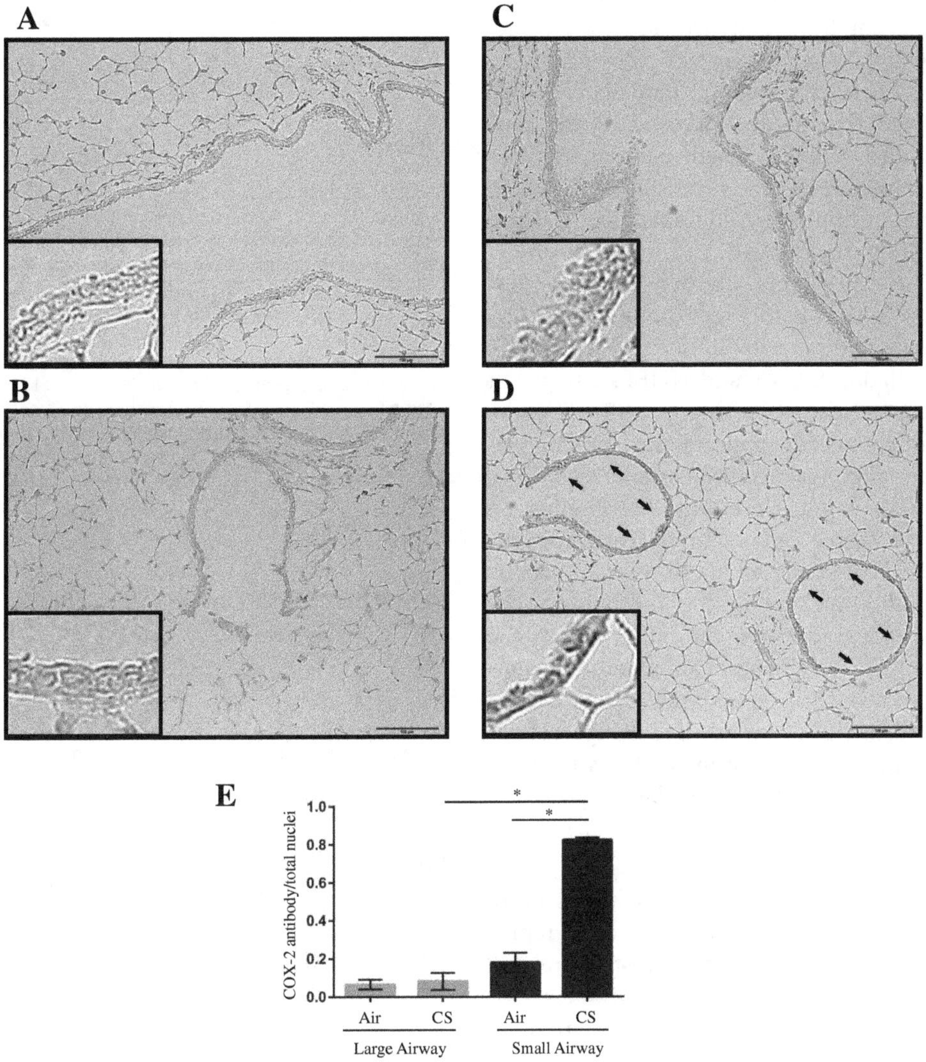

Fig. 4 Effects of CS exposure on COX-2 expression in the lungs of C57BL/6 J mice. Mice were exposed to either 3.5% CS or fresh air (control) for 30 min/day for 5 days. Representative immunohistochemistry images of (**a**) the large-airway area in a control lung, (**b**) the small-airway area in a control lung, (**c**) the large-airway area in a CS-exposed lung, and (**d**) the small-airway area in a CS-exposed lung. Brown color indicates COX-2-positive airway epithelial cells (*arrows*). Scale bar, 100 μm. *Insets* are high magnification views of airway epithelial cells. **e** The ratio of COX-2-positive nuclei to the total count of nuclei present in a field at 400× magnification and determined in 10 different areas of the lung per mouse. Values are shown as the mean ± SEM ($n = 3$/group). *$p < 0.001$. CS, cigarette smoke; COX-2, cyclooxygenase-2

study, using primary lung fibroblasts from patients with COPD and smokers without COPD (controls), demonstrated that following stimulation with inflammatory cytokines, fibroblasts from COPD subjects produced higher PGE_2 levels relative to those from control subjects, and that elevated PGE_2 levels were the result of an increase in COX-2 expression due to alterations in mRNA stability caused by weak induction of microRNA-146a [17]. More recently, Zago et al. demonstrated that expression of RelB, a component of the non-canonical NF-κB pathway, and the aryl hydrocarbon receptor, are both reduced in fibroblasts from COPD patients and regulate COX-2 protein levels by altering mRNA stability [26–29]. These findings suggest that the regulation of COX-2 is critical to controlling abnormal inflammation associated with COPD pathogenesis, and that its targeting could be a promising strategy for COPD therapeutics. Interestingly, a recent study suggested that mesenchymal stem cells attenuated airway inflammation and emphysema in CS-exposed rats through the downregulation of COX-2 and PGE_2 [30].

This study had several limitations. First, we did not use primary cells from COPD patients to evaluate the direct contribution of the current findings to the disease condition. Second, the SAECs and NHBEs used in the current study were not from matched donors. Instead, we confirmed COX-2 expression in the lungs of CS-exposed mice as an experimental model of COPD. Thirdly, we used different media approved by the supplier for SAECs and NHBEs. Their components are almost identical; however, there is a possibility that they influenced the current findings. Additionally, we did not perform air-liquid interface (ALI) culture to promote differentiation. The phenotypes of each cell type observed under non-differentiating conditions could be affected by contamination with different cell types. Therefore, differentiating SAECs and NHBEs using ALI culture system first and then exposing to CSE will make experimental findings more applicable to human airways. However, our findings were consistent with those from a previous study using ALI culture [22], indicating that commercially available cells cultured using conventional methods can be suitable for these types of experiment. Lastly, we did not define the mechanisms by which inflammation spreads from the initial site to the whole lung, leading to development of pulmonary emphysema. Further investigation of the transition of COX-2 expression in the airways, following various durations of CS exposure, and the interactions between small-airway cells and other cells will be beneficial.

Conclusions

This study demonstrated that the small airway is more susceptible to CS than the large airway and might represent an initial target site for development of CS-related respiratory diseases, such as COPD. These findings support the results of previous pathological investigations.

Additional file

Additional file 1: Table S1. A list of 44 probes upregulated by CSE exposure in both NHBEs and SAECs. **Table S2.** A list of 72 probes upregulated by CSE exposure only in SAECs. **Table S3.** A list of 39 probes upregulated by CSE exposure only in NHBEs. **Table S4.** A list of 23 probes downregulated by CSE exposure in both NHBEs and SAECs. **Table S5.** A list of 55 probes downregulated by CSE exposure only in SAECs. **Table S6.** A list of 71 probes downregulated by CSE exposure only in NHBEs.

Abbreviations

ALI: Air-liquid interface; COPD: Chronic obstructive pulmonary disease; COX-2: Cyclooxygenase-2; CS: Cigarette smoke; CSE: Cigarette smoke extract; GO: Gene ontology; GSEA: Gene set enrichment analysis; KEGG: Kyoto Encyclopedia of Genes and Genomes; NF-κB: Nuclear factor-κB; NHBE: Normal human bronchial epithelial cells; PBS: Phosphate-buffered saline; PG: Prostaglandin; PGE_2: Prostaglandin E_2; PTGS2: Prostaglandin-endoperoxide synthase 2; SAEC: Small airway epithelial cells; SEM: Standard error of the mean; TNF: Tumor necrosis factor

Acknowledgments

The authors wish to thank Mr. Dai Ogura for excellent support with microarray analysis.

Funding

This work was supported in part by JSPS KAKENHI Grant Number 26461199 (T. Sato) and the Institute for Environmental and Gender-Specific Medicine, Juntendo University Graduate School of Medicine, Grant Number E2920 (T. Sato). The funder had no role in the design of the study and collection, analysis, and interpretation of data and in writing the manuscript.

Authors' contributions

Conception and experimental design: HB, TS, and KT; data analysis and interpretation: HB and KS; animal experiments: KK and AM; microarray analysis: TS and FT; molecular studies: FN and MK; immunohistochemistry: HB and YS; western blot analysis: NA and YK; and drafting of the manuscript: HB and TS. All authors read and approved the final manuscript.

Consent for publication

Not applicable.

Competing interests

The authors have no competing interests to declare.

Author details

[1]Department of Respiratory Medicine, Juntendo University Graduate School of Medicine, 3-1-3 Hongo, Bunkyo-ku, Tokyo 113-8431, Japan. [2]Department of Pulmonology and Respiratory Medicine, Universitas Indonesia Faculty of Medicine, Jalan Persahabatan Raya No. 1, Rawamangun, Jakarta 13230, Indonesia.

References

1. Lin JL, Thomas PS. Current perspectives of oxidative stress and its measurement in chronic obstructive pulmonary disease. COPD. 2010;7:291–306.
2. Vogelmeier CF, Criner GJ, Martinez FJ, Anzueto A, Barnes PJ, Bourbeau J, et al. Global strategy for the diagnosis, management, and prevention of chronic obstructive lung disease 2017 report. GOLD Executive Summary. Am J Respir Crit Care Med. 2017;195:557–82.
3. Rennard SI, Daughton DM. Smoking cessation. Clin Chest Med. 2014;35:165–76.
4. Rennard SI, Drummond MB. Early chronic obstructive pulmonary disease: definition, assessment, and prevention. Lancet. 2015;385:1778–88.
5. Anthonisen NR, Connett JE, Murray RP. Smoking and lung function of lung health study participants after 11 years. Am J Respir Crit Care Med. 2002;166:675–9.
6. Lee W, Thomas PS. Oxidative stress in COPD and its measurement through exhaled breath condensate. Clin Transl Sci. 2009;2:150–5.
7. Barnes PJ. Cellular and molecular mechanisms of chronic obstructive pulmonary disease. Clin Chest Med. 2014;35:71–86.
8. Hogg JC, Macklem PT, Thurlbeck WM. Site and nature of airway obstruction in chronic obstructive lung disease. N Engl J Med. 1968;278:1355–60.
9. Hogg JC, Chu F, Utokaparch S, Woods R, Elliott WM, Buzatu L, et al. The nature of small-airway obstruction in chronic obstructive pulmonary disease. N Engl J Med. 2004;350:2645–53.
10. Hogg JC. Pathophysiology of airflow limitation in chronic obstructive pulmonary disease. Lancet. 2004;364:709–21.

11. McDonough JE, Yuan R, Suzuki M, Seyednejad N, Elliott WM, Sanchez PG, et al. Small-airway obstruction and emphysema in chronic obstructive pulmonary disease. N Engl J Med. 2011;365:1567–75.
12. Kasagi S, Seyama K, Mori H, Souma S, Sato T, Akiyoshi T, et al. Tomato juice prevents senescence-accelerated mouse P1 strain from developing emphysema induced by chronic exposure to tobacco smoke. Am J Physiol Lung Cell Mol Physiol. 2006;290:L396–404.
13. Sato T, Seyama K, Sato Y, Mori H, Souma S, Akiyoshi T, et al. Senescence marker protein-30 protects mice lungs from oxidative stress, aging, and smoking. Am J Respir Crit Care Med. 2006;174:530–7.
14. Koike K, Ishigami A, Sato Y, Hirai T, Yuan Y, Kobayashi E, et al. Vitamin C prevents cigarette smoke-induced pulmonary emphysema in mice and provides pulmonary restoration. Am J Respir Cell Mol Biol. 2014;50:347–57.
15. Suzuki Y, Sato T, Sugimoto M, Baskoro H, Karasutani K, Mitsui A, et al. Hydrogen-rich pure water prevents cigarette smoke-induced pulmonary emphysema in SMP30 knockout mice. Biochem Biophys Res Commun. 2017;492:74–81.
16. Togo S, Holz O, Liu X, Sugiura H, Kamio K, Wang X, et al. Lung fibroblast repair functions in patients with chronic obstructive pulmonary disease are altered by multiple mechanisms. Am J Respir Crit Care Med. 2008;178:248–60.
17. Sato T, Liu X, Nelson A, Nakanishi M, Kanaji N, Wang X, et al. Reduced miR-146a increases prostaglandin E2 in chronic obstructive pulmonary disease fibroblasts. Am J Respir Crit Care Med. 2010;182:1020–9.
18. Domej W, Oettl K, Renner W. Oxidative stress and free radicals in COPD – implications and relevance for treatment. Int J Chron Obstruct Pulmon Dis. 2014;9:1207–24.
19. O'Donnell DE, Laveneziana P, Webb K, Neder JA. Chronic obstructive pulmonary disease: clinical integrative physiology. Clin Chest Med. 2014;35:51–69.
20. Battaglia S, Mauad T, van Schadewijk AM, Vignola AM, Rabe KF, Bellia V, et al. Differential distribution of inflammatory cells in large and small airways in smokers. J Clin Pathol. 2007;60:907–11.
21. Mercer BA, Lemaitre V, Powell CA, D'Armiento J. The epithelial cell in lung health and emphysema pathogenesis. Curr Respir Med Rev. 2006;2:101–42.
22. Yang J, Zuo WL, Fukui T, Chao I, Gomi K, Lee B, et al. Smoking-dependent distal-to-proximal Repatterning of the adult human small airway epithelium. Am J Respir Crit Care Med. 2017;196:340–52.
23. Montuschi P, Macagno F, Parente P, Valente S, Lauriola L, Ciappi G, et al. Effects of cyclo-oxygenase inhibition on exhaled eicosanoids in patients with COPD. Thorax. 2005;60:827–33.
24. Xaubet A, Roca-Ferrer J, Pujols L, Ramirez J, Mullol J, Marin-Arguedas A, et al. Cyclooxygenase-2 is up-regulated in lung parenchyma of chronic obstructive pulmonary disease and down-regulated in idiopathic pulmonary fibrosis. Sarcoidosis Vasc Diffuse Lung Dis. 2004;21:35–42.
25. Roh GS, Yi CO, Cho YJ, Jeon BT, Nizamudtinova IT, Kim HJ, et al. Anti-inflammatory effects of celecoxib in rat lungs with smoke-induced emphysema. Am J Physiol Lung Cell Mol Physiol. 2010;299:L184–91.
26. Zago M, Sheridan JA, Nair P, Rico de Souza A, Gallouzi IE, Rousseau S, et al. Aryl hydrocarbon receptor-dependent retention of nuclear HuR suppresses cigarette smoke-induced cyclooxygenase-2 expression independent of DNA-binding. PLoS One. 2013;8:e74953.
27. Zago M, Rico de Souza A, Hecht E, Rousseau S, Hamid Q, Eidelman DH, et al. The NF-kappaB family member RelB regulates microRNA miR-146a to suppress cigarette smoke-induced COX-2 protein expression in lung fibroblasts. Toxicol Lett. 2014;226:107–16.
28. Sheridan JA, Zago M, Nair P, Li PZ, Bourbeau J, Tan WC, et al. Decreased expression of the NF-kappaB family member RelB in lung fibroblasts from smokers with and without COPD potentiates cigarette smoke-induced COX-2 expression. Respir Res. 2015;16:54.
29. Zago M, Sheridan JA, Traboulsi H, Hecht E, Zhang Y, Guerrina N, et al. Low levels of the AhR in chronic obstructive pulmonary disease (COPD)-derived lung cells increases COX-2 protein by altering mRNA stability. PLoS One. 2017;12:e0180881.
30. Gu W, Song L, Li XM, Wang D, Guo XJ. Xu WG. Mesenchymal stem cells alleviate airway inflammation and emphysema in COPD through down-regulation of cyclooxygenase-2 via p38 and ERK MAPK pathways. Sci Rep. 2015;5:8733.

9

Genome-wide association study identifies loci and candidate genes for non-idiopathic pulmonary hypertension in Eastern Chinese Han population

Caiyong Yin[1,2†], Kai Li[1†], Yanfang Yu[1], Huijie Huang[1], Youjia Yu[1], Zhongqun Wang[3], Jinchuan Yan[3], Yan Pu[4], Zheng Li[1], Ding Li[1], Peng Chen[1*] and Feng Chen[1,5*]

Abstract

Background: Pulmonary hypertension (PH) is a rare disease characterized by proliferation and occlusion of small pulmonary arterioles, which has been associated with a high mortality rate. The pathogenesis of PH is complex and incompletely understood, which includes both genetic and environmental factors that alter vascular structure and function.

Methods: Thus we aimed to reveal the potential genetic etiology of PH by targeting 143 tag SNPs of 14 candidate genes. Totally 208 individuals from Chinese Han population were enrolled in the present study, including 109 non-idiopathic PH patients and 99 healthy controls.

Results: The data revealed that 2 SNPs were associated with PH overall susceptibility at $p < 3\times10^{-4}$ after Bonferroni correction. The top hit was rs6557421 ($p = 4.5\times10^{-9}$), located within *Nox3* gene on chromosome 6. Another SNP rs3744439 located in *Tbx4* gene, also showed evidence of association with PH susceptibility ($p = 1.2\times10^{-6}$). The distribution of genotype frequencies of rs6557421 and rs3744439 have dramatic differences between PH patients and controls. Individuals with rs6557421 TT genotype had a 10.72-fold/14.20-fold increased risk to develop PH when compared with GG or GG/GT carriers in codominant or recessive model, respectively (TT versus GG: 95%CI = 4.79–24.00; TT versus GG/GT: 95%CI = 6.65–30.33). As for rs3744439, AG genotype only occurred in healthy controls but has not been observed in PH patients. We further validated the result by using 26 different populations from five regions around the globe, including African (AFR), American (AMR), East Asian (EAS), European (EUR), and South Asian (SAS). In consistent with the present case-control study's results, significantly different genotype frequencies of the observed SNPs existed between PH patients and healthy individuals from all over the world.

Conclusions: The results suggested that rs6557421 variant in *Nox3* and rs3744439 variant in *Tbx4* might have potential effect on individual susceptibility to pulmonary hypertension, which could lead to therapeutic or diagnosis approaches in PH.

Keywords: Pulmonary hypertension, Nox3, Tbx4, GWAS

* Correspondence: chenpeng@njmu.edu.cn; fchen@njmu.edu.cn
†Caiyong Yin and Kai Li contributed equally to this work.
[1]Department of Forensic Medicine, Nanjing Medical University, Nanjing, Jiangsu 211166, People's Republic of China
Full list of author information is available at the end of the article

Table 1 Summarized 14 genes that were analyzed in the present study

Gene name	The (potential) relationship between the studied genes and PH occurrence.
Solute carrier family 4 member 4 (SLC4A4, also known as NBCe1)	*SLC4A4* encodes NBCe1 which is the first eukaryotic Na^+ – coupled transporter. The transporter is a member of the anion exchange family belonging to the second largest secondary carrier superfamily (APC). A previous GWAS study have revealed that SLC4A4 was hypertension susceptibility gene [12].
NADPH oxidase 3 (Nox3)	Nox3 is a member of the NADPH oxidase (Nox) family of oxidant-generating enzymes. After its original cloning and detection in fetal tissues and inner ear, studies remain limited and its function mostly limited to gravity perception. However, several studies have also reported the physiologic role of Nox3 induction in lungs and lung endothelial cells [7, 13].
Interleukin 6 (IL6)	Interleukin 6 (IL6) is a pleiotropic cytokine with a wide range of biologic function on hematopoiesis, inflammation, immune regulation and oncogenesis. The increasing levels of IL-6 in lung and serum are associated with PH [3].
Transcription factor EC (TFEC)	Transcription factor EC (TFEC) most likely acts as a transcriptional repressor in heterodimers with other microphthalmia-TFE (MiT) family members. The expression of murine TFEC is restricted to macrophages (mTFEC). mTFEC as a macrophage-specific transcription factor plays a critical role in macrophage-specific gene regulation [3]. Considering the activities of macrophages in PH development, TFEC might have potential connection with PH.
Caveolin-1	Caveolin-1, which is a major protein constituent of caveolae, interacts with a variety of signaling molecules implicated in PH. Disruption and progressive loss of endothelial caveolin-1 with reciprocal activation of proliferative pathways occur before the onset of PH, and the rescue of caveolin-1 inhibits proliferative pathways and attenuates PH [4].
NADPH oxidase 4 (Nox4)	NADPH oxidase 4 is the major NADPH oxidase homolog expressed in human PASMCs and its expression both at the mRNA and protein level is significantly increased in lungs from patients with PH, which suggests a correlation between Nox4 and the onset of PH [5, 6]. Additionally, Nox4 acts as a primary source of ROS, contributes to the proliferation and remodeling of PH [7, 8].
Oxidized low density lipoprotein receptor 1 (OLR-1)	Oxidized low density lipoprotein receptor 1 (OLR-1), the receptor for oxidized low-density lipoprotein, is expressed in endothelial cells, macrophages or smooth muscle cells. Recent studies have shown that OLR-1 is involved in the lung inflammation and injury [3].
Thrombospondin 1 (THBS1)	Thrombospondin 1 (THBS1) is a kind of matricellular protein, which is a secreted molecular that has both extracellular matrix and cell surface receptor. In animals, pulmonary THBS1 is upregulated rapidly following hypoxic challenge. Additionally, clinical studies of plasma THBS1 and mutations of THBS1 in PH have been reported [4].
ATPase phospholipid transporting 8B4 (ATP8B4)	ATPase phospholipid transporting 8B4 (ATP8B4) activity is important in ATP biosynthesis and phospholipid transport via a variety of potential mechanisms. A recent whole-exome sequencing research identified that ATP8B4 gene is strongly associated with the risk of development of PH [5].
NADPH oxidase 5 (Nox5)	NADPH oxidase 5 (Nox5) is the last NOX family member to be identified. Caveolin-1 binds directly to Nox5 and suppresses the activity of Nox5. Although the direct connection between Nox5 and PH has not been reported, dysregulation of caveolin-1 has been documented with PH states.
T-box4 (Tbx4)	T-box4 (Tbx4) is a transcription factor in the T-box gene family, which is expressed in variety of organs including mesenchyme of the lung and trachea. Tbx4 has been shown to be involved in lung growth and branching. The function mutations in Tbx4 have been previously reported to be associated with PH [3].
Chromobox 7 (CBX7)	Chromobox 7 (CBX7) is one of the five mammalian orthologues of Drosophila Polycomb. CBX7 was recognized as the main orthologue of Drosophila Polycomb implicated in maintaining the self-renewal of embryonic stem cells. Until now, litter is known about the potential correlation of CBX7 to PH.
Cytochrome b-245 beta chain (CYBB)	The *Cytochrome b-245 beta chain (CYBB)* gene encodes membrane protein Nox2, which plays a crucial role in stromal interaction molecular 1 (STIM1) activation and in the control of the cytosolic oscillations that drive murine pulmonary microvascular endothelial cells (MPMVECs) activation [4]. Our recent research has also revealed the role of STIM1 during the acute lung intoxication [5].
Galectin-3 (Gal-3)	Galectin-3 (Gal-3) is a β-galactoside binding lectin that regulates multiple pathways. Our recent study has revealed the effectiveness of genetic and pharmacological strategies targeting Gal-3 in halting the progression of PH remodeling and development of experimental PH [1].

Background

Pulmonary hypertension (PH) is a rare disease characterized by proliferation and occlusion of small pulmonary arterioles, leading to progressive elevation of pulmonary artery pressure, pulmonary vascular resistance, and right ventricular failure [1]. There are 3 subtypes of PH according to the National Organization for Rare Disorders (NORD), including heritable pulmonary hypertension (HPH), idiopathic pulmonary arterial hypertension (IPH) and associated pulmonary hypertension (APH) [2]. More than half of the PH patients are non-idiopathic PH, which are also known as secondary PH. During the present study, we focused on the genetic susceptibility of non-idiopathic PH. Revealing the genetic etiology of non-idiopathic PH would facilitate diagnosis and development of novel therapies in the future. During the present study, we reviewed and screened several candidate genes that are potentially or directly associated with PH occurrence (Table 1).

In summary, these genes were shown to be associated or potentially related with PH development though the molecular mechanism had not been well understood. To further clarify the association and reveal the candidate functional variants, we conducted the limited scale genome wide association study. One hundred forty-three tag SNPs were screened from the sequences between the upstream and downstream 2Kb of the 14 studied genes. The screening population data are from Chinese Han population in Beijing (CHB) of the Hapmap Project (NCBI build 36, dbSNPb126) and the candidate SNPs were screened by using Haploview software.

Methods

Samples

Totally 208 individuals were enrolled in the present study, including 109 non-idiopathic PH patients and 99 healthy controls. Patients were consecutively recruited from the Affiliated Hospital of Jiangsu University between May 2014 and July 2016. Clinical information was obtained from medical records, including gender, age, drink, smoke and coronary artery disease (CAD) history and so on. Baseline profiles of the studied population were summarized in Table 2. None of the patients have connective tissue diseases, HIV infection, portal hypertension, congenital heart diseases or thyroid dysfunction. The control subjects were collected from healthy volunteers who visited the Sir Run Run Hospital Nanjing Medical University for medical examination during the same period. The study was performed with the approval of the ethics committee of the Nanjing Medical University and the informed consent was obtained from each participant.

Experimental design and Genotyping

Genomic DNA was extracted from 200 μl EDTA-anticoagulated peripheral blood using a commercial extraction kit (Tiangen Biotech Corporation, Beijing, China) according to the instruction manual. The 143 tag SNPs in 109 PH patients were firstly genotyped by using Illumina X-10 platform, and the sequencing was done by commercial company (Decode Genomics Bio-Tech Co., Ltd, Nanjing, China). The genotyping results were then compared with healthy individuals from Southern Han Chinese (CHS) population of 1000G database. And 2 SNPs emerged at a significant level ($P < 3\times10^{-4}$) (Fig. 1). To confirm the finding, we further genotyped 2 SNPs in 99 healthy individuals from Nanjing, Jiangsu by performing fluorescent PCR and Ligase detection reaction (LDR). The primers were designed by using Primer 3 online software version 0.4.0 (http://frodo.wi.mit.edu/) and Oligo software version 6.3.1 (Molecular Biology Insights, USA). The SNPs were amplified in a final volume of 20 μl that contained 50 ng of DNA, 2 μl 1×buffer, 0.6 μl 3 mM Mg2+, 2 μl 2 mM dNTP, 0.2 μl Taq DNA polymerase (1 unit/μl) and appropriate concentrations of primers. The PCR reaction

Table 2 Demographic and clinical characteristics of the subjects

	Patients	Controls
Sex		
Male	50 (0.46)	63 (0.62)
Female	59 (0.54)	36 (0.38)
Age (y)	74.07 ±12.86	37.26±9.18
Systolic PAP (mmHg)	60.67 ± 12.73	
Drink		
Yes	6 (0.06)	
No	103 (0.94)	
Smoke		
Yes	16 (0.15)	
No	93 (0.85)	
Coronary heart disease		
Yes	66 (0.60)	
No	43 (0.40)	
Heart failure (HF)		
Yes	17 (0.15)	
No	92 (0.84)	
Echocardiogram		
LA (mm)	48.62 ± 10.58	
LvIDd (mm)	52.18 ± 9.77	
IVSD (mm)	10.60 ± 4.80	
LVEF (%)	57.85 ± 15.40	

PAP pulmonary artery pressure, *LA* atrial diameter, *LvIDd* left ventricular end diastolic diameter, *IVST* interventricular septal thickness, *LVEF* left ventricular ejection fraction

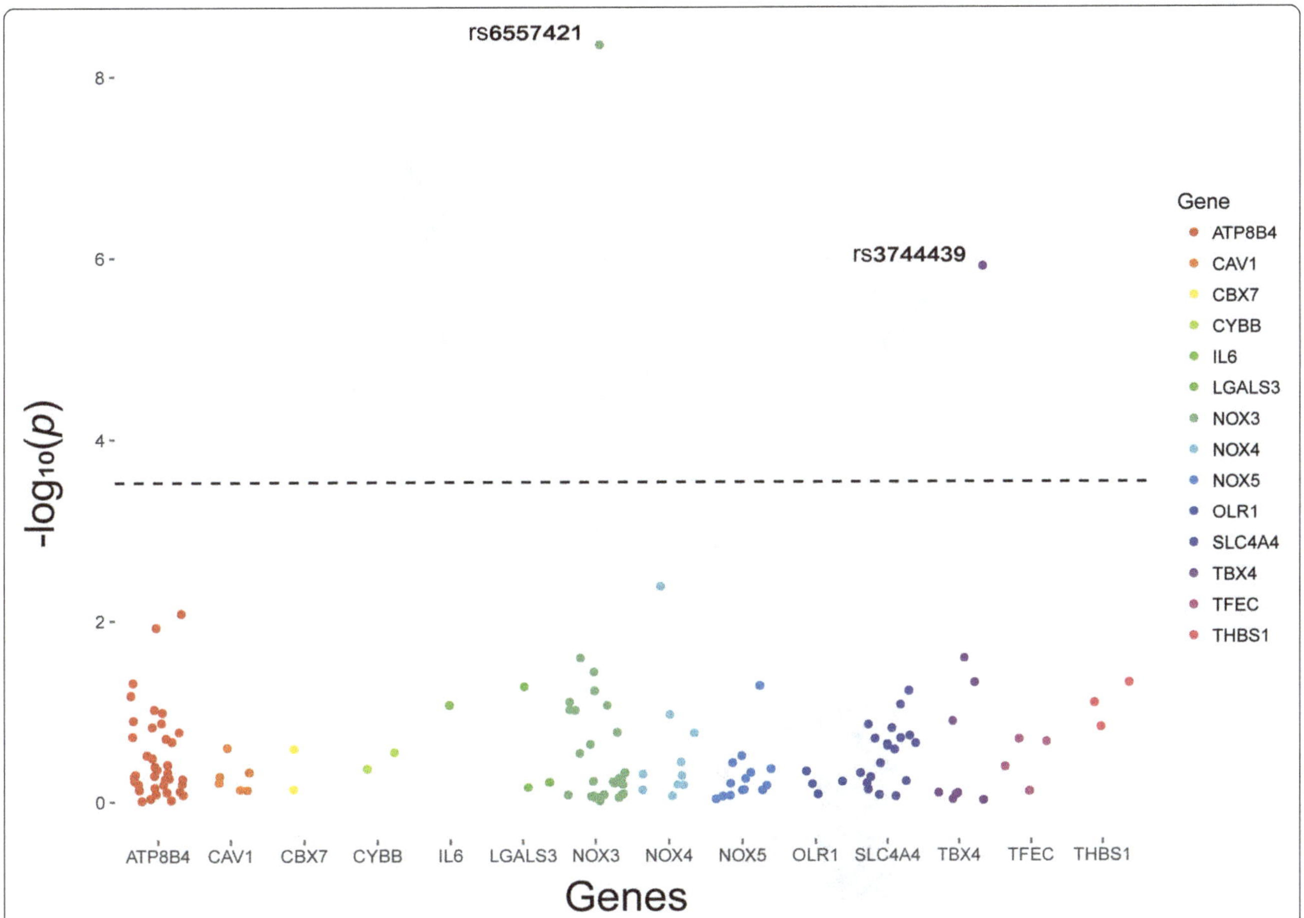

Fig. 1 Manhattan plot for SNPs in the different genes ($n = 143$)

was subjected to an initial denaturation at 95 °C for 2 min, followed by 40 cycles of amplification consisting of denaturation at 94 °C for 30 s, annealing at 53 °C for 90 s, extension at 65 °C for 30 s, followed by final extension at 65 °C for 10 mim. The LDR was carried out on the PRISM 3730 DNA analyzer (Thermo Fisher Scientific, USA). The LDR were performed in a total volume of 10 μl that contained 4 μl PCR production, 1 μl 1×buffer, 1 μl probe mix, 0.05 μl Taq DNA polymerase (2 unit/μl). The LDR condition was 95 °C for 2 mim, followed by 40 cycles of 15 s at 94 °C and 25 s at 50 °C. The SNPs were further genotyped by using Genemapper.

Statistical analysis

All data were analyzed by using SPSS 19 (SPSS Inc., Chicago, IL). Genotype frequencies of SNPs were obtained by directed computing. Genotypic association analyses in a case-control pattern assuming codominant, dominant, recessive and overdominant genetic models were performed using SNPstats [3]. Odds ratio (OR) and respective 95% confidence interval were reported to evaluate the effects of any differences between allele and genotype frequencies.

Results

Candidate SNP selection

Totally 143 SNPs were successfully genotyped in 109 PH patients. After comparing the genotyping results with the data generated from 105 individuals from Southern Han Chinese population in 1000G database, the results demonstrated that 2 SNPs were associated with PH with overall susceptibility at $p < 3\times10^{-4}$ after Bonferroni adjustment. The related analysis was shown in Fig. 1. The top hit was rs6557421 ($p = 4.5\times10^{-9}$), which is located in *Nox3* gene on chromosome 6. Another SNP rs3744439 located in *Tbx4* gene, also showed evidence of association with PH susceptibility ($p = 1.2\times10^{-6}$).

We further genotyped the 2 SNPs in 99 healthy control subjects. The distribution of genotype frequencies of rs6557421 and rs3744439 was illustrated in Fig. 2. Dramatic differences existed between PH patients and controls. As shown in Table 3, individuals with rs6557421 TT genotype had a 10.72-fold/14.20-fold increased risk to develop PH when compared with GG or GG/GT carriers in codominant or recessive model, respectively (TT versus GG: 95%CI = 4.79–24.00; TT versus GG/GT:

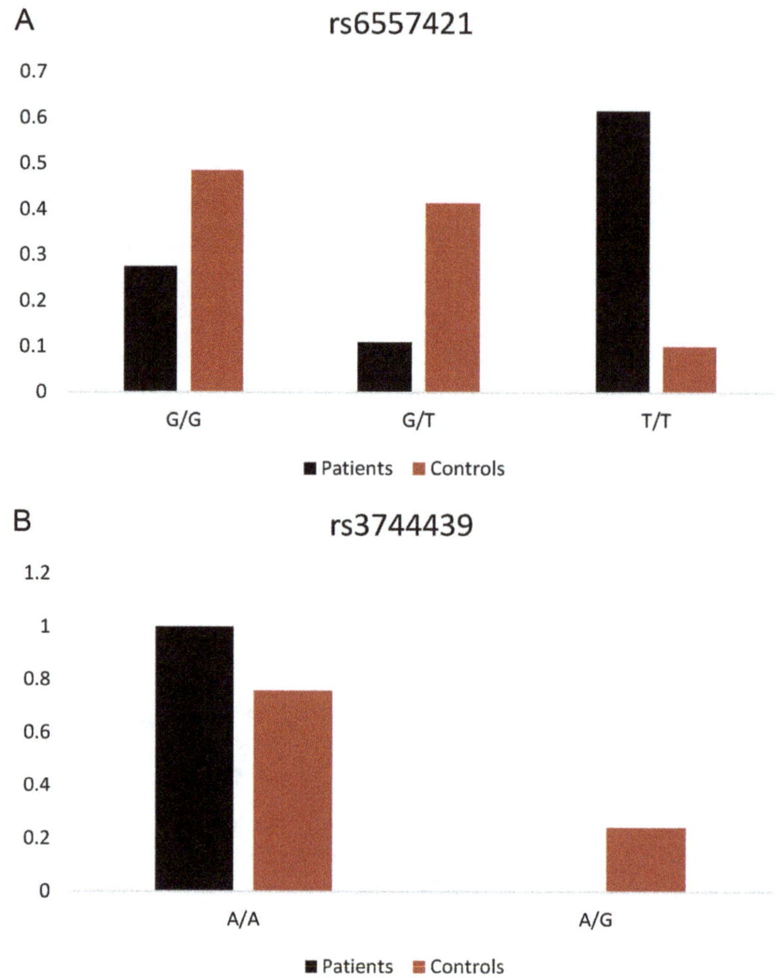

Fig. 2 The distribution of genotype frequencies of *Nox3* rs6557421 (**a**) and *Tbx4* rs3744439 (**b**) among PH patients and healthy controls

Table 3 Genotype frequencies of rs6557421 in *Nox3* gene among PH patients and controls

Genetic model	Genotype	Patients	Controls	Logistic regression		Logistic regression (adjusted)	
		N = 109 (%)	*N* = 99 (%)	OR (95%CI)	*P*-value	OR[c] (95%CI)	*P*-value
Codominant	GG	30 (27.5)	48 (48.5)	1.00		1.00	
	GT	12 (11)	41 (41.4)	0.47 (0.21–1.03)	**< 0.0001**	0.22 (0.03–1.66)	**0.0001**
	TT	67 (61.5)	10 (10.1)	**10.72 (4.79–24.00)**		**9.66 (1.82–51.28)**	
Dominant	GG	30 (27.5)	48 (48.5)	1		1.00	
	GT/TT	79 (72.5)	51 (51.5)	**2.48 (1.39–4.41)**	**0.0018**	2.02 (0.53–7.74)	0.3
Recessive	GG/GT	42 (38.5)	89 (89.9)	1.00		1.00	
	TT	67 (61.5)	10 (10.1)	**14.20 (6.65–30.33)**	**< 0.0001**	**17.29 (3.60–83.02)**	**0.0001**
Overdominant	GG/TT	97 (89)	58 (58.6)	1.00		1.00	
	GT	12 (11)	41 (41.4)	**0.18 (0.09–0.36)**	**< 0.0001**	**0.08 (0.01–0.48)**	**0.0013**

Bold-faced values indicate a significant difference at the 5% level; [c]adjusted by sex and age

95%CI = 6.65–30.33). In dominant model, significantly increased PH susceptibility was associated with GT/TT genotypes compared with GG genotype (OR = 2.48, 95%CI = 1.39–4.41). Furthermore, dramatically decreased PH risk was associated with GT genotype when compared with GG/TT genotypes in an overdominant model.

As shown in Fig. 2b and Table 4, rs3744439 AG genotype only occurred in healthy controls which had not been observed in PH patients.

Stratification analysis was also performed, and PH patients were divided into three groups according to the *Nox3* rs6557421 genotypes. The distribution of patients' left atrial diameter (LA), left ventricular end diastolic diameter (LvIDd), interventricular septal thickness (IVST), left ventricular ejection fraction (LVEF) and systolic pulmonary artery pressure (PAP) were compared between each groups (Fig. 3). No significant differences were observed among different genotyping groups.

Comparison between different populations around globe

We further validated the observation by using 26 different populations from five regions around the globe, including African (AFR), American (AMR), East Asian (EAS), European (EUR), and South Asian (SAS). As illustrated in Fig. 4a and b, the distribution of rs6557421 and rs3744439 genotypes' frequencies of control group from Chinese Han population was quite similar to which from Asian populations. In consistent to the present case-control study's results, significantly different genotype frequencies existed between PH Patients and healthy individuals from all over the world (Fig. 4a and b).

Discussion

Among NADPH oxidases, Nox3 seems to have the most restricted expression pattern in the mammalian organism. Nox3 is specifically localized to the inner ear. Thus the previous studies mostly focused on the unique function of Nox3 involving in the biogenesis of otoconia/otolith [4]. However, few studies have revealed the potential critical role of Nox3 in the pathophysiological process of PH development. Nox3 is the predominant source of palmitate-induced ROS generation [5]. Nox3 activation during ischemia-reperfusion injury may contribute to the development of primary graft dysfunction after lung transplantation [6]. Upregulated Nox3 leads to increased oxidant generation and elastolytic activity, resulting in increased oxidant injury and death in mice and lung endothelial cells [7]. Treatment of $Tlr^{-/-}$ mice or endothelial cells with *Nox3* siRNA or chemical NADPH inhibitors could reverse the phenotype [7]. Overall, the studies identified that Nox3 could be a potential therapeutic target in the lungs.

The present case-control study revealed that a *Nox3* tagSNP rs6557421 had a significantly association with the PH susceptibility. When random individuals carry rs6557421 TT genotype, they have nearly 10-fold increased risk to develop PH when compared with GG or GG/GT carriers. Moreover, GT genotype carriers have a significantly decreased PH risk compared with GG/TT genotype carriers. To further investigate the racial disparities, we enrolled 26 populations from 1000G to make a comparison. All the populations from different continents possessed relatively low frequency of TT genotype (AFR = 0.006, AMR = 0.052, EAS = 0.113, EUR = 0.056, SAS = 0.08, Han in present = 0.101). On the contrary, the proportion of TT genotype carriers in PH patients reached 0.615. The data indicated that TT genotype might be associated with increased PH in different races.

Mutations in *Tbx4* have been proved to be associated with PH onset [8]. Tbx4 shows high specific expression in lung fibroblasts and broadly regulates fibroblast-related pathway that partly contributes to super-enhancer-mediated transcriptional programs [9]. Decreased Tbx4 in the pulmonary mesenchyme during fetal lung development may lead to the decrease or arrest of airway branching, thus contributing to PH [10]. Tbx4 was also regarded as a mesenchymal transcription factor that drove myofibroblasts accumulation and the development of lung fibrosis [11].

Our research revealed that *Tbx4* rs3744439 had a significant association with PH risk. The frequencies of AG genotype in present control Chinese Han population and other 26 populations around the globe are all over than 0.10 (Han in present = 0.24, AFR = 0.23, AMR = 0.19, EAS = 0.17, EUR = 0.10, SAS = 0.14). Interestingly, during the PH patients, AG and GG genotype frequencies were 0. The data suggested that

Table 4 Genoetype frequencies of rs3744439 in *Tbx4* gene among *PH* patients and controls

Genetic model	Genotype	Patients	Controls	Logistic regression		Logistic regression (adjusted)	
		N = 109 (%)	*N* = 99 (%)	OR (95%CI)	*P*-value	OR[c] (95%CI)	*P*-value
	AA	109 (100)	75 (75.8)	1.00		1.00	
	AG	0 (0)	24 (24.2)	0.00 (0.00-NA)	**< 0.0001**	0.00 (0.00-NA)	**0.0013**

Bold-faced values indicate a significant difference at the 5% level; [c]adjusted by sex and age

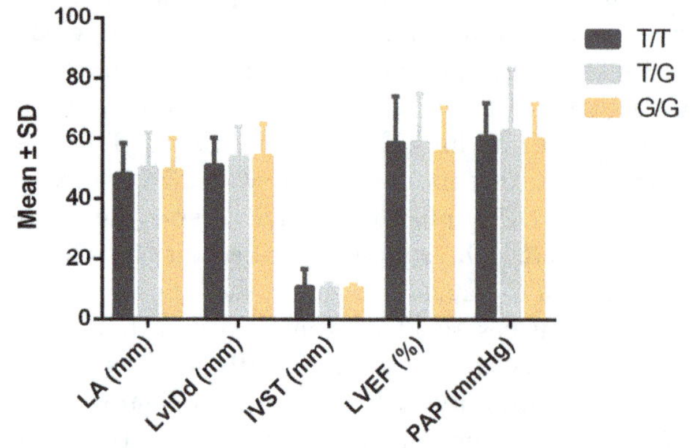

Fig. 3 The distribution of patients' left atrial diameter (LA), left ventricular end diastolic diameter (LvIDd), interventricular septal thickness (IVST), left ventricular ejection fraction (LVEF) and systolic pulmonary artery pressure (PAP) among different genotypes of *Nox3* rs6557421

AG genotype could be a protective factor for the PH development.

The present study has an obvious limitation. As noted in the Methods section that the ages of patients and controls are significantly different. The controls are younger, and they might develop PH in the future. Considering the relative low incidence of PH, we believe the results are reliable. To further validate the results, healthy independent individuals from 1000G database were also included. And the results were consistent.

Conclusions

In summary, it is biologically plausible that rs6557421 variant in *Nox3* and rs3744439 variant in *Tbx4* may have potential effects on individual susceptibility to pulmonary hypertension, which could lead to therapeutic or diagnosis approaches in PH.

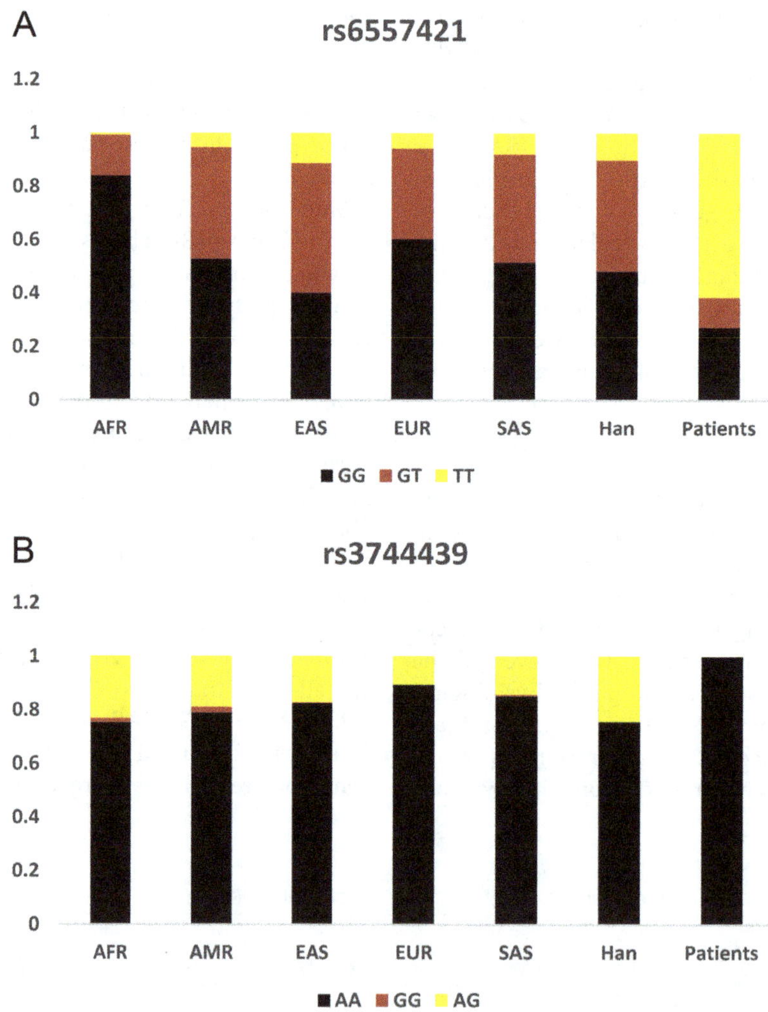

Fig. 4 The distribution of genotype frequencies of *Nox3* rs6557421 (**a**) and *Tbx4* rs3744439 (**b**) among the studied population and 26 populations from 1000G

Abbreviations

ATP8B4: ATPase phospholipid transporting 8B4; CHX7: Chromobox 7; CYBB: Cytochrome b-245 beta chain; IL6: Interleukin 6; NORD: National Organization for Rare Disorders; Nox3: NADPH oxidase 3; Nox4: NADPH oxidase 4; Nox5: NADPH oxidase 5; OLR-1: Oxidized low density lipoprotein receptor 1; PH: Pulmonary hypertension; SLC4A4: Solute carrier family 4 member 4; Tbx4: T-box4; TFEC: Transcription factor EC; THBS1: Thrombospondin 1

Funding

This work was supported by the National Natural Science Foundation of China (No.81570378, No.81772020 and No.81801879), the Science and Technology of Jiangsu Province China (BK20170048 and BK20161034), and Jiangsu Specially-Appointed Professor program. The National Natural Science Foundation of China, the Science and Technology of Jiangsu Province China and Jiangsu Specially-Appointed Professor program played no role in the design of the study and collection, analysis, and interpretation of data and in writing the manuscript.

Authors' contributions

FC and PC designed the study and were major contributors in writing the manuscript. KL, ZQW and JCY collected samples of patients and controls. YFY, HJH and YJY performed the experiments. CYY, YP, ZL and DL analyzed and interpreted the data. All authors read and approved the final manuscript.

Consent for publication

Not applicable.

Competing interests

The authors declare that they have no competing interests.

Author details

[1]Department of Forensic Medicine, Nanjing Medical University, Nanjing, Jiangsu 211166, People's Republic of China. [2]MOE Key Laboratory of Contemporary Anthropology, Department of Anthropology and Human Genetics, School of Life Sciences, Fudan University, Shanghai 200438, People's Republic of China. [3]Department of Cardiology, Affiliated Hospital of Jiangsu University, Zhenjiang, Jiangsu 212001, People's Republic of China. [4]School of Medicine, Southeast University, Nanjing, Jiangsu 210009, People's Republic of China. [5]Key Laboratory of Targeted Intervention of Cardiovascular Disease, Collaborative Innovation Center for Cardiovascular Disease Translational Medicine, Nanjing Medical University, Nanjing, Jiangsu 211166, People's Republic of China.

References

1. Barman SA, Chen F, Li X, Haigh S, Stepp DW, Kondrikov D, Mahboubi K, Bordan Z, Traber P, Su Y, Fulton DJR. Galectin-3 promotes vascular remodeling and contributes to pulmonary hypertension. Am J Respir Crit Care Med. 2018;197:1488–92.
2. Soubrier F, Chung WK, Machado R, Grunig E, Aldred M, Geraci M, Loyd JE, Elliott CG, Trembath RC, Newman JH, Humbert M. Genetics and genomics of pulmonary arterial hypertension. J Am Coll Cardiol. 2013;62:D13–21.
3. Sole X, Guino E, Valls J, Iniesta R, Moreno V. SNPStats: a web tool for the analysis of association studies. Bioinformatics. 2006;22:1928–9.
4. Zhang X, Shan P, Jiang G, Cohn L, Lee PJ. Toll-like receptor 4 deficiency causes pulmonary emphysema. J Clin Invest. 2006;116:3050–9.
5. Garcia-Redondo AB, Aguado A, Briones AM, Salaices M. NADPH oxidases and vascular remodeling in cardiovascular diseases. Pharmacol Res. 2016;114:110–20.
6. Cantu E, Shah RJ, Lin W, Daye ZJ, Diamond JM, Suzuki Y, Ellis JH, Borders CF, Andah GA, Beduhn B, et al. Oxidant stress regulatory genetic variation in recipients and donors contributes to risk of primary graft dysfunction after lung transplantation. J Thorac Cardiovasc Surg. 2015;149:596–602.
7. Zhang Y, Shan P, Srivastava A, Jiang G, Zhang X, Lee PJ. An endothelial Hsp70-TLR4 axis limits Nox3 expression and protects against oxidant injury in lungs. Antioxid Redox Signal. 2016;24(17):991–1012.
8. Zhu N, Gonzaga-Jauregui C, Welch CL, Ma L, Qi H, King AK, Krishnan U, Rosenzweig EB, Ivy DD, Austin ED, et al. Exome sequencing in children with pulmonary arterial hypertension demonstrates differences compared with adults. Circ Genom Precis Med. 2018;11:e001887.
9. Horie M, Miyashita N, Mikami Y, Noguchi S, Yamauchi Y, Suzukawa M, Fukami T, Ohta K, Asano Y, Sato S, et al. TBX4 is involved in the super-enhancer-driven transcriptional programs underlying features specific to lung fibroblasts. Am J Physiol Lung Cell Mol Physiol. 2018;314:L177–l191.
10. Takahashi T, Friedmacher F, Zimmer J, Puri P. Expression of T-box transcription factors 2, 4 and 5 is decreased in the branching airway mesenchyme of nitrofen-induced hypoplastic lungs. Pediatr Surg Int. 2017; 33:139–43.
11. Xie T, Liang J, Liu N, Huan C, Zhang Y, Liu W, Kumar M, Xiao R, D'Armiento J, Metzger D, et al. Transcription factor TBX4 regulates myofibroblast accumulation and lung fibrosis. J Clin Invest. 2016;126:3063–79.
12. Yang HC, Liang YJ, Chen JW, Chiang KM, Chung CM, Ho HY, Ting CT, Lin TH, Sheu SH, Tsai WC, Chen JH, Leu HB, Yin WH, Chiu TY, Chern CL, Lin SJ, Tomlinson B, Guo Y, Sham PC, Cherny SS, Lam TH, Thomas GN, Pan WH. Identification of IGF1, SLC4A4, WWOX, and SFMBT1 as hypertension susceptibility genes in Han Chinese with a genome-wide gene-based association study. Plos One. 2012;7(3):e32907.
13. Wang H, Albadawi H, Siddiquee Z, Stone JM, Panchenko MP, Watkins MT, Stone JR. Altered vascular activation due to deficiency of the NADPH oxidase component p22phox. Cardiovasc Pathol. 2014;23(1):35-42.

10

Pleural infection: a retrospective study of clinical outcome and the correlation to known etiology, co-morbidity and treatment factors

Christian Niels Meyer[1,2*], Karin Armbruster[3], Michael Kemp[4], Trine Rolighed Thomsen[5], Ram Benny Dessau[6] for The Danish Pleural Empyema group

Abstract

Background: We explored the hypothesized importance of early knowledge of microbiological etiology in patients with pleural infection, including comorbidity and treatment factors in the outcome analyses.

Methods: Data from the medical records of a large cohort of 437 consecutive patients in 9 hospitals in East-Denmark were included retrospectively.

Results: Microbiology, co-morbidity, therapy and outcome are described in detail. Patient groups with microbiology negative and known bacterial etiology had a similar 30-day and 90-day mortality. There were no differences in initial antibiotic treatment regimens, antibiotic treatment duration, rate of intra-pleural fibrinolysis treatment, surgical referral rate, and ICU admittance rate. Patients with microbiology negative etiology were younger (60.8 vs 64.3 years) and fewer had predisposing risk factors (59% vs 71%), but pleural drainage was more often delayed (49% vs 36%). Mortality was similar in patients treated with either of the two nationally recommended initial antibiotic regimens. However, higher 90-day mortality (22.5% vs 9.7%), disease severity (31.5% vs 6.2%), and ICU admittance rate (21.3% vs 2.9%) was observed in a sub-group with initial broad-spectrum treatment compared to patients receiving the nationally recommended initial treatments, irrespective of knowledge of etiology. Several factors correlated independently to 90-day mortality, including age, predisposing risk factors, surgical referral (Odds-Ratios > 1), drainage delay and intra-pleural fibrinolysis (ORs < 1).

Conclusions: No difference was found between patients with microbiology negative and known bacterial etiology regarding outcome or treatment parameters. Treatment factors and predisposing factors independently relating to mortality were found in the cohort. Broad-spectrum antibiotics were initially used for treatment of patients with more severe illness and poorer outcome.

Keywords: Empyema, Pleural, Infection, Pleural disease, Pyothorax, Respiratory tract infection

* Correspondence: cnm@regionsjaelland.dk
[1]Department of Internal Medicine, Zealand University Hospital Roskilde, Sygehusvej 10, 4000 Roskilde, Denmark
[2]Department of Clinical Medicine, University of Copenhagen, Copenhagen, Denmark
Full list of author information is available at the end of the article

Background

Pleural bacterial infection is most often a complication to pneumonia, but with an increased morbidity and mortality. Recommended treatment consists of antibiotics and pleural drainage. Surgical therapy with thoracoscopy and debridement or decortication may be needed in a minority of patients to obtain clinical stabilization and treatment success [1]. An adequate initial antibiotic regimen takes into account the locally expected spectrum of bacterial etiology and the antibiotic susceptibility, but this specific information may not be present in up to 47% of cases with microbiology negative etiology due to recent outpatient antibiotic treatment or due to delayed in-hospital sampling [2–4]. An antibiotic treatment duration of 3–6 weeks has been recommended for pleural infection [1]. In observational studies, the presence of underlying diseases, predisposing risk factors, and treatment factors have been associated with outcome [1, 4]. In randomized controlled trials, treatment factors such as active pleural drain irrigation or intra-pleural treatment with a fibrinolytic agent plus DNase without routine use of active drain irrigation correlated to outcome [5, 6]. With a limited number of patients included at individual participating centers and not including all consecutive patients in trials, the possibility of patient selection bias cannot be excluded [6].

The aim of the study was to investigate whether patients without verified bacterial etiology differed from patients with known etiology with regard to outcome in a large cohort of consecutive patients with pleural infection. In addition, the role of predisposing risk factors, initial antibiotic treatment regimens and other treatment factors was investigated.

Methods

Study population

All consecutive adult patients ($n = 437$) admitted with pleural infection at nine hospitals in Eastern Denmark without an in-house thoracic surgery department in a 3.5 year period (2008–2011) were included in the Danish Pleural Empyema Project, geographically covering a population of 1.96 million adults (36% of the Danish population). No patients with pleural infection were admitted directly to the only tertiary hospital with in-house thoracic surgery in the region, as patients could only be referred from satellite hospitals as the actual practice of patient visitation. Patients were identified using three complementary strategies in order to include all patients and to counteract selection: combining the trial related prospective collection of microbiological samples with the databases of the departments of clinical microbiology, combined with the ICD-10 codes DJ860 and DJ869 in the hospital codes of diagnosis at discharge. Microbiological data was routinely collected and included microscopy, culture, and antibiotic susceptibility. The intention in the study protocol was prospectively to obtain samples from all relevant patients in the participating centers and to freeze samples for later possible bacterial identification by PCR-technology. Successful freeze samples were obtained from 72 patients of the cohort, thus adding microbiological information to few poly-microbial samples.

Clinical data included symptoms, history of predisposing risk factors, clinical findings, radiology, biochemical findings, treatment before and after hospital admission, timing of and type of therapy, length of hospital stay (LOS), intensive care unit (ICU) admittance, and all-cause mortality at day 30 and at day 90.

Two patients who were not treated with antibiotics, according to the patient's wish or by order of the attending physician, were excluded from the study. Six patients had missing data on antibiotic treatment and were excluded.

One medical record was missing. Thirteen cases of pleural infection with attempted but unsuccessful thoracocentesis sampling and with no other positive microbiological sample were included in the analysis of the whole cohort, but were not included in statistical analyses regarding knowledge of etiology. The 13 patients with no successful pleural sample for microbiology had a trend to higher 90 day mortality (29% vs 11.7%, $p = 0.054$) but did not differ significantly in length of antibiotic treatment, proportion of nosocomial infection, pre-admission antibiotic treatment, predisposing risk factor or 30 day mortality (all $p > 0.19$), when compared to the rest of the cohort. Length of hospital stay was shorter (7.6 vs 17 days).

Definitions

Nosocomial or hospital associated infection was defined according to the Center for Disease Control and Prevention criteria (CDC) [7].

Severe illness

Hypotension with systolic blood pressure < 95 mmHg, heart rate > 150 beats/min, nasal oxygen-flow above 4 L/min, other abnormities of severe sepsis, or need for ICU treatment.

Intra-pleural fibrinolytic treatment

The national guideline at the time from the Danish Society of Pulmonary Medicine (which had BTS guidelines as a reference) mentioned the possibility of 3 days treatment with either streptokinase or tissue plasminogen activator (t-PA). Treatment did not include DNase for any patients, as the study-period was prior to 2012, when superiority of the combination tissue plasminogen activator (t-PA) plus DNase compared to placebo was demonstrated, with a similar but non-significant difference with t-PA alone compared to placebo [6].

Predisposing risk factors or conditions

Alcoholism (ethanol intake > 50 g/day), cancer within the recent 5 years, hematologic malignancy, severe liver or renal disease, COPD, immune-deficiency, HIV, diabetes, aspiration tendency caused by neurologic disease, active or treated rheumatologic disease.

Pleural drainage

The techniques and drain types and sizes used and the type of medical persons performing the pleural drainage varied between the 9 participating centers, and at the individual center varied during the time of the day or weekends. The chosen drain size presumably varied according to the treating physician's judgement of the individual patients need, though the national guideline suggested using a minimum 10–14 F drain. According to the national guideline, flushing of the drain with minimum 100 ml saline twice daily was recommended.

Delay in thoracocentesis and in pleural drainage

Number of days from detection of pleural effusion on chest X-ray or CT-scan.

Antibiotic regimens

In the study period, the national and regional Danish recommendations for initial treatment regimens for pleural infection (which were adopted from and inspired by the current 2003 and 2010 BTS guidelines) were cefuroxime +/− metronidazole (CEFU) or penicillin/aminopenicillin +/− metronidazole (PENI), in accordance with the national clinical microbiological findings and antibiotic susceptibility. We defined broad-spectrum treatment (BROAD) as these initial antibiotic regimens with further antibiotics added (most often a quinolone or a macrolide), or the use of other broad-spectrum regimens (most often meropenem or piperacillin/tazobactam). Each case was categorized according to the predominant antibiotic treatment (given > 50% of the time) during the first 3 days of treatment.

Bacterial etiology sub-groups

Cases were categorized as streptococci, *Staphylococcus aureus*, mixed infection, anaerobes only, enterobacteriaceae, other bacterial etiology, or microbiology negative etiology. This subgroup division was chosen according to our earlier publications [3, 4] and was included in the estimation and decision on sample size of the study.

Statistical analysis

All statistical analyses were performed using Statistica 7 ® (StatSoft, Tulsa OK, USA), R-statistics (www.r-project.org), SPSS (ver 23, IBM Cooperation) or Statcalc (EpiInfo 7.2, CDC, Atlanta GA, USA). T-test or Mann-Whitney U test was used for continuous data. Chi-square or Kruskal-Wallis test was used for categorical data, backward logistic regression for multivariate outcome analyses. The individual parameters were chosen from the clinically relevant factors in the univariate analyses (from biological plausible importance and earlier publications) and the planned number of included parameters in the model according to the estimations of sample size, and estimated outcome frequency in the study design. Interaction analyses were performed as parts of the analyses. $P < 0.05$ was considered statistically significant.

Results

The main results focus on differences in outcome or other important variables between cases with microbiology negative etiology and cases with known etiology, and are presented in Tables 1 and 2.

For the whole cohort ($n = 429$), mean age was 62.6 years (SD 14.8), 11.6% of the patients were severely ill (see Definitions) at admittance, with 6.6% admitted to the ICU. Length of ICU stay was median 6 days (range 1–25). The infection was hospital associated in 14% of cases, and 43% of the patients were treated with antibiotics before hospital admittance. Antibiotic treatment was started before thoracocentesis in 77.8% of the cases. Median duration of antibiotic treatment after hospital admission was 35 days. Intra-pleural fibrinolysis treatment was given to 30.2% of patients. Median length of hospital stay was 17 days (IQR = 11–25), 30-day mortality was 8.7%, 90-day mortality was 13% and the surgical referral rate was 11.7%.

The categorized bacterial etiology sub-groups consisted of pleural effusions with streptococci (23%), *Staphylococcus aureus* (3.7%, all were MSSA), mixed infection (11%, mostly including anaerobes), anaerobes only (1.8%), enterobacteriaceae (1.8%), other bacterial etiology (8.2%), and microbiology negative (51%).

Among the 437 consecutive patients with pleural infection, a categorized initial antibiotic regimen was administered to 200 with microbiology negative bacterial etiology, to 216 with known etiology, and to 13 with no successfully obtained pleural samples (Tables 1 and 2). The remaining eight patients could not fulfill the criteria of initial antibiotic regimen sub-groups.

Descriptives and demographics

Patients with microbiology negative etiology were marginally younger (60.8 vs 64.3 years, $p = 0.02$), were more often treated with antibiotics prior to thoracocentesis (89.1% vs 76.4%, $p < 0.001$), and fewer had pre-defined risk factors (59% vs 71%, $p < 0.01$) compared to patients with known etiology, but had similar length of hospital stay (16 vs 18 days, $p = 0.22$) (Table 1).

The other recorded severity factors did not differ significantly between patients with microbiology negative and known bacterial etiology: The proportions of patients with severe disease, with nosocomial infection, or

Table 1 Clinical factors, predisposing risk factors, severity factors, treatment factors, and outcome in pleural infection, in patients with microbiology negative or known etiology according to the initial antibiotic regimen

	Microbiology Negative					Known Etiology					$p=$[§]
	PENI	CEFU	broad	All	$p=$[*]	PENI	CEFU	broad	All	$p=$[*]	
n=, (%)	62 (31)	101 (49)	37 (20)	200		57 (26)	106 (49)	49 (23)	216		
Age (years)	59.7	62.9	57.7	60.8	0.27	63.5	65.5	62.5	64.3	0.37	0.02
para-pneumonic (%)	93.5	89	92	90.5	0.90	86	90.7	85.7	88.4	0.01	0.43
Nosocomial (%)	8.0	12	13.5	10.9	0.51	10.5	20	18.4	17.2	0.24	0.06
Risk factors (%)	44[#]	68[#]	54	59	0.22	59	73	80	71	0.45	0.009
AB before hospital admittance (%)	48	57	36	50.3	0.61	39	40	51	42.5	0.44	0.13
Severely ill (%)	4.8	5.0	37	11.1	< 0.001	10.7	5.7	32	13.2	0.0001	0.90
Thoracocentesis delay, median / mean (days)	4.5 /6.3	1 /3.6	2 /2.9	2.5 /4.7	0.01	2 /4.7	1 /2.9	1 /3.4	1/3.5	0.07	0.004
AB before thoracocentesis (%)	97[#]	80[#]	91	89.1	0.37	81	75	78	76.4	0.70	0.0008
AB treatment, median days	38.5	34	34.5	35	0.48	38	39.5	36.5	38	0.49	0.30
Pleural drainage delay > 2 days (%)	57	48	40	49	0.33	45	30	39	36	0.11	0.02
Fibrinolysis intrapleural (%)	27	33	28	30	0.71	40	31	31	34	0.45	0.43
ICU admittance (%)	4.8	2.0	18.9	5.9	< 0.001	5.3	1.9	25	7.9	< 0.0001	0.45
Mortality 30-day (%)	1.6	8.0	18.9	7.9	0.025	7.0	7.5	12.2	8.8	0.55	0.76
Mortality 90-day (%)	3.2	9.9	21.6	10.3	0.03	12.3	10.4	22.4	14.4	0.12	0.21
Surgery referral (%)	8.1	14.9	10.8	14.3	0.41	15.8	7.5	20.4	14.8	0.06	0.88
LOS, median (days)	15.5	15	19.5	16	0.25	19	18	19	18	0.49	0.22

AB antibiotics, *ICU* intensive care unit, *LOS* length of hospital stay
[*]comparing three treatment regimens. [§]comparing all etiology-negatives and etiology-positives

Table 2 Clinical factors, predisposing risk factors, severity factors, treatment factors, and outcome in the whole cohort[a] of patients with pleural infection according to initial antibiotic regimen

	PENI	CEFU	Broad	All[a]	[*]*p*-value
n=, (%)	125 (29)	215 (50)	89 (21)	429	
Age (years)	61.4	63.9	60.7	62.6	0.12
Pneumonic (%)	90.4	89.8	88.8	89.7	0.12
Nosocomial (%)	8.8[#]	16.2[#]	15.7	14	0.09
Predisposing risk factors (%)	53.6[#]	70.7[#]	68.6	65.6	0.01
Antibiotics before hospital admittance (%)	40.8	45.6	42.7	43	0.62
Severely ill (%)	8.8	5.1	31.5	11.6	< 0.0001
Thoracocentesis delay, median /mean (days)	3 / 5.5	1 / 3.1	1 / 3.9	1 / 4.0	0.0003
Antibiotics before thoracocentesi (%)	87.2[#]	74.9[#]	77	77.6	0.24
Antibiotic treatment, median (days)	38.5	35	35.5	35	0.79
Pleural drainage delay > 2 days (%)	38.4	29.8	29.2	31.6	0.22
Fibrinolysis intrapleural (%)	32	30.7	28.1	30.2	0.96
ICU admittance (%)	4.8	1.9	21.3	6.6	< 0.0001
Mortality 30-day (%)	4.8	7.9	14.6	8.7	0.06
Mortality 90-day (%)	8	10.7	22.5	13	0.006
Surgery referral (%)	11.2	10.7	14.6	11.7	0.75
LOS, median	16	16	19	17	0.15

[a] incl 13 patients with no successful thoracocentesis [*] comparing three treatment regimens. [#] $= p < 0.05$ for PENI vs CEFU

the proportion treated with antibiotics before hospital admission were comparable (all $p > 0.21$) (Table 1).

For the whole cohort, patients with broad-spectrum initial treatment regimens were more often severely ill (31.5% vs 6.2%) and more frequently admitted to the ICU (21.3% vs 2.9%) than patients treated with the nationally recommended initial regimens PENI or CEFU, all $p < 0.0001$ (Table 2). This was also demonstrated separately in each patient sub-category of microbiology negative or known etiology, all $p < 0.001$ (Table 1).

Therapy

The nationally recommended initial antibiotic regimens PENI (29%) or CEFU (50%) dominated over broad spectrum therapy (21%), and the distribution of these three regimens were similar in patients with known and microbiology negative etiology, (Tables 1 and 2). Patients with microbiology negative and known etiology had a comparable median duration of antibiotic therapy (35 vs 38 days, $p = 0.30$), proportion of intrapleural fibrinolytic treatment (30% vs 34%, $p = 0.43$), and a similar proportion of surgical referral (14.3% vs 14.8%, $p = 0.88$) (Table 1). Patients with microbiology negative etiology had a longer delay until thoracocentesis (median 2.5 days vs 1 day, $p <$ 0.01) and more often a delay in drainage > 2 days (49% vs 36%, $p = 0.02$).

Outcome

The length of hospital stay (LOS), 30-day mortality, 90-day mortality, need for surgical referral, or ICU-admittance did not differ between patients with microbiology negative and known etiology (all $p > 0.20$) (Table 1).

In the univariate analyses, 30-day and 90-day mortality did not differ significantly between the six microbiological sub-groups of known etiology (7.9% vs 6.3% vs 0% vs 12.5% vs 12.5% vs 8.3% $p = 0.85$; 9.9% vs 18.8% vs 12.5% vs 14.6% vs 25% vs 19.4% $p = 0.65$). When including microbiologic sub-groups in a logistic regression model (203 cases with known etiology) with age, predisposing risk factor status, nosocomial status, pleural drain delay > 2 days, and intra-pleural fibrinolysis, the microbiologic sub-group parameter was not independently correlated to 30-day or 90-day mortality ($p = 0.63$ and, $p = 0.90$, respectively).

Comparing patients treated with the two recommended initial therapy regimens (PENI group vs CEFU group), there were no significant differences in LOS, 30-day mortality, 90-day mortality, surgical referral, or ICU admittance, neither in the whole cohort or separately in patients with microbiology negative or known etiology (all $p > 0.11$) (Tables 1 and 2).

Patients treated with a broad-spectrum initial regimen trended to have a higher 30-day (14.6% vs 6.8%, $p =$ 0.06), and had a higher 90-day mortality (22.5% vs 9.7%, $p < 0.01$) compared to patients receiving PENI or CEFU, in the whole cohort (Table 2) and separately in the group with microbiology negative etiology, with a similar trend not reaching statistical significance in the group with known etiology (Table 1).

In univariate analyses, 30-day and 90-day mortality in the whole cohort (the actual direction and size of odds-ratios (OR) and the 95% confidence intervals (CI) are presented in Table 3) correlated to mean age (71 vs 61.3 years and 72 vs 61.7 years, respectively; both $p <$ 0.001), pre-disposing risk factors (OR = 4.4 [1.5–12.7] and 5.7 [2.2–14.5], both $p < 0.003$), intra-pleural fibrinolysis (OR = 0.17 [0.05–0.58] and 0.35 [0.16–0.72], both $p < 0.006$). In addition, the 90-day mortality correlated to nosocomial infection (OR = 2.3 [1.16–4.5], $p = 0.01$), pleural drainage delay > 2 days (OR = 0.40 [0.20–0.83], $p < 0.02$), but did not reach significantly correlation to referral for surgery (OR = 2.0 [0.97–4.2], $p = 0.055$).

The multivariate outcome analyses included age, predisposing risk factors, nosocomial infection, pleural drainage delay > 2 days, intra-pleural fibrinolysis, and referral to surgery in the model (direction and size of ORs and CIs are presented in Table 3). The 30-day mortality correlated independently to age (OR = 1.06 [1.03–1.10], $p < 0.0001$), intra-pleural fibrinolysis (OR = 0.19 [0.04–0.54], $p = 0.007$), predisposing risk factors (OR = 3.3 [1.3–11.9], $p = 0.03$), and pleural drainage delay (OR = 0.33 [0.16–0.92], $p = 0.04$). The 90-day mortality correlated independently to age (OR = 1.06 [1.04–1.09], $p <$ 0.0001), predisposing risk factors (OR = 4.2 [1.7–12.6], $p =$ 0.004), referral to surgery (OR = 3.1 [1.2–7.3], p = 0.01) with ORs > 1, and pleural drainage delay (OR = 0.33 [0.15–0.68], $p = 0.005$), intra-pleural fibrinolysis (OR = 0.35 [0.14–0.77], $p = 0.01$) with OR < 1. (Table 3).

Discussion

In this study, there were 200 or more patients with pleural infection in each of the two etiology groups, and the bacterial findings were similar to recent European studies [1].

The more severe illness and poorer outcome in the group of patients initially treated with broad-spectrum antibiotics most probably reflects clinical decisions based on the severity of the condition at admission to hospital. But because the rate of fibrinolysis or the rate of referral to surgery were not significantly different in this broad-spectrum group, the detrimental outcome may rather be due to a systemic sepsis effect of the disease.

By definition, change in antibiotic treatment within a few days according to results of susceptibility testing is not an option in cases with microbiology negative etiology and this may theoretically affect outcome. In our study, patients with microbiology negative etiology were more often treated with antibiotics before thoracocentesis, and the effect of antibiotics before microbiological

Table 3 Outcome analyses

	90-day mortality				30-day mortality			
	Uni-variate		Multi-variate		Uni-variate		Multi-variate	
	OR	95% CI	OR	95% CI	OR	95% CI	OR	95% CI
Age	–	–	1.06	1.04–1.09	–	–	1.06	1.03–1.10
Intrapleural fibrinolysis	0.35	0.16–0.72	0.35	0.14–0.77	0.17	0.05–0.58	0.19	0.04–0.54
Nosocomial infection	2.3	1.16–4.5			0.94	0.35–2.5		
Pleural drainage delay > 2 days	0.40	0.20–0.83	0.33	0.15–0.68	0.52	0.23–1.2	0.33	0.16–0.92
Surgery referral	2.0	0.97–4.2	3.1	1.2–7.3	0.64	0.19–2.2		
Predisposing Risk factors	5.7	2.2–14.5	4.2	1.7–12.6	4.4	1.5–12.7	3.3	1.3–11.9

The correlation of 90-day and 30-day mortality to hypothesized important categorical factors among 437 patients with pleural infection, in uni-variate and multivariate analyses

sampling may account for this fact. In clinical practice, the physician's motivation for swift pleural drainage may also depend on the presumed effusion volume and of disease severity in the individual patient; apart from the possible delay caused by lack in recognition of the condition. The slightly younger age, lower rate of predisposing risk factors (underlying diseases), and the trend towards fewer nosocomial infections in patients with microbiology negative etiology could bias prognosis towards a better outcome. On the other hand, the delay in initiating pleural drainage theoretically could result in a poorer outcome. Even though all other medical and surgical treatment measures and severity measures in this study were similar between patients with known and microbiology negative etiology, we were pleased to find that all outcome measures were comparable in the two groups. Thus, we could not confirm a hypothesized difference in outcome according to whether etiology was known or microbiologically negative.

In the literature, not many large studies (with more than 150 patients) have been published regarding pleural infection in adults, and, to our knowledge, none focused on the correlation between knowledge of etiology and clinical outcome. Compared to a large randomized controlled British study (MIST-1) [8] of intra-pleural streptokinase treatment in 430 patients with pleural infection, the patients in our cohort were of similar age (62.5 vs 60.5 years) and had similar outcomes with regard to 3 month's mortality (13% vs 15%), referral rate for surgery (11.7% vs 15%), and LOS (17 day vs 12.5 days). In the MIST-1 trial, disease severity or outcome was not reported according to microbiology negative or known etiology, and a direct comparison to our cohort is therefore not possible [8]. The randomized MIST-2 trial cohort with 193 included patients reported a similar age (59 vs 62.5 years) and referral rate for surgery (16% vs 11.7%), but a lower 3 month's mortality (8% vs 13%) and a similar length of hospital stay (20 vs 17 days) [6]. In the MIST-2 trial, outcomes were reported according to the four intra-pleural treatment randomization arms and were not categorized or reported according to knowledge of etiology [6]. A Danish study of 158 patients from a 9 year period just prior to our study period reported only cases of verified etiology. Compared to the present study, patients had similar age (63 years vs 62.5), a higher mortality (27% vs 13%), a longer hospital stay (29 days vs 17 days), a higher ICU-admittance rate (17% vs 6.6%) and more referrals to surgery (34% vs 11.7%) [4]. Further publications with large cohorts of patients with pleural empyema were not found for possible comparison with our study regarding the main question of disease severity or outcome according to knowledge of etiology.

The outcome analyses in our study demonstrated independent correlations between mortality and high age, referral to surgery, predisposing risk factors (OR > 1), and delayed pleural drainage more than 2 days, and intra-pleural fibrinolysis (OR < 1). Because the treatment factors were not randomized in this retrospective study, the causal relations will be rather hypothetical, despite controlling for factors included in the multivariate analysis. One can expect, that the attending physicians have judged the need for and the possibility of some interventions (f.ex. intentional or unintentional delay in drainage, referral for surgery, or intra-pleural fibrinolysis) differently according to disease acuteness, disease severity, the frailness of the patient, and the sufficient or the insufficient improvement in the individual patient. Also, lack of timely recognition of the condition may be a factor in some cases.

Regarding a possible improvement in outcome using initial treatment with early thoracoscopic debridement, a few small studies have demonstrated promising results of reduced length of hospital stay compared to initial treatment with pleural drainage [9, 10]. Larger and better powered randomized trials are needed in order to clarify the potential role of early pleural debridement in the adult population. However, early thoracoscopic debridement was not a therapeutic option in our hospitals.

In analogy with PSI, CURB-65, SOFA and other prognostic scores in pneumonia, the RAPID-score (**r**enal failure, **a**ge, non-**p**urulence, (hospital acquired) **i**nfection source, **d**ietary factors (=low albumin)) was recently developed as a prognostic score in patients with pleural infection and includes 5 non-interventional factors [11]. The renal parameter used (blood urea nitrogen) was not routinely assessed at admission to our hospitals, and thus, the RAPID-score could not be evaluated in our cohort. In our study-cohort, we did find association of mortality to the available RAPID parameters age and nosocomial infection, but we did not separate out renal insufficiency or malnutrition as individual factors (from the predisposing factors) in our multi-variate analyses. Recently, the RAPID-score was validated in a not very typical study-cohort of all ages with a large number of *Staphylococcus aureus* infections (40%) and nosocomial infections (41%) among 187 culture-positive patients, assessing stratified mortality risk at 3 months, but also at 1 year, 3 year and 5 year [12]. The stratification power was more pronounced at 3 months and in the sub-group of patients treated with invasive surgery [12].

The main strengths of our study are the sample size and the completeness of the cohort using several strategies for patient inclusion. Although we used the databases of clinical microbiology and the national clinical diagnosis register, and attempted prospective inclusion, we cannot rule out the possibility of missing cases due to mislabeling in the national clinical diagnosis register in culture-negative cases of pleural infection. Our study has inborn limitations (including some missing data) due to the predominantly retrospective mode of data collection.

As the occurrence of the time-dependent covariates (f.ex. delayed drainage > 2 days, referral to surgery) are possible always in the surviving sub-group but may only be possible in some patients in the dying group (if the intended intervention is not delayed before the outcome of death), the immortal time bias is a possible limitation in the logistic regression mortality analysis. Among the 56 dying patients in our cohort with four patients dying within 2 days, two were drained and the two others were left to palliative care without drainage. The referral to surgery factor was not documented as an unfulfilled intention in the medical charts in any of the dying patients, but missing documentation cannot be ruled out. Thus, we suggest that the covariate delayed drainage > 2 days did not suffer from immortal time bias of clinical importance. A potential shortcoming of the analysis in our database is that the possible immortal time bias could not be estimated for the covariate referral to surgery, and therefore effect estimates of referral to surgery should be interpreted with caution.

Conclusion

This study adds outcome results, clinical data and treatment information regarding the serious and often complicated condition of pleural infection from a large patient cohort. Comparing patients with microbiology negative and known bacterial etiology, no differences were found in observed mortalities, in underlying disease severity, initial antibiotic treatment type, total treatment duration, or in the rate of surgical referral. Thus, lack of data on etiology and antibiotic susceptibility in many of the patients did not signal a change in outcome in a geographical area with expectedly well-functioning health-care facilities and limited problems of antibiotic resistance, though the limitations of a retrospective design precludes from conclusions on causation.

Abbreviations

AB: Antibiotic; CDC: Center for Disease Control and Prevention; CEFU: Cefuroxime +/− metronidazole; COPD: Chronic obstructive pulmonary disease; DNA: Deoxyribonucleic acid; ICD: International Classification of Diseases; ICU: Intensive care unit; LOS: Length of hospital stay; OR: Odds ratio; PCR: Polymerase chain reaction; PENI: Penicillin/aminopenicillin +/− metronidazole; t-PA: Tissue plasminogen activator

Acknowledgements

Danish pleura empyema group (DPEG) members:
Christian N Meyer, ZUH-Roskilde, DK
Thomas Ringbæk, Hvidovre Hospital, DK
Karin Armbruster, Gentofte Hospital, DK
Torben Evald, Allergi-klinikken, København, DK
Asbjørn Høegholm, Næstved Hospital, DK
Alan Victor, Bispebjerg Hospital, DK
Lars C Laursen, Herlev Hospital, DK
Thyge L Nielsen, Hillerød Hospital, DK
Mogens Kappel, Gentofte Hospital, DK
Henriette Enevoldsen, Allergi- og Lungeklinikken Charlottenlund, DK
Erik Munch, Holbæk Sygehus, DK
Signe Rosenlund, Køge Sygehus, DK
Jannie Broberg, Psykiatrisk Center Amager, DK
Alice Friis-Møller, Hvidovre Hospital, DK
Michael Kemp, Odense University Hospital, DK
Ram BC Dessau, Slagelse Hospital, DK
Michael Pedersen, Herlev Hospital, DK
Britta Bruun, Hillerød Hospital, DK
Trine R Thomsen, Danish Technological Institute/Aalborg University, DK
Per H Nielsen, Aalborg University, DK
Oli J Dalsgard, Hvidovre hospital, DK; Bo Broberg, Herlev Hospital, DK; Uffe Bødtger, Næstved hospital, DK; Jette Bangsborg, Herlev Hospital, DK; Ina Sleimann Petersen, Slagelse hospital, DK, are all thanked for participation in the retrieval of patient- or microbiologic data.

Funding

Regions Sjællands Sundhedsvidenskabelige Forskningsfond supported the DNA-technology assays in relation to the DPEG-project. No further funding source was used for this study.

Authors' contributions

Conception and design by CNM and the members of DPEG; Analysis and interpretation by CNM, KA, RBD, MK, TRT. Drafting the manuscript for important intellectual content: CNM, KA, MK, TRT, RBD. All authors read and approved the final manuscript.

Consent for publication
No individual patient data is presented in this study. Thus consent to publication is not applicable.

Competing interests
The authors declare that they have no competing interests.

Author details
[1]Department of Internal Medicine, Zealand University Hospital Roskilde, Sygehusvej 10, 4000 Roskilde, Denmark. [2]Department of Clinical Medicine, University of Copenhagen, Copenhagen, Denmark. [3]Department of Respiratory Medicine, Copenhagen University Hospital Gentofte, Gentofte, Denmark. [4]Department of Clinical Microbiology, Odense University Hospital, University of Southern Denmark, Odense, Denmark. [5]Danish Technological Institute, Life Science, Århus and Section of Biotechnology, Aalborg University, Aalborg, Denmark. [6]Department of Clinical Microbiology, Slagelse Hospital, Slagelse, Denmark.

References
1. Davies HE, Davies RJ, Davies CW. Management of pleural infection in adults: British Thoracic Society pleural disease guideline 2010. Thorax. 2010; 65(Suppl 2):ii41–53.
2. Maskell NA, Batt S, Hedley EL, Davies CW, Gillespie SH, Davies RJ. The bacteriology of pleural infection by genetic and standard methods and its mortality significance. Am J Respir Crit Care Med. 2006;174:817–23.
3. Meyer CN, Rosenlund S, Nielsen J, Friis-Moller A. Bacteriological aetiology and antimicrobial treatment of pleural empyema. Scand J Infect Dis. 2011; 43:165–9.
4. Nielsen J, Meyer CN, Rosenlund S. Outcome and clinical characteristics in pleural empyema: a retrospective study. Scand J Infect Dis. 2011;43:430–5.
5. Hooper CE, Edey AJ, Wallis A, Clive AO, Morley A, White P, et al. Pleural irrigation trial (PIT): a randomised controlled trial of pleural irrigation with normal saline versus standard care in patients with pleural infection. Eur Respir J. 2015;46:456–63.
6. Rahman NM, Maskell NA, West A, Teoh R, Arnold A, Mackinlay C, et al. Intrapleural use of tissue plasminogen activator and DNase in pleural infection. N Engl J Med. 2011;365:518–26.
7. Garner JS, Jarvis WR, Emori TG, Horan TC, Hughes JM. CDC definitions for nosocomial infections, 1988. Am J Infect Control. 1988;16:128–40.
8. Maskell NA, Davies CW, Nunn AJ, Hedley EL, Gleeson FV, Miller R, et al. U.K. controlled trial of intrapleural streptokinase for pleural infection. N Engl J Med. 2005;352:865–74.
9. Bilgin M, Akcali Y, Oguzkaya F. Benefits of early aggressive management of empyema thoracis. ANZ J Surg. 2006;76:120–2.
10. Wait MA, Sharma S, Hohn J, Dal NA. A randomized trial of empyema therapy. Chest. 1997;111:1548–51.
11. Rahman NM, Kahan BC, Miller RF, Gleeson FV, Nunn AJ, Maskell NA. A clinical score (RAPID) to identify those at risk for poor outcome at presentation in patients with pleural infection. Chest. 2014;145:848–55.
12. White HD, Henry C, Stock EM, Arroliga AC, Ghamande S. Predicting long-term outcomes in pleural infections. RAPID score for risk stratification. Ann Am Thorac Soc. 2015;12:1310–6.

11

Epidemiology of pulmonary disease due to nontuberculous mycobacteria in Southern China, 2013–2016

Yaoju Tan[1†], Biyi Su[1†], Wei Shu[2], Xingshan Cai[1], Shaojia Kuang[1], Haobin Kuang[1], Jianxiong Liu[1*] and Yu Pang[2*]

Abstract

Background: Pulmonary nontuberculous mycobacteria (NTM) disease is of increasing public health concern in China. Information is limited regarding risk factors associated with this disease in China. The objective of this study was to describe the epidemiology of pulmonary disease due to NTM in Southern China.

Methods: We retrospectively reviewed the medical records of pulmonary NTM patients registered in the Guangzhou Chest Hospital with positive mycobacterial cultures during 2013–2016. We described sex, age, residence, treatment history, laboratory examination results and comorbidities of pulmonary NTM patients.

Results: Among the 607 NTM cases, the most prevalent species were *Mycobacterium avium* complex (44.5%), *Mycobacterium abscessus* complex (40.5%), *Mycobacterium kansasii* (10.0%) and *Mycobacterium fortuitum* (2.8%). The male:female ratio was significantly lower among patients infected with rapidly growing mycobacteria (RGM) than among those with slowly growing mycobacteria (SGM). The risk of developing SGM disease significantly increased with advancing age. In addition, pulmonary RGM diseases were more common in migrant population than resident population. Notably, patients with pulmonary RGM diseases were significantly more likely to have bronchiectasis underlying noted than those with SGM diseases. No significant difference was observed in in vitro drug susceptibility among NTM species.

Conclusion: Our data illustrate that the *M. avium* complex is the most predominant causative agent of pulmonary NTM disease in Southern China. Female, migrant population, the presence of bronchiectasis are independent risk factors for pulmonary diseases due to RGM. In addition, the prevalence of SGM increases significantly with advancing age.

Keywords: Nontuberculous mycobacteria, Epidemiology, Slowly growing mycobacteria, Rapidly growing mycobacteria, Comorbidity

Background

Nontuberculous mycobacteria (NTM) are a heterogeneous group of species other than the *Mycobacterium tuberculosis* complex and *Mycobacterium leprae* [1]. As the etiologic agents, NTM have been found in a variety of environmental sources, such as soil, water and aerosols [2]. Despite being less pathogenic than *M. tuberculosis*, these environmental bacteria are associated with a wide array of clinical diseases, especially in HIV-infected patients or those with immunodeficiencies [3]. Notably, NTM disease incidence has increased significantly during the past decade [3], while this emerging disease is given a lower public health priority as compared with tuberculosis due to lack of definitive evidence of person-to-person transmission of NTM [4]. The most available data on NTM infections come from sentinel laboratory–based surveillance studies [5, 6], which makes it difficult to distinguish between colonizers and causative pathogens among these positive mycobacteria

* Correspondence: Ljxer64@qq.com; pangyupound@163.com
†Yaoju Tan and Biyi Su contributed equally to this work.
[1]Department of Clinical Laboratory, Guangzhou Chest Hospital, State Key Laboratory of Respiratory Disease, No. 62, Hengzhigang Road, Yuexiu District, Guangzhou, Guangdong Province 510095, People's Republic of China
[2]National Clinical Laboratory on Tuberculosis, Beijing Key laboratory on Drug-resistant Tuberculosis Research,, Beijing Chest Hospital, Beijing Tuberculosis and Thoracic Tumor Institute, No. 9, Beiguan Street, Tongzhou District, Beijing 101149, People's Republic of China

cultures [7]; consequently, the exact distribution of mycobacteria species among patients is not well known, especially in high-TB-burden settings.

Although China has achieved impressive reductions in TB prevalence and mortality over the past 20 years [8], NTM infections have become a serious issue, accounting for about one quarter of mycobacterial patient isolates according to the national population-based data [9], triggering public health concerns. More importantly, NTM prevalence varies greatly across China, and Southern China has a significantly higher proportion of NTM infection [1]. In addition, national epidemiological data have revealed that NTM species distribution differs significantly by region, reflecting the diversity of species distribution in the local environment [3]. Given that NTM species differ significantly in pathogenicity and drug susceptibility profiles, understanding this regional diversity is a major priority for optimizing appropriate treatment regimen. Unfortunately, previous reports regarding this issue are lacking, and few laboratory data were mainly on the basis of NTM isolates from microbiology laboratory, which made it difficult to differentiate NTM diseases from host respiratory colonization [1, 10]. Furthermore, information is limited regarding risk factors associated with this disease, thereby hampering attempts to implement effective infection control programmes. The objective of this study was to describe the prevalence of NTM species among pulmonary NTM patients in regional tuberculosis clinical centre in Southern China between 2013 and 2016. We also aimed to identify demographic and clinical factors associated with pulmonary NTM diseases between slowly growing mycobacteria (SGM) and rapidly growing mycobacteria (RGM).

Methods

Study design and population

This study was conducted at the Guangzhou Chest Hospital, an 800-bed regional tuberculosis clinical centre in Southern China. We retrospectively reviewed the medical records of pulmonary NTM patients registered in the hospital with positive mycobacterial cultures during 2013–2016. Factors that were assessed in this study included demographic and clinical characteristics, such as sex, age, residence, treatment history, laboratory examination results and comorbidities. The definition of NTM lung disease met the criteria established by the American Thoracic Society (ATS) in 2007 [11], including clinical symptoms and abnormal chest radiograph suggestive of pulmonary TB or NTM diseases; isolation of the same NTM species from more than two sputum specimens collected at different time points; and exclusion of other differential diagnoses. In addition, the residents were defined as individuals with the local household registration of Guangzhou, while the migrants were defined as individuals without local household registration of Guangzhou.

Laboratory examination

Media supplied with paranitrobenzoic acid was used for differential identification of *Mycobacterium tuberculosis* (MTB) complex and NTM. The NTM strains identified by conventional biochemical method were subcultured on the Löwenstein-Jensen (L-J) medium [1]. Colonies were scraped from the surface of L-J medium, and transferred to 500 µL Tris-EDTA (TE) buffer. The was heated at 95 °C for 30 min in a water bath, and the supernatant was used as DNA template for PCR amplification. The commercial Biochip test was performed for species identification of mycobacterium according to the manufacturer's instructions [12]. In addition, the isolates identified as *Mycobacterium chelonae-Mycobacterium abscessus* group by Biochip were further divided into subspecies with the sequencing of multiple genes, including 16S rRNA, *hsp65*, *rpoB*, and 16S–23S rRNA internal transcribed spacer (ITS) sequence as previously reported [9]. The PCR products were sent to Ruibo Company (Beijing, China) for DNA sequencing service. Nucleotide sequences were aligned with the homologous sequences of the reference mycobacteria strains by using multiple sequence alignments via the BLAST web pages (http://www.ncbi.nlm.nih.gov/BLAST).

Drug susceptibility testing

The in vitro drug susceptibility of *M. abscessus* complex was determined with a broth microdilution method based on the guidelines from the Clinical and Laboratory Standards Institute (CLSI) [13]. Eight antimicrobial agents were enrolled in this study, including amikacin, clarithromycin, linezolid, tobramycin, cefoxitin, ciprofloxacin, doxycycline and imipenem. The breakpoint values to distinguish susceptibility and resistance for drugs were followed as recommendation from CLSI [13]. For *M. avium* and *M. intracellulare* isolates, three agents were selected for MIC assessment, including clarithromycin, moxifloxacin and linezolid. The in vitro drug susceptibility for these drugs were evaluated with a broth microdilution method, and their breakpoint values were followed the recommendation from CLSI [13].

Statistical analysis

All collected data were entered using Epi Data version 3.1 (EpiData Association, Odense, Denmark). Each entry was cross checked independently to ensure the data quality. The predictor variables of age, sex, residence, previous history for tuberculosis, and comorbidity were tested for association with various NTM diseases using univariate and multivariate logistic analysis. The level of significance of univariate analysis was 0.05, and that for inclusion in the multivariate model was 0.15. Association between NTM diseases and predictor variables was calculated using adjusted odds ratio and 95% confidence interval. In addition, comparison of rate of drug resistance between different NTM species was evaluated by chi-square and Fisher's exact tests. Differences were considered to be statistically significant at $P < 0.05$. We conducted analyses by using SPSS version 20.0 (SPSS Inc., Chicago, USA).

Results

Proportion of different NTM species

A total of 607 pulmonary NTM patients were enrolled during January 1, 2013-December 31, 2017. Among the 607 NTM cases, the most prevalent species were *M. avium* complex (MAC, 270 isolates, 44.5%), *M. abscessus* complex (MABC, 246 isolates, 40.5%), *M. kansasii* (61 isolates, 10.0%) and *M. fortuitum* (17 isolates, 2.8%). These four groups accounted for 97.9% of all mycobacteria identified. Of 270 *M. avium* complex isolates, there were 171 *M. intracellulare* (63.3%, 171/270) and 99 *M. avium* (36.7%, 99/270) isolates, respectively. In addition, 58.9% (145/246) of *M. abscessus* complex isolates were *M. abscessus subspecies abscessus*, and the remining 41.1% (101/246) belonged to *M. abscessus subspecies massiliense* (Fig. 1).

Factors associated with SGM and RGM infections

Comparison in demographic and clinical characteristics of NTM patients between SGM and RGM is summarized in Table 1. The male:female ratio was significantly lower among patients infected with RGM than among those with SGM [adjusted odds ratio (aOR): 0.526, 95% confidence interval (95% CI): 0.429–0.862; $P = 0.005$]. In addition, the risk of developing RGM disease significantly decreased with advancing age. Compared with patients with SGM, the adjusted odds ratios were 0.488 (95% CI: 0.287–0.827) for 40–60 years group and 0.395 (95% CI: 0.235–0.666) for > 60 years group, respectively. We also found that the prevalence of infection caused by RGM and SGM differed significantly in resident and migrant population, and pulmonary RGM diseases were more common in migrant population than resident population (aOR: 1.551; 95% CI: 1.092–2.202; $P = 0.014$). Notably, patients with pulmonary RGM diseases were significantly more likely to have bronchiectasis underlying noted than those with SGM diseases (aOR: 1.521; 95% CI: 1.064–2.176; $P = 0.021$). In contrast, there were no other differences regarding TB history or comorbidities noted between SGM and RGM, respectively ($P > 0.05$).

In vitro drug susceptibility profiles of MAC and MABC

We further analysed the in vitro drug susceptibility profiles of *M. avium* complex and *M. abscessus* complex. As shown in Table 2, clarithromycin was the most highly active agent against *M. avium* complex, and the percentages of resistant strains were 4.2% (4/95) for *M. avium* and 3.8% (6/159) for *M. intracellulare*, respectively. Moxifloxacin and linezolid also showed potent activity against *M. avium* complex. There were 5 (5.3%) *M. avium* isolates and 8 (5.0%) *M. intracellulare* isolates resistant to moxifloxacin. For linezolid, the proportions of resistant isolates were 11.6% (11/95) for *M. avium* and 8.2% (13/159) for *M. intracellulare*, respectively. Of the antimicrobial agents tested, amikacin, clarithromycin, linezolid and tobramycin showed highly active against *M. abscessus* complex, and less than 5% of *M.*

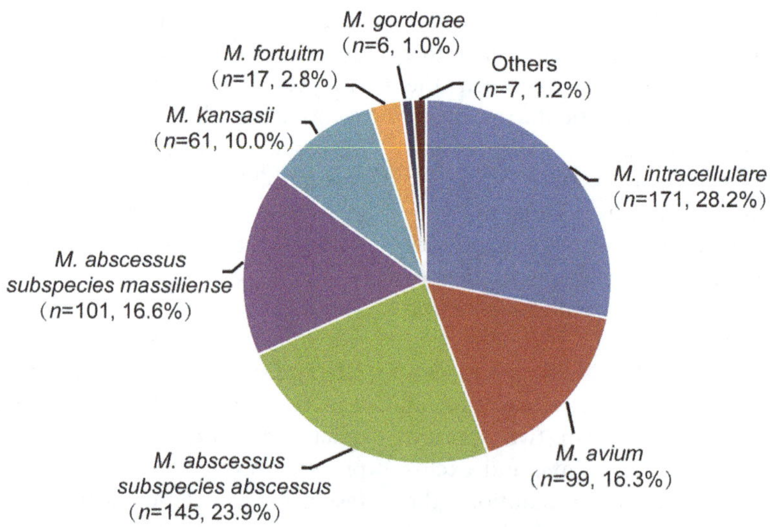

Fig. 1 Distribution of nontuberculous mycobacteria species isolated from pulmonary NTM patients in South China

Table 1 Comparison in demographic and clinical characteristics of NTM patients between slowly growing mycobacteria and rapidly growing mycobacteria at Guangzhou Chest Hospital, China, January 1, 2013 to December 31, 2017

Characteristics	No. of pulmonary NTM cases (%)		Univariate analysis		Multivariate analysis	
	SGM ($n = 344$)	RGM ($n = 263$)	OR (95% CI)	*P* value	OR (95% CI)	*P* value
Gender						
Female	170 (49.4)	171 (65.0)	0.526 (0.378–0.731)	< 0.001	0.608 (0.429–0.862)	0.005
Male	174 (50.6)	92 (35.0)	1.000	–	1.000	–
Age group (years)						
18–40	34 (9.9)	53 (20.2)	1.000	–	1.000	–
40–60	122 (35.5)	106 (40.3)	0.557 (0.337–0.922)	0.023	0.488 (0.287–0.827)	0.008
> 60	188 (54.7)	104 (39.5)	0.355 (0.217–0.581)	< 0.001	0.395 (0.235–0.666)	< 0.001
TB history						
No	149 (43.8)	96 (36.5)	1.000	–		
Yes	195 (57.4)	167 (63.5)	1.329 (0.953–1.852)	0.093		
Population						
Residence	168 (48.8)	89 (33.8)	1.000	–	1.000	–
Migration	176 (51.2)	174 (66.2)	1.855 (1.331–2.585)	< 0.001	1.551 (1.092–2.202)	0.014
Diabetes						
No	328 (95.3)	252 (95.8)	1.000	–		
Yes	16 (4.7)	11 (4.2)	0.895 (0.408–1.962)	0.895		
Bronchiectasis						
No	158 (45.9)	93 (35.4)	1.000	–	1.000	–
Yes	186 (54.1)	170 (64.6)	1.553 (1.116–2.16)	0.009	1.521 (1.064–2.176)	0.021
COPD						
No	326 (94.8)	256 (97.3)	1.000	–		
Yes	18 (5.2)	7 (2.7)	0.495 (0.204–1.204)	0.121		
Tumor						
No	321 (93.3)	251 (95.4)	1.000	–		
Yes	23 (6.7)	12 (4.6)	0.667 (0.326–1.367)	0.269		

SGM slowly growing mycobacteria, *RGM* rapidly growing mycobacteria, *COPD* chronic obstructive pulmonary disease, *OR* odds ratio, *95% CI* 95% confidence interval

avium and *M. intracellulare* were resistant to each drug, respectively. In addition, cefoxitin had moderate activity against *M. abscessus* complex, and the percentages of cefoxitin -resistance were observed in 33.8% (46/136) of *M. abscessus subspecies abscessus* and 25.3% (24/95) of *M. abscessus subspecies massiliense* isolates. Statistical analysis revealed that there were no significant differences in the drug resistant rate between *M. abscessus subspecies abscessus* and *M. abscessus subspecies massiliense* ($P > 0.05$) (Table 3).

Table 2 Comparison of in vitro drug susceptibility profiles between *M. intracellulare* and *M. avium* isolates

Antimicrobial agents	No. of resistant isolates (%)		*P* value
	M. avium ($n = 95$)	*M. intracellulare* ($n = 159$)	
Clarithromycin	4 (4.2)	6 (3.8)	1.000
Moxifloxacin	5 (5.3)	8 (5.0)	1.000
Linezolid	11 (11.6)	13 (8.2)	0.370

The breakpoints to establish susceptibility and resistance for clarithromycin, moxifloxacin and linezolid were followed as recommendation from Clinical and Laboratory Standards Institute (CLSI-M24-A2)

Discussion

Pulmonary NTM disease is of increasing public health concern worldwide [6]. This study firstly describes the demographic and clinical characteristics of patients with pulmonary NTM disease in Southern China. Our study has demonstrated that the most common NTM that causes pulmonary disease in Southern China is *M. avium* complex, accounting for 44.5% of pulmonary NTM disease burden in this study, which is consistent with its predominance in other parts of the world, including the United States (85%) [14], Denmark (81%)

Table 3 Comparison of in vitro drug susceptibility profiles between *M. abscessus subspecies abscessus* and *M. abscessus subspecies massiliense* isolates

Antimicrobial agents	No. of resistant isolates (%)		*P* value
	M. abscessus subspecies abscessus (*n* = 136)	*M. abscessus subspecies massiliense* (*n* = 95)	
Amikacin	3 (2.2)	2 (2.1)	1.000
Clarithromycin	6 (4.4)	3 (3.2)	0.740
Linezolid	6 (4.4)	2 (2.1)	0.476
Tobramycin	6 (4.4)	2 (2.1)	0.476
Cefoxitin	46 (33.8)	24 (25.3)	0.164
Ciprofloxacin	86 (63.2)	68 (71.6)	0.186
Doxycycline	127 (93.4)	94 (98.9)	0.050
Imipenem	134 (98.5)	95 (100.0)	1.000

The breakpoints to establish susceptibility and resistance for drugs were followed as recommendation from Clinical and Laboratory Standards Institute (CLSI-M24-A2)

[15] and South Korea (48%) [16]. The second most frequently identified NTM specie is *M. abscessus* complex. Despite occurring less frequently in Northern America and Europe [14, 15], this species was found to generally cause > 30% of pulmonary NTM infections in India [17], Taiwan [18] and South Korea [16]. The marked geographic variation in mycobacteria species could reflect the diversity of species composition of NTM in environmental niches [3]. Interestingly, all the regions with high isolation frequency of *M. abscessus* are in Asia; we thus speculate that Asian persons may also be more susceptible to *M. abscessus* infection. In line with our hypothesis, Adjemian and colleagues found that Asian persons have an increased risk for infection with *M. abscessus* than other ethnics [19]. Hence, the ethnic factors contributing to susceptibility to different NTM species may also play an important role in the diverse geographic NTM patterns across world regions.

Another interesting finding of this study is that the frequency of NTM species from pulmonary patients differs significantly from the observations from a recent laboratory-based study in Guangzhou [1]. First, *M. avium* complex exceeds *M. abscessus* complex as the predominant causative agent of pulmonary NTM disease, which reflects the inherent difference in NTM prevalence between pulmonary diseases and colonization. The species difference of pulmonary NTM colonization may partly determine the frequency and manifestations of pulmonary NTM disease [3]. However, the variation of pathogenicity among distinct NTM species could greatly contribute to the prevalence of diseases due to NTM species [20]. A population-based study of patients with respiratory NTM isolates from the Netherlands revealed that differences in clinical relevance exist among NTM species [20]. Similar results were noted in a systematic review in Eastern Asian that *M. avium* complex was clinically more relevant than *M. abscessus* complex among patients meeting the ATS diagnostic criteria [21]. Although experimental evidences are limited, there is no doubt that the relative greater pathogenicity of *M. avium* complex compared with *M. abscessus* complex would increase the risk from NTM colonization to active disease in respiratory tract.

Second, *M. gordonae* was the third frequently isolates species in South China on the basis of previous data, accounting for 22.5% of NTM isolates [1]. In contrast, only 1% of pulmonary NTM diseases was caused by *M. gordonae* in the present study. This finding confirms that this species is a rarely isolated weak pathogen, majorly contributing to patient colonization and culture contamination rather than patient disease [3].

Third, several rare geographically restricted NTM species identified by previous study was not associated with NTM diseases [1]. Although for these species the small number of isolates decrease the reliability of conclusions, the disappearance of previous laboratory isolation of these rare species among NTM patients may reflect NTM colonization due to their weak pathogenicity for human individuals. Therefore, the significant change in the prevalence of NTM species between pulmonary diseases and colonization indicates that the pathogenicity differs by species, thereby leading to the difference in clinical relevance of the various NTM species, which should be taken into consideration in formulating the diagnostic criteria for pulmonary NTM diseases.

Pulmonary NTM disease is not uncommon, particularly among elderly females [22]. Our results demonstrate that female is more likely to be associated with the acquisition of NTM diseases caused by RGM than SGM. In agree with our observation, an early study from the United States suggested that *M. avium* complex lung disease was more common among males than females

[23]. The gender difference in the NTM diseases may reflect differences in the immune responses during infection between RGM and SGM [24]. Generally, females exhibit greater cell-mediated immune responses to infection and vaccination than males [25], which is also important in host defense against mycobacteria. We therefore hypothesize that this instinct immunological difference may affect in SGM infections more than RGM infections.

Numerous studies have documented that pulmonary NTM infection more frequently affect elderly patients [6, 25]. In this study, we found that the prevalence of SGM increased significantly with advancing age. Furthermore, half of SGM diseases occurred in patients > 60 years of age. On one hand, the immunity in elderly persons is less able to produce an effective immune response after challenges with mycobacteria than the young [26]. This condition would result in greater incidence or reactivation of mycobacteria. On the other hand, the high incidence of co-morbidities presumed to affect the immune response in this population, such as diabetes, kidney failure, and immunosuppressive therapy, may favor the progression of pulmonary NTM infection. More studies are need to evaluate the relative contribution of each factor to the increased risk of pulmonary SGM diseases.

The association between bronchiectasis and NTM disease has been described by several reports [27–29]. We found that the presence of bronchiectasis appears to be more closely associated with RGM than SGM. It has been hypothesized that the impaired secretion clearance due to bronchiectasis enables NTM airway colonization and increases the risk of infection [29]. A recent report by Williams et al. compared the biofilm formation between RGM and SGM, demonstrating that *M. avium* complex is better equipped to grow in low-nutrient conditions than RGM by the development of more culturable biofilm [30]. Although the exact reason remains unknown, the reduced capability in the synthesis of biofilm of RGM allows these species prefer to inhabit in architectural-defected airway rather than normal airway, offering an explanation for the greater occurrence of bronchiectasis among pulmonary RGM cases.

This study is subject to several limitations. First, HIV infection has been regarded as an independent risk factor for NTM infections [31], while the HIV-positive patients were not included in this study because the HIV-positive patients with were transferred to another hospital receiving antiviral treatment. Given that *M. avium* infections are frequently encountered in AIDS patients [31], we may underestimate the prevalence of *M. avium* isolates in Southern China. Second, the clinical outcomes of pulmonary NTM patients were not collected in this study, because patients are not under follow-up for NTM diseases in China. As a consequence, we only analysed in vitro antibiotic susceptibility of NTM isolates rather than its correlation with treatment results. Therefore, further study is urgently needed to investigate the correlation between in vitro drug susceptibility and clinical outcomes among NTM patients. Third, another important explanation for poor response to macrolide-based chemotherapy for *M. abscessus* infections is the inducible macrolide resistance phenotype. Unfortunately, the routine detection of drug susceptibility for RGM only incubates 96-well microtiter plates for 3 days, whereas the detection of inducible resistance requires an extended incubation of plates with reading after 14 days of incubation. As a consequence, the resistance to clarithromycin for *M. abscessus* would be underestimated. Fourth, although cavitary is another major category regarding NTM pulmonary diseases, the radiological characteristics were not collected in this study due to the limited information in the medical records of patients. Nevertheless, this study provides important hints to help clinicians interpret laboratory results and recognize the risk factors associated with various NTM species.

Conclusion

In conclusion, our data illustrate that the *M. avium* complex is the most predominate causative agent of pulmonary NTM disease in Southern China. Female, migrant population, the presence of bronchiectasis are independent risk factors for pulmonary diseases due to RGM. In addition, the prevalence of SGM increases significantly with advancing age. In view of the growing public health concern, further studies will be carried out to determine the association between in vitro susceptibility and treatment outcome among these NTM patients, which is essential to help clinicians select effective regimens for the treatment of NTM infections.

Acknowledgments

We thank all staffs from Guangzhou Chest Hospital for their help in carrying out this study.

Funding

This research was supported by the Guangzhou Collaborative Innovation Major Project on Health and Medicine (201604020019), National Key Project (2015ZX10003003) and the Beijing Municipal Administration of Hospitals' Youth Programme (QML20171601).

Authors' contributions

YT, BS, WS, XC, SK, HK, JL, and YP: Substantial contributions to conception and design of, or acquisition of data or analysis and interpretation of data. YT, BS, JL, and YP: Drafting the article or revising it critically for important intellectual content. All authors read and approved the final manuscript.

Consent for publication

Not applicable.

Competing interests

The authors declare that they have no competing interests.

References

1. Pang Y, Tan Y, Chen J, Li Y, Zheng H, Song Y, Zhao Y. Diversity of nontuberculous mycobacteria in eastern and southern China: a cross-sectional study. Eur Respir J. 2017;49(3):1601429.
2. Falkinham JO III. Epidemiology of infection by nontuberculous mycobacteria. Clin Microbiol Rev. 1996;9(2):177–215.
3. Hoefsloot W, van Ingen J, Andrejak C, Angeby K, Bauriaud R, Bemer P, Beylis N, Boeree MJ, Cacho J, Chihota V, et al. The geographic diversity of nontuberculous mycobacteria isolated from pulmonary samples: an NTM-NET collaborative study. Eur Respir J. 2013;42(6):1604–13.
4. Bryant JM, Grogono DM, Greaves D, Foweraker J, Roddick I, Inns T, Reacher M, Haworth CS, Curran MD, Harris SR, et al. Whole-genome sequencing to identify transmission of Mycobacterium abscessus between patients with cystic fibrosis: a retrospective cohort study. Lancet. 2013;381(9877):1551–60.
5. Grubek-Jaworska H, Walkiewicz R, Safianowska A, Nowacka-Mazurek M, Krenke R, Przybylowski T, Chazan R. Nontuberculous mycobacterial infections among patients suspected of pulmonary tuberculosis. Eur J Clin Microbiol Infect Dis. 2009;28(7):739–44.
6. McShane PJ, Glassroth J. Pulmonary disease due to nontuberculous mycobacteria: current state and new insights. Chest. 2015;148(6):1517–27.
7. Hernandez-Garduno E, Elwood RK. Increasing incidence of nontuberculous mycobacteria, Taiwan, 2000-2008. Emerg Infect Dis. 2010;16(6):1047 author reply 1047-1048.
8. Wang L, Zhang H, Ruan Y, Chin DP, Xia Y, Cheng S, Chen M, Zhao Y, Jiang S, Du X, et al. Tuberculosis prevalence in China, 1990-2010; a longitudinal analysis of national survey data. Lancet. 2014;383(9934):2057–64.
9. Zhang Z, Pang Y, Wang Y, Cohen C, Zhao Y, Liu C. Differences in risk factors and drug susceptibility between Mycobacterium avium and Mycobacterium intracellulare lung diseases in China. Int J Antimicrob Agents. 2015;45(5):491–5.
10. Shao Y, Chen C, Song H, Li G, Liu Q, Li Y, Zhu L, Martinez L, Lu W. the epidemiology and geographic distribution of nontuberculous mycobacteria clinical isolates from sputum samples in the eastern region of China. PLoS Negl Trop Dis. 2015;9(3):e0003623.
11. Griffith DE, Aksamit T, Brown-Elliott BA, Catanzaro A, Daley C, Gordin F, Holland SM, Horsburgh R, Huitt G, Iademarco MF, et al. An official ATS/IDSA statement: diagnosis, treatment, and prevention of nontuberculous mycobacterial diseases. Am J Respir Crit Care Med. 2007;175(4):367–416.
12. Zhu L, Jiang G, Wang S, Wang C, Li Q, Yu H, Zhou Y, Zhao B, Huang H, Xing W, et al. Biochip system for rapid and accurate identification of mycobacterial species from isolates and sputum. J Clin Microbiol. 2010; 48(10):3654–60.
13. Clinical and Laboratory Standards Institute. Susceptibility testing of mycobacteria, nocardia, and other aerobic actinomycetes; approved standard, 2nd ed; CLSI document M24-A2. Clinical and Laboratory Standards Institute, Wayne. (2011).
14. Cassidy PM, Hedberg K, Saulson A, McNelly E, Winthrop KL. Nontuberculous mycobacterial disease prevalence and risk factors: a changing epidemiology. Clin Infect Dis. 2009;49(12):e124–9.
15. Andrejak C, Thomsen VO, Johansen IS, Riis A, Benfield TL, Duhaut P, Sorensen HT, Lescure FX, Thomsen RW. Nontuberculous pulmonary mycobacteriosis in Denmark: incidence and prognostic factors. Am J Respir Crit Care Med. 2010;181(5):514–21.
16. Koh WJ, Kwon OJ, Jeon K, Kim TS, Lee KS, Park YK, Bai GH. Clinical significance of nontuberculous mycobacteria isolated from respiratory specimens in Korea. Chest. 2006;129(2):341–8.
17. Prevots DR, Marras TK. Epidemiology of human pulmonary infection with nontuberculous mycobacteria: a review. Clin Chest Med. 2015;36(1):13–34.
18. Chien JY, Lai CC, Sheng WH, Yu CJ, Hsueh PR. Pulmonary infection and colonization with nontuberculous mycobacteria, Taiwan, 2000-2012. Emerg Infect Dis. 2014;20(8):1382–5.
19. Adjemian J, Frankland TB, Daida YG, Honda JR, Olivier KN, Zelazny A, Honda S, Prevots DR. Epidemiology of nontuberculous mycobacterial lung disease and tuberculosis, Hawaii. USA Emerg Infect Dis. 2017;23(3):439–47.
20. van Ingen J, Bendien SA, de Lange WC, Hoefsloot W, Dekhuijzen PN, Boeree MJ, van Soolingen D. Clinical relevance of non-tuberculous mycobacteria isolated in the Nijmegen-Arnhem region. The Netherlands Thorax. 2009;64(6):502–6.
21. Simons S, van Ingen J, Hsueh PR, Van Hung N, Dekhuijzen PN, Boeree MJ, van Soolingen D. Nontuberculous mycobacteria in respiratory tract infections. eastern Asia Emerg Infect Dis. 2011;17(3):343–9.
22. Winthrop KL, McNelley E, Kendall B, Marshall-Olson A, Morris C, Cassidy M, Saulson A, Hedberg K. Pulmonary nontuberculous mycobacterial disease prevalence and clinical features: an emerging public health disease. Am J Respir Crit Care Med. 2010;182(7):977–82.
23. O'Brien RJ, Geiter LJ, Snider DE Jr. The epidemiology of nontuberculous mycobacterial diseases in the United States. Results from a national survey Am Rev Respir Dis. 1987;135(5):1007–14.
24. vom Steeg LG, Klein SL. SeXX matters in infectious disease pathogenesis. PLoS Pathog. 2016;12(2):e1005374.
25. Klein SL, Jedlicka A, Pekosz A. The Xs and Y of immune responses to viral vaccines. Lancet Infect Dis. 2010;10(5):338–49.
26. Solana R, Pawelec G, Tarazona R. Aging and innate immunity. Immunity. 2006;24(5):491–4.
27. Fowler SJ, French J, Screaton NJ, Foweraker J, Condliffe A, Haworth CS, Exley AR, Bilton D. Nontuberculous mycobacteria in bronchiectasis: prevalence and patient characteristics. Eur Respir J. 2006;28(6):1204–10.
28. Reich JM. Genesis of the nodular bronchiectasis phenotype of pulmonary disease due to nontuberculous mycobacteria. Chest. 2016;149(4):1113.
29. Cook JL. Nontuberculous mycobacteria: opportunistic environmental pathogens for predisposed hosts. Br Med Bull. 2010;96:45–59.
30. Williams MM, Yakrus MA, Arduino MJ, Cooksey RC, Crane CB, Banerjee SN, Hilborn ED, Donlan RM. Structural analysis of biofilm formation by rapidly and slowly growing nontuberculous mycobacteria. Appl Environ Microbiol. 2009;75(7):2091–8.
31. Guthertz LS, Damsker B, Bottone EJ, Ford EG, Midura TF, Janda JM. Mycobacterium avium and Mycobacterium intracellulare infections in patients with and without AIDS. J Infect Dis. 1989;160(6):1037–41.

12

Paraneoplastic syndrome as the presentation of limited stage small cell carcinoma

Kia Nikoomanesh[1*], Julian Choi[2] and Sarkis Arabian[2]

Abstract

Background: Small cell lung carcinoma (SCLC) is one of the deadliest forms of lung cancer due to its poor prognosis upon diagnosis, rapid doubling time, and affinity for metastasis. As 60–70% of patients with SCLC have disseminated disease upon presentation, it is imperative to determine the extent of disease burden for treatment. As a neuroendocrine carcinoma, clinicians must pay close attention to abnormal findings in a smoker that could lead to earlier diagnosis and better prognostication.

Case presentation: A 64 year-old 20-pack year smoker presented to the emergency department with nausea and vomiting for 3 days. No inciting events were elicited. History and review of symptoms were negative including symptoms most-commonly associated with malignancy such as fevers and weight loss. He also denied any pulmonary symptoms. Physical examination was benign except for right lung end-expiratory wheezing. Our patient was clinically euvolemic. Initial blood laboratories showed a sodium 110, serum osmolarity 227, and urine osmolarity of 579. Fluid restriction led to normalization of his sodium and resolution of nausea & vomiting. Chest radiography was obtained to follow-up on the wheezing, which was read as no acute cardiopulmonary disease by radiology. Due to high suspicion of SIADH from malignancy, a CT of the chest was performed which showed a conglomerate of nodules and opacities in the right upper lobe. Biopsy revealed SCLC. At outpatient follow-up, patient had a PET-CT showing one active mediastinal lymph node as the only site of metastasis. He received three round of chemotherapy, chest and prophylactic cranial radiation, and deemed in remission by oncology.

Discussion and conclusions: Due to its affinity for metastases, 70% of patients with SCLC present with symptoms related to the spread of cancer to affected organ systems. Given the aggressive nature of this disease, screening measures have been implemented to help diagnose limited stage SCLC. Unfortunately, in our patient and many others, screening guidelines may fail to identify appropriate patients to scan. It is therefore imperative to use our clinical index of suspicion and identify any early presentations (including paraneoplastic syndromes) which may tip off the beginning stages of SCLC. This could improve survival rates by up to 45%.

Keywords: Small cell lung carcinoma, Paraneoplastic syndrome, Syndrome of inappropriate ADH secretion, Hyponatremia

Background

Small cell lung cancer (SCLC) is a highly aggressive form of pulmonary malignancy which accounts for 15–20% of lung cancer cases [1]. SCLC is well known for its rapid doubling time, tendency to metastasize, and its affinity for relapsing. Nearly 60–70% of patients with SCLC present with disseminated disease [1], and early diagnosis improves outcomes. Typical presentations include cough, dyspnea, and weight loss. However, SCLC can present in more atypical ways.

Paraneoplastic syndromes such as syndrome of inappropriate antidiuretic hormone secretion (SIADH), Lambert-Eaton myasthenic syndrome, hypercalcemia, and Cushing's syndrome are some atypical presentations. Up to 10% of patients with lung cancer develop a paraneoplastic syndrome during the course of their disease progression [2]. An even smaller number of patients have paraneoplastic syndromes as their presenting feature. It is

* Correspondence: kianikoomanesh@gmail.com
[1]Department of Internal Medicine, Arrowhead Regional Medical Center, Colton, California, USA
Full list of author information is available at the end of the article

therefore not surprising that abnormal laboratory values can be misinterpreted as isolated findings when there is no obvious evidence of malignancy.

SCLC has almost an exclusive association with cigarette smoking. In one study, smoking was associated in 100 and 97.9% of cases in men and women, respectively [3]. With this strong of a relationship, SCLC should be considered in current and past smokers with evidence of abnormal laboratories or symptoms consistent with paraneoplastic syndromes. The following case depicts how identifying a paraneoplastic syndrome helped uncover an underlying SCLC and improve one patient's prognosis.

Case discussion

A 64 year-old caucasian male presented with a chief complaint of nausea and vomiting. These episodes occurred three-to-four times per day for the past 3 days and were non-bilious, non-bloody, mostly foodstuff. There were no precipitating factors or associated symptoms including abdominal pain or diarrhea. He did not complain of any recent pulmonary symptoms such as cough, hemoptysis, dyspnea, or chest pain, and denied any fevers, night sweats, or weight loss. He had no past medical history except for hypercholesterolemia controlled with atorvastatin. His only family history included Hodgkin's lymphoma. Smoking history revealed 20 pack years and quit 3 months prior to his visit. Vital signs upon presentation were unremarkable. Physical examination revealed mild right upper lung field end-expiratory wheezing, no clubbing of his digits, no jugular venous distention, no lower extremity edema, was euvolemic, and had unremarkable abdominal findings.

An anterior-posterior chest plain film (Fig. 1) was performed in the emergency department, and read by the radiologist as having no evidence of acute cardiopulmonary disease. Laboratories drawn on admission revealed hyponatremia in the context of a low serum osmolality and a high urine osmolality (Table 1). Given these laboratory findings, SIADH ranked high in our differential diagnoses.

Treatment with fluid restriction was initiated and sodium levels gradually improved (Table 1). The patient's nausea and vomiting had resolved as his sodium levels improved, which later was attributed to his hyponatremia from SIADH. Potential etiologies for SIADH (i.e. infectious, cerebral, medications, endocrinopathies) were further investigated and were unremarkable. Due to the patient's significant smoking history, unilateral end-expiratory wheeze, initial poor quality chest imaging, and high-index of suspicion, a CT chest was ordered. It revealed the presence of a conglomeration of nodules and opacities measuring 3.0 × 1.9 cm in the inferior segment of the right upper lobe of the lung with ipsilateral mediastinal lymphadenopathy. Subsequent CT-guided percutaneous biopsy was performed. Biopsy specimen stained positive for CK, CD56, NSE, BcL2, Synaptophysin, PAX-5, and TTF-1, but negative for Chromogranin, CD57, and NFP; consistent with small cell carcinoma. Further metastatic workup including CT abdomen and pelvis along with brain MRI was performed, which showed no evidence of metastasis.

He was subsequently discharged with an appointment with an outside oncologist near his home as he lived far from our institution. A follow-up telephone conversation occurred 4 weeks from discharge. The patient's oncologist had ordered a whole-body PET scan within 1 week of hospital discharge and it revealed uptake in one ipsilateral mediastinal lymph node. He was classified as having limited stage small cell lung cancer (LS-SCLC) and was undergoing chemotherapy with plans for subsequent prophylactic cranial irradiation. At 4 months follow-up, he had completed three chemotherapy sessions and

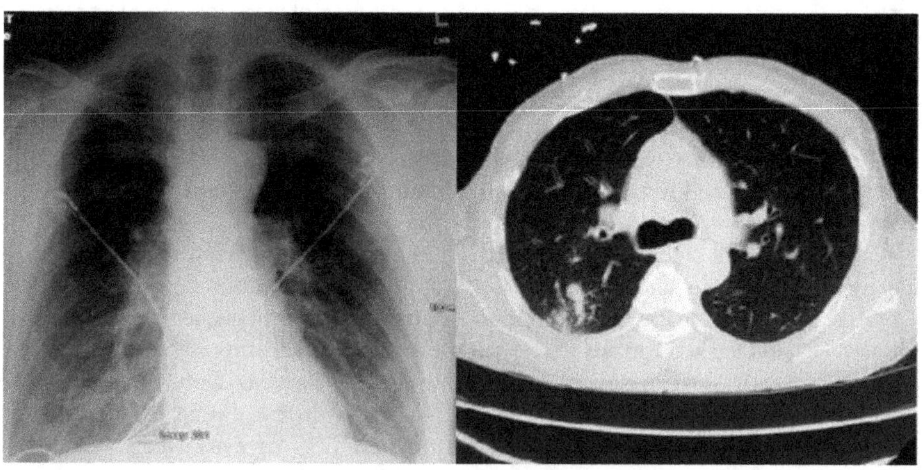

Fig. 1 Left: AP chest plain film read as no acute cardiopulmonary disease. Right: CT chest showing a conglomeration of nodules and opacities measure 3.0 × 1.9 cm of the inferior portion of the right upper lobe

Table 1 Blood laboratories from day 1, 2, and 6

Laboratory Studies	Day 1	Day 2	Day 6
Sodium (mEq/L)	110	119	130
Blood Urea Nitrogen (mg/dL)	7	9	16
Creatinine (mg/dL)	0.5	0.5	0.6
Serum osmolality (mOsm/kg)	227	237	
Urine osmolality (mOsm/kg)	579		
Urine sodium (mEq/L)	126		
Adrenocorticotropic hormone (pg/mL)	15		
Total cortisol (ug/dL)	16.55		
Thyroid stimulating hormone (mIU/mL)	1.59		

prophylactic cranial irradiation. His oncologist had deemed him to be in remission and undergoing continued surveillance.

Discussion and conclusions

SCLC can present with three possible manifestations: pulmonary, metastatic, and endocrinologic/neurologic paraneoplastic syndromes. The most common of these three manifestations is metastatic as approximately 70% of patients with SCLC present with metastatic disease [4]. This is a clear testament to the highly aggressive nature of this disease process. For this reason, screening measures have been implemented to help identify SCLC at an earlier stage. Current US Preventive Services Task Force (USPSTF) guidelines recommend screening individuals between 55 and 80 years old with at least a 30 pack year smoking history for lung cancer. The screening modality recommended is a low dose CT scan of the chest. This guideline has been supported by trials such as the national lung screening trial (NLST) which showed a 20% reduction in mortality in patients who met criteria and were screened appropriately.

Unfortunately, as seen in our patient, screening based on age and pack year history alone can lead to missed diagnoses.More recent studies suggest that a screening model using individual risk factors could be superior to the current established guideline. One study investigated the efficacy of nine different screening models based on various risk factors [5]. Risk factors in these screening models included: gender, race, ethnicity, education, body mass index, chronic obstructive pulmonary disease, emphysema, personal history of cancer, personal history of pneumonia, and family history of lung cancer. Results from this study suggest increased sensitivity and specificity for risk factor based screening groups in comparison to NLST guideline based groups. However, both the USPSTF guidelines, and risk factor based screening models have the potential to miss early diagnoses. Our case outlines a patient who does not fit the USPSTF guidelines for screening and does not fit perfectly into any risk factor based screening model.

Therefore, it continues to be a diagnostic challenge to detect early stage lung cancer such as SCLC. The aggressive nature of SCLC leaves physicians with a narrow window for discovering LS-SCLC. Despite advances in screening guidelines and modalities patients often fail to meet criteria and therefore go unnoticed before they present with metastatic disease. Given the possible shortcomings of screening modalities, physicians must rely on their clinical index of suspicion to help discover early disease. This includes a holistic approach to each patient, correlating possible early symptoms of presentation with abnormal lab values that could indicate a possible paraneoplastic syndrome. Identifying these underlying paraneoplastic syndromes may be the key to discovering a LS-SCLC in a patient who otherwise appears asymptomatic. This could significantly alter a patient's disease course and improve a 5 year survival rate by nearly 45% [5].

Abbreviations

BUN/Cr: Blood urea nitrogen/creatinine ratio; ES-SCLC: Extensive-stage small-cell lung carcinoma; LS-SCLC: Limited-stage small-cell lung carcinoma; mEq/L: Milli-equivalents per liter; mg/dL: Milligram per deciliter; mg/L: Milligram per liter; mIU/mL: milli-international units per milliliter; mOsm/kg: milliosmoles per kilogram; pg/mL: Nanogram per milliliter; SCLC: Small cell lung carcinoma; SIADH: Syndrome of inappropriate antidiuretic hormone secretion; ug/dL: Microgram per deciliter; USPSTF: US Preventive Services Task Force

Acknowledgements

Not applicable

Funding

No funding was involved in this case study.

Authors' contributions

KN, JC, and SA spearheaded the original idea of the case report. KN and JC wrote the manuscript with help from SA in ideas or the direction the case report should follow. KN, JC, and SA all proofread the case report and helped make appropriate edits to final product. All authors read and approved the final manuscript.

Consent for publication

Written informed consent was obtained from the patient for publication of this case report and any accompanying images.

Competing interests

The authors declare that they have no competing interests.

Author details

[1]Department of Internal Medicine, Arrowhead Regional Medical Center, Colton, California, USA. [2]Department of Pulmonary and Critical Care Medicine, Arrowhead Regional Medical Center, Colton, California, USA.

References

1. Huber RM, Tufman A. Update on small cell lung cancer management. Breathe. 2012;8:314–30. https://doi.org/10.1183/20734735.013211.
2. Kanaji N, Watanabe N, Kita N, Bandoh S, Tadokoro A, Ishii T, Dobashi H, Matsunaga T. Paraneoplastic syndromes associated with lung cancer. World J Clin Oncol. 2014;5(3):197–223.
3. Pesch B, Kendzia B, Gustavsson P, et al. Cigarette smoking and lung cancer – relative risk estimates for the major histological types from a pooled analysis of case-control studies. Int J Cancer. 2012;131(5):1210–9. https://doi.org/10.1002/ijc.27339.
4. Molina JR, Yang P, Cassivi SD, Schild SE, Adjei AA. Non-small cell lung cancer: epidemiology, risk factors, treatment, and survivorship. Mayo Clin Proc. 2008;83(5):584–94.
5. Ten Haaf K, Jeon J, Tammemägi MC, Han SS, Kong CY, Plevritis SK, et al. Risk prediction models for selection of lung cancer screening candidates: a retrospective validation study. PLoS Med. 2017;14(4):e1002277.

13

Circulating serotonin levels in COPD patients

Pietro Pirina[1,2*], Elisabetta Zinellu[1], Panagiotis Paliogiannis[3], Alessandro G. Fois[2], Viviana Marras[2], Salvatore Sotgia[3], Ciriaco Carru[3] and Angelo Zinellu[3]

Abstract

Background: Chronic obstructive pulmonary disease (COPD) is a major and increasing global health problem. Serotonin is a neurotransmitter that participates in several pulmonary functions and it has been involved in oxidative stress, which plays essential roles in the pathogenesis of COPD. The current study aimed at establishing the levels of circulating serotonin in COPD, and investigating eventual relations between serotonin and oxidative stress markers.

Methods: Whole blood serotonin was assessed in 43 consecutive patients with stable COPD and in 43 age and sex-matched healthy controls.

Results: Serotonin blood levels were significantly higher in COPD patients than in controls (median 0.81 μmol/L, IQR: 0.61–4.02 vs 0.65 μmol/L, IQR: 0.53–1.39, $p = 0.02$). The univariate logistic regression analysis evidenced that serotonin levels are independently associated with presence of COPD (crude OR = 7.29, 95% CI: 1.296–41.05, $p = 0.003$) and such an association was confirmed also after adjusting for several confounders (OR 21.92, 95% CI 2.02–237.83; $p = 0.011$).

Conclusions: Our study showed higher levels of circulating serotonin in COPD and an inverse correlation with the worsening of airway obstruction. Future studies are necessary to investigate the clinical utility of this finding.

Keywords: COPD, Oxidative stress, Serotonin, Markers

Background

COPD is an increasing global health problem that nowadays represents the third leading cause of death in the world [1, 2]. It is a chronic progressive disease characterized by a not fully reversible airflow limitation, associated with a chronic inflammation of the lungs and small airways [3, 4]. Although cigarette smoking represents the most known risk factor, in-door and out-door pollution, second-hand smoking and genetic conditions, such as α_1 antitrypsin deficiency, are considered important additional risk factors [5–7]. The noxious compounds present in cigarette smoke and in environmental pollution, trigger the inflammatory response of the airways and the lungs in susceptible subjects, causing epithelial injury with subsequent production of reactive oxygen species (ROS) [8, 9]. The increased amount of oxidants together with the depletion of antioxidant defenses, results in oxidative stress. It is now recognized that oxidative stress is involved in the pathogenesis of COPD [9, 10] and, in this regard, several biomarkers have been evaluated [11].

Serotonin (5-hydroxytyptamine, 5-HT) is a ubiquitous neurotransmitter that plays important roles in pulmonary functions, being involved in the modulation of respiratory rhythm and in pulmonary vasoconstriction [12, 13]. Furthermore, serotonin has been implicated in the pathogenesis of some of the main comorbidities of COPD, like depression [14, 15] despite the relation between serotonin, COPD and depression is still to be verified.

Moreover, serotonin has been reported to induce oxidative stress via monoamine oxidase-dependent pathway in human heart valves [16] and in mesenchymal

* Correspondence: pirina@uniss.it
[1]Department of Respiratory Diseases, University Hospital Sassari (AOU), Sassari, Italy
[2]Department of Clinical and Experimental Medicine, University of Sassari, Sassari, Italy
Full list of author information is available at the end of the article

stem cells [17] indicating that serotonin metabolism may be involved in oxidative stress. Its role in the genesis and maintenance of oxidative stress in COPD patients is not well-established. In this pilot study we focused on the assessment of blood serotonin levels in COPD patients compared to healthy controls and in relation to airway obstruction severity; we have also evaluated potential associations between serotonin and oxidative stress markers, like thiobarbituric acid reactive substances (TBARS) and protein sulfhydryl groups (PSH), which have been demonstrated in previous studies to be altered in patients with COPD [18, 19].

Methods

Subjects

This case–control pilot study involved 43 consecutive patients with stable COPD (mean age 74.8 ± 5.9 years, range 52–85 years), treated at the Respiratory Unit of the University of Sassari.

The diagnosis of COPD was made in accordance with the Global Initiative for Chronic Obstructive Lung Disease criteria [20]. The patients enrolled did not have a previous diagnosis of COPD and they were not under treatment with long- or short-acting β-agonists, or long-acting muscarinic antagonists, as well as with inhaled corticosteroids at least within 4 weeks prior to enrollment. Each patient performed respiratory function tests and underwent physical examination, blood tests and chest radiographs. The functional diagnosis of COPD was based on the presence of not fully reversible airflow limitation, defined by a post-bronchodilator ratio of forced expiratory volume in 1 s to forced vital capacity (FEV1/FVC) < 70% of the predicted value [4]. In order to collect demographic and clinical data, including smoking history and information about occupational and/or in-door and out-door pollutants exposure, a structured questionnaire was administered. In particular, patients who were never smokers, had been exposed to other COPD risk factors: half of them were women exposed to second-hand smoke, three of them had worked as miners and therefore exposed to silica powders and two of them had been exposed to indoor pollutants (biomass heating, etc).

A group of 43 age- and sex-matched healthy controls, with no medical history, was also included. Subjects with severe concomitant diseases, such as heart diseases, kidney and liver diseases, systemic inflammatory diseases, patients with severe COPD and patients with a history of asthma and atopic diseases, were excluded from the study. The study was approved by the Institutional Local Ethics Committee (Azienda Sanitaria Locale n°1 di Sassari (Italy) (prot. 2175/CE del 21/04/2015). The subjects who decided to participate, signed a written informed consent before enrollment.

Biochemical analysis

The levels of serotonin in whole blood of COPD subjects and healthy controls were determined according to a method previously described [21]. The inter-assay CV was < 8%. The oxidative stress indices TBARS and PSH were measured as previously reported [22, 23]. TBARS assay was employed to measure malondialdehyde (MDA) and other aldehydes produced by lipid peroxidation induced by reactive oxygen species. TBARS were determined by measuring the absorbance at 535 nm after reaction with thiobarbituric acid. A calibration curve was obtained using MDA as reference standard. Plasma PSH determination was performed by spectrophotometry with 5,5′-dithiobis-2-nitrobenzoic acid (DTNB) as titrating agent by measuring the absorbance of conjugate at 405 nm. Concentration in samples was determined from a GSH standard curve. ROS can oxidize protein SH to disulfide or sulfenic acid, leading to a reduction in –SH groups.

Statistical analysis

The results are expressed as mean (mean ± SD) or median values (median and IQR). The distribution of variables was evaluated by means of Shapiro-Wilk test. The statistical comparisons between groups were assessed by means of unpaired Student's t-test or Mann-Whitney rank sum test, as appropriate. Correlations between variables were estimated using Spearman's or Pearson's correlation, as appropriate. In order to verify the presence of association between variables potentially implicated in disease development, logistic regression analysis was performed. Receiver operating characteristics (ROC) curve analysis was used to test the ability of serotonin to predict COPD, alone and in combination with TBARS and PSH. ROC curves were obtained with calculation of the area under the curve (AUC). Optimal cut-off maximizing sensitivity and specificity was selected according to the Youden Index.

Statistical analyses were performed using MedCalc for Windows, version 15.4 64 bit (MedCalc Software, Ostend, Belgium) and SPSS for Windows, version 14.0 32 bit (IBM Corporation; Armonk, NY, USA).

Results

Table 1 reports the demographic and clinical characteristics in controls and COPD patients. As expected, COPD patients showed a reduced FEV_1 and FEV_1/FVC ratio. There were no between-group differences in smoking status or BMI. Serotonin blood levels were significantly higher in COPD patients (median 0.81 μmol/L, IQR: 0.61–4.02) than in controls (median 0.65 μmol/L, IQR: 0.53–1.39), $p = 0.02$ (Fig. 1). As previously reported TBARS concentrations significantly increased, and PSH

Table 1 Clinical and functional parameters of healthy subjects and COPD patients

	Controls ($n = 43$)	COPD ($n = 43$)
Age (years)	73 ± 7	75 ± 6
Gender (F/M)	9/34	9/34
BMI (kg/m^2)	26 ± 4	27 ± 4
Never smoked	14 (33%)	10 (23%)
Current smokers	3 (7%)	3 (7%)
Ex smokers	26 (60)	30 (70%)
FEV1 (L)	2.8 ± 0.6	2.0 ± 0.6**
FEV1 (% predicted)	112 ± 14	80 ± 18**
FVC (L)	3.4 ± 0.7	2.9 ± 0.8*
FVC (% predicted)	108 ± 15	88 ± 15**
FEV1/FVC	80.4 ± 3.9	66.6 ± 4.8**
RV (L)	2.0 ± 0.5	3.4 ± 0.9**
RV (% predicted)	105 ± 12	137 ± 32**
TLC (L)	6.0 ± 1.1	6.4 ± 1.1
TLC (% predicted)	107 ± 10	108 ± 14
RV/TLC (%)	32 ± 3	53 ± 9**

FEV1 Forced Expiratory Volume in the 1st second, *FVC* Forced Vital Capacity, *FEV1/FVC* Tiffeneau index (calculated as LLN)
*$p < 0.01$, **$p < 0.001$ obtained by Student's t-test

concentrations significantly decreased, according to COPD presence [18]. However, no significant correlations were observed between serotonin blood levels and oxidative stress indices. As reported in Fig. 2, Spearman's correlations in the whole study population indicated that serotonin blood values are inversely associated with FEV_1 (rho = – 0.25, $p = 0.023$) and FVC (rho = – 0.26, $p = 0.017$). Table 2 summarizes the results of the univariate logistic regression analysis, which evidenced that serotonin levels were independently associated with presence of COPD (crude OR = 7.29, 95% CI: 1.296–41.05, $p = 0.003$). This association remained significant also after adjusting for age, gender, BMI, smoking status, and oxidative stress indices (OR 21.92, 95% CI 2.02–237.83; $p = 0.011$).

ROC curve analysis was performed to evaluate the sensitivity, specificity, and diagnostic accuracy of serum serotonin levels alone, or in combination with PSH and TBARS, in distinguishing COPD from healthy subjects (Fig. 3 and Table 3). Serotonin alone, with a cut-off of 0.78 μmol/L discriminated COPD from controls with 53.5% sensitivity and 74.4% specificity (AUC = 0.647, 95% CI 0.537–0.747, $p = 0.014$). Serotonin in combination with PSH and TBARS produced the best result, with an AUC of 0.830 (95% CI 0.733–0.902, $p < 0.0001$), sensitivity 76.7% and specificity 74.4%. Pairwise comparison of ROC curves indicated that the combination of serotonin, PSH and TBARS yield a significant increase in AUC (+ 0.183, $p = 0.0035$) compared to AUC obtained with serotonin alone.

Discussion

Serotonin is a biogenic amine known for its role as a neurotransmitter. It is synthesized from L-tryptophan within the central nervous system (CNS), where it is stored in the presynaptic neurons. Serotonin synthesis outside the CNS is limited to enterochromaffin cells, while platelets take up serotonin from plasma representing a further major storing site for serotonin [24]. The main metabolic pathway of serotonin is the

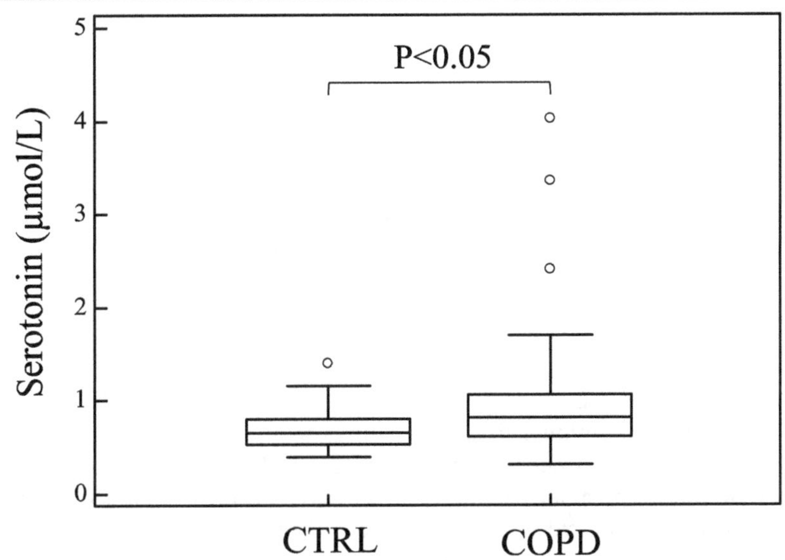

Fig. 1 Blood levels of serotonin in healthy subjects ($n = 43$) and in the totality of COPD patients ($n = 43$). The central horizontal line on each box represents the median, the ends of the boxes are 25 and 75 percentiles and the error bars 5 and 95%. *P*-values derived from Student's t-test

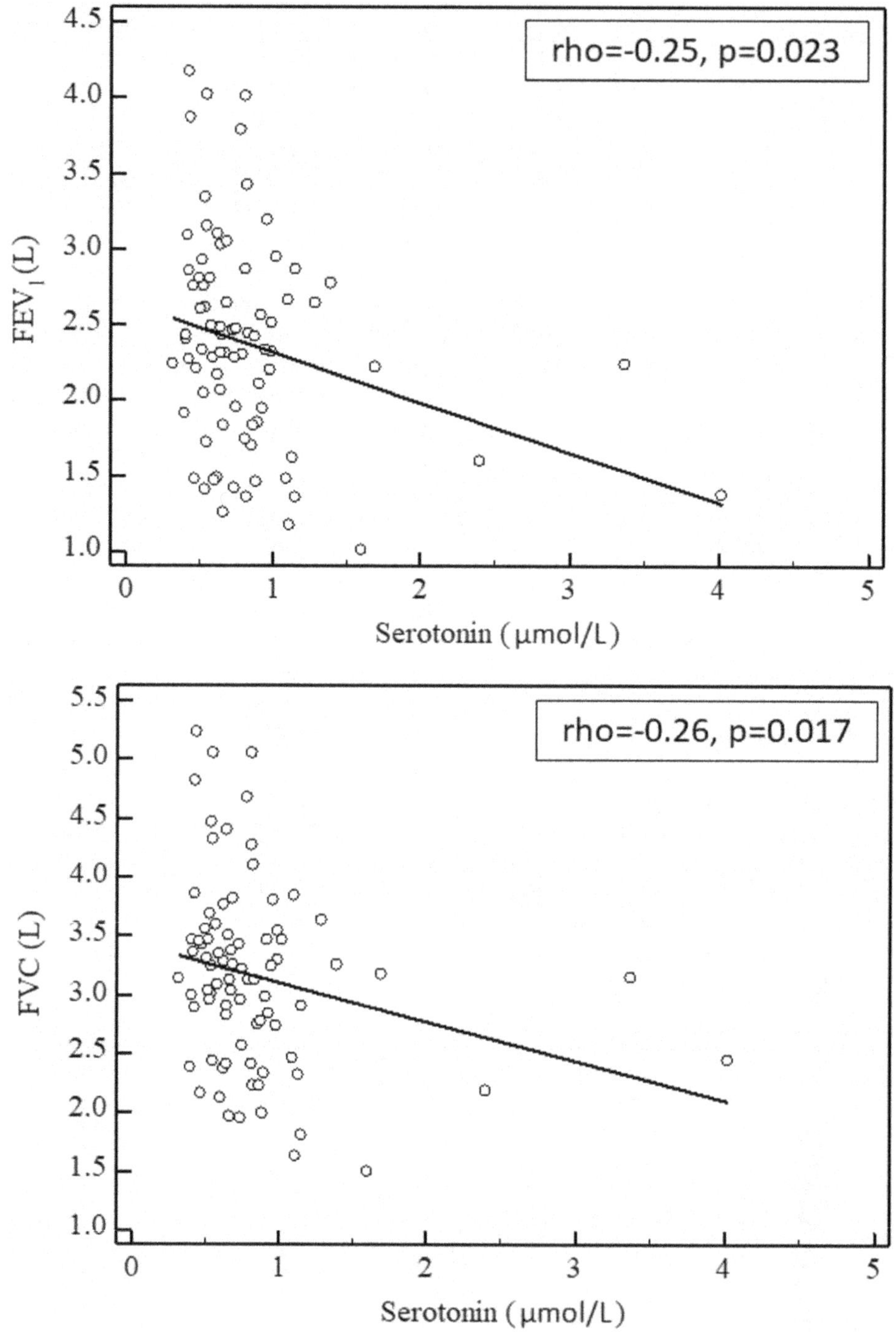

Fig. 2 Correlation between FEV1 and FVC with blood serotonin in COPD patients

metabolism by monoamine oxidase (MAO) that catalyses the oxidative deamination of the amine substrate, with production of its aldehyde intermediate and hydrogen peroxide as a by-product. The aldehyde intermediate is then rapidly oxidized by aldehyde dehydrogenase to 5-hydroxyindoleacetic acid [24, 25].

It is known that lung represent an important site in which removal and metabolism of serotonin take place [26]. The ability of the endothelial cells of the lungs to metabolise amines may be reduced in disease states, and this could explain their increased levels in the circulation. Elevated circulating levels of serotonin have been reported in respiratory diseases such as asthma [27] and lung cancer [28]. COPD has also been associated with a variation of a transporter gene involved in serotonin re-uptake [29] and metabolites

Table 2 Predicting factors for chronic obstructive pulmonary disease

Factor	Univariate analysis			Multivariate analysis		
	Crude OR	95%CI	*p*-value	OR	95%CI	*p*-value
Age	1.035	0.967–1.109	0.749	0.998	0.917–1.088	0.978
Gender	1.000	0.368–2.720	0.061	1.567	0.341–7.203	0.563
BMI	1.076	0.953–1.216	0.692	1.108	0.942–1.303	0.217
Smoking status	1.404	0.551–3.581	1.000	0.516	0.144–1.854	0.319
PSH	0.427	0.258–0.705	0.0001	0.289	0.144–0.580	0.0005
TBARS	1.816	1.053–3.131	0.02	2.947	1.322–6.570	0.008
Serotonin	7.294	1.296–41.05	0.003	21.92	2.02–237.83	0.011

BMI body mass index, *PSH* protein sulfhydryl groups, *TBARS* thiobarbituric acid reactive substances, *OR* odds ratio, *CI* confidence interval

of the serotonin pathway have been associated with adverse outcome in exacerbated COPD [30]. Furthermore, it is now recognized that oxidative stress is involved in the pathogenesis of COPD [9, 10] and it has been reported that serotonin induces oxidative stress via MAO-dependent pathway in human heart valves [16] and in mesenchymal stem cells [17]. Moreover, it has been described that cigarette smoke, a major COPD risk factor, inhibit MAO in different species in vitro [31]. Such evidences suggest that serotonin may play relevant roles in the pathogenesis of COPD.

Our study has evidenced a significant increase in serotonin levels in COPD patients compared to controls. Spearman's correlations indicated that blood serotonin values are inversely associated with FEV1 and FVC, to confirm an association of serotonin levels not only with the presence of COPD, but also with the severity of airway obstruction. The univariate logistic regression analysis has shown that serotonin levels were independently associated with presence of COPD also after adjusting for age, gender, BMI, smoking status, and oxidative stress indices.

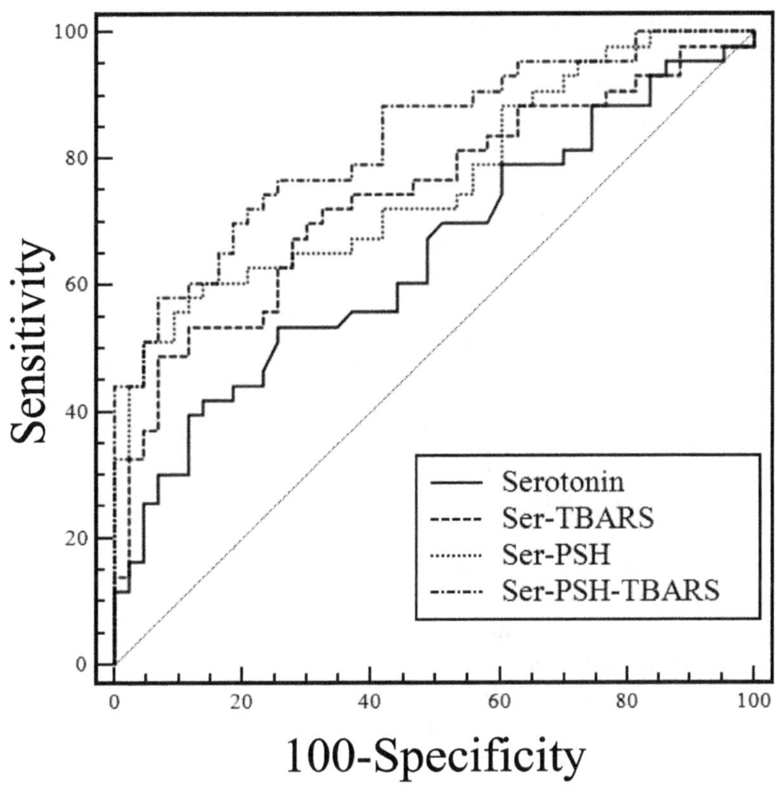

Fig. 3 The area under receiver operating characteristic curves of serotonin

Table 3 Prognostic accuracy of serotonin alone or in combination with TBARS and MDA

Marker	AUC	95%CI	*p* value	Cut-off	Sensib	Specif
Serotonin	0.647	0.537–0.747	0.014	> 0.780	53.5%	74.4%
Ser-TBARS	0.741	0.635–0.829	< 0.0001	> 0.543	53.5%	88.4%
Ser-PSH	0.764	0.660–0.849	< 0.0001	> 0.569	60.5%	86.1%
Ser-PSH-TBARS	0.830	0.733–0.902	< 0.0001	> 0.460	76.7%	74.4%

PSH protein sulfhydryl groups, *TBARS* thiobarbituric acid reactive substances, *MDA* malondialdehyde, *AUC* area under the curve, *CI* confidence interval

Lau et al. [32], investigated the role of serotonin in the pathogenesis of COPD and found higher levels of circulating serotonin in patients compared to healthy controls. Unlike us, they examined only male COPD subjects who were significantly older than controls, and found a positive correlation between serotonin levels and age in pathological subjects. Moreover, in their analysis they prevalently included moderate to very severe COPD cases, finding no differences in serotonin levels according to disease progression. In our study, we confirmed the presence of higher blood serotonin levels in COPD compared to age- and sex-matched controls. As opposed to the study of Lau et al., our patients had a mild-moderate degree of airway obstruction (FEV1 > 50%). From this point of view these patients can be considered in the early phase of the disease. In fact, they were all newly diagnosed patients who had not yet started a treatment. These data support the hypothesis that serotonin could be a predictive marker of the onset of COPD. Moreover, the inverse correlation that we found between serotonin levels and FEV1 and FVC, suggests a relation of this molecule with the worsening of airway obstruction.

The ROC curve analysis for serotonin significantly discriminate patients with COPD from those without COPD and showed that the diagnostic accuracy is higher when serotonin is combined with TBARS and PSH. In particular, the triple combination of serotonin, TBARS and PSH increased significantly the AUC of the ROC curve. Although it is an interesting result, its clinical validity and usefulness needs to be further investigated. Moreover, Spearman's correlation analysis failed to find a relationship between serotonin and oxidative stress biomarkers. This could be due to the low number of subjects involved, in particular to the absence of severe COPD subjects. The small number of cases, and the lack of advanced stage COPD patients represent the main limitations of our work. On the other hand, our study is the first to investigate blood serotonin levels in a cohort of early COPD cases and has several strengths, like its prospective case-match design, the accurate statistical analysis, and the research of associations with other well-established biomarkers of oxidative stress.

Conclusions

Our study confirms literature data showing an involvement of serotonin in the pathogenesis of COPD, demonstrating a statistically significant increase of circulating serotonin levels in an early phase of the disease, and a relation with the worsening of the airway obstruction. Given the need of biomarkers useful to detect and monitor COPD and its response to treatments, this seems to be a promising result that need to be further investigated.

Abbreviations

5-HT: Serotonin; AUC: Area under the curve; BMI: Body mass index; CNS: Central nervous system; COPD: Chronic obstructive pulmonary disease; FEV1: Forced expiratory volume in the 1st second; FVC: Forced vital capacity; MAO: Monoamine oxidase; MDA: Malondialdehyde; PSH: Protein sulfhydryl groups; ROC: Receiver operating characteristics; TBARS: Thiobarbituric acid reactive substances

Acknowledgements

Not applicable.

Funding

This research did not receive any specific grant from funding agencies in the public, commercial, or not-for-profit sectors.

Authors' contributions

PP1 participated in the design of the study and drafted the manuscript. EZ helped to draft the manuscript and contributed to the biochemical analysis. PP2 and AGF helped to draft the manuscript. VM and SS contributed to the biochemical analysis. CC contributed to the statistical analysis. AZ conceived and designed the study, was responsible for data extraction and performed statistical analysis. All authors have critically revised the manuscript and have approved the final version.

Consent for publication

Not applicable.

Competing interests

The author Pietro Pirina is currently acting as an Associate Editor for BMC Pulmonary Medicine. All other authors declare that they have no competing interests.

Author details

[1]Department of Respiratory Diseases, University Hospital Sassari (AOU), Sassari, Italy. [2]Department of Clinical and Experimental Medicine, University of Sassari, Sassari, Italy. [3]Department of Biomedical Sciences, University of Sassari, Sassari, Italy.

References

1. López-Campos JL, Tan W, Soriano JB. Global burden of COPD. Respirology. 2016;21(1):14–23.
2. Lozano R, Naghavi M, Foreman K, Lim S, Shibuya K, Aboyans V, Abraham J, Adair T, Aggarwal R, Ahn SY, Alvarado M, Anderson HR, Anderson LM, Andrews KG, Atkinson C, et al. Global and regional mortality from 235 causes of death

for 20 age groups in 1990 and 2010: a systematic analysis for the Global Burden of Disease Study 2010. Lancet. 2012;380(9859):2095–128.

3. Decramer M, Janssens W, Miravitlles M. Chronic obstructive pulmonary disease. Lancet. 2012;379:1341–51.
4. Vogelmeier CF, Criner GJ, Martinez FJ, Anzueto A, Barnes PJ, Bourbeau J, Celli BR, Chen R, Decramer M, Fabbri LM, Frith P, Halpin DM, López Varela MV, Nishimura M, Roche N, Rodriguez-Roisin R, Sin DD, Singh D, Stockley R, Vestbo J, Wedzicha JA, Agusti A. Global Strategy for the Diagnosis, Management, and Prevention of Chronic Obstructive Lung Disease 2017 Report: GOLD Executive Summary. Eur Respir J. 2017;49(3). https://doi.org/10.1183/13993003.00214-2017.
5. Mannino DM, Buist AS. Global burden of COPD: risk factors, prevalence, and future trends. Lancet. 2007;370:765–73.
6. Eisner MD, Anthonisen N, Coultas D, Kuenzli N, Perez-Padilla R, Postma D, Romieu I, Silverman EK, Balmes JR, Committee on Nonsmoking COPD, Environmental and Occupational Health Assembly. An official American Thoracic Society public policy statement: novel risk factors and the global burden of chronic obstructive pulmonary disease. Am J Respir Crit Care Med. 2010;182:693–718.
7. Gooptu B, Ekeowa UI, Lomas DA. Mechanisms of emphysema in alpha1-antitrypsin deficiency: molecular and cellular insights. Eur Respir J. 2009;34:475–88.
8. Larsson K. Aspects on pathophysiological mechanisms in COPD. J Intern Med. 2007;262(3):311–40.
9. Kirkham PA, Barnes PJ. Oxidative stress in COPD. Chest. 2013;144(1):266–73.
10. Santus P, Corsico A, Solidoro P, Braido F, Di Marco F, Scichilone N. Oxidative stress and respiratory system: pharmacological and clinical reappraisal of N-acetylcysteine. COPD. 2014;11(6):705–17.
11. Zinellu E, Zinellu A, Fois AG, Carru C, Pirina P. Circulating biomarkers of oxidative stress in chronic obstructive pulmonary disease: a systematic review. Respir Res. 2016;17(1):150.
12. Hilaire G, Voituron N, Menuet C, Ichiyama RM, Subramanian HH, Dutschmann M. The role of serotonin in respiratory function and dysfunction. Respir Physiol Neurobiol. 2010;174(1–2):76–88.
13. Morecroft I, Loughlin L, Nilsen M, Colston J, Dempsie Y, Sheward J, Harmar A, MacLean MR. Functional interactions between 5-hydroxytryptamine receptors and the serotonin transporter in pulmonary arteries. J Pharmacol Exp Ther. 2005;313(2):539–48.
14. Blier P, El Mansari M. Serotonin and beyond: therapeutics for major depression. Philos Trans R Soc Lond Ser B Biol Sci. 2013;368(1615):20120536.
15. Yohannes AM, Alexopoulos GS. Depression and anxiety in patients with COPD. Eur Respir Rev. 2014;23(133):345–9.
16. Peña-Silva RA, Miller JD, Chu Y, Heistad DD. Serotonin produces monoamine oxidase-dependent oxidative stress in human heart valves. Am J Physiol Heart Circ Physiol. 2009;297(4):H1354–60.
17. Trouche E, Mias C, Seguelas MH, Ordener C, Cussac D, Parini A. Characterization of monoamine oxidases in mesenchymal stem cells: role in hydrogen peroxide generation and serotonin-dependent apoptosis. Stem Cells Dev. 2010;19(10):1571–8.
18. Zinellu A, Fois AG, Sotgia S, Sotgiu E, Zinellu E, Bifulco F, Mangoni AA, Pirina P, Carru C. Arginines plasma concentration and oxidative stress in mild to moderate COPD. PLoS One. 2016;11(8):e0160237.
19. Zinellu A, Fois AG, Sotgia S, Zinellu E, Bifulco F, Pintus G, Mangoni AA, Carru C, Pirina P. Plasma protein thiols: an early marker of oxidative stress in asthma and chronic obstructive pulmonary disease. Eur J Clin Investig. 2016; 46(2):181–8.
20. Global Strategy for the Diagnosis, Management, and Prevention of Chronic Obstructive Lung Disease 2017 Report. GOLD Executive Summary. Am J Respir Crit Care Med. 2017;195(5):557–82.
21. Zinellu A, Sotgia S, Deiana L, Carru C. Reverse injection capillary electrophoresis UV detection for serotonin quantification in human whole blood. J Chromatogr B Anal Technol Biomed Life Sci. 2012;895–896:182–5.
22. Esterbauer H, Cheeseman KH. Determination of aldehydic lipid peroxidation products: malonaldehyde and 4-hydroxynonenal. Methods Enzymol. 1990; 186:407–21.
23. Ellman GL. Tissue sulfhydryl groups. Arch Biochem Biophys. 1959;82(1):70–7.
24. Mohammad-Zadeh LF, Moses L, Gwaltney-Brant SM. Serotonin: a review. J Vet Pharmacol Ther. 2008;31(3):187–99.
25. Lewis A, Miller JH, Lea RA. Monoamine oxidase and tobacco dependence. Neurotoxicology. 2007;28(1):182–95.
26. Block ER, Stalcup SA. Metabolic functions of the lung. Of what clinical relevance? Chest. 1982;81(2):215–23.
27. Lechin F, van der Dijs B, Orozco B, Lechin M, Lechin AE. Increased levels of free serotonin in plasma of symptomatic asthmatic patients. Ann Allergy Asthma Immunol. 1996;77(3):245–53.
28. Takahashi C, Goto E, Taira S, Kataoka N, Nishihara M, Katsumata T, Goto I, Takiuchi H. Serotonin syndrome in a patient with small cell lung cancer. Gan To Kagaku Ryoho. 2013;40(8):1059–61.
29. Ishii T, Wakabayashi R, Kurosaki H, Gemma A, Kida K. Association of serotonin transporter gene variation with smoking, chronic obstructive pulmonary disease, and its depressive symptoms. J Hum Genet. 2011;56(1):41–6.
30. Meier MA, Ottiger M, Vögeli A, Steuer C, Bernasconi L, Thomann R, Christ-Crain M, Henzen C, Hoess C, Zimmerli W, Huber A, Mueller B, Schuetz P. Activation of the serotonin pathway is associated with poor outcome in COPD exacerbation: results of a long-term cohort study. Lung. 2017;195(3): 303–11.
31. Khalil AA, Davies B, Castagnoli N Jr. Isolation and characterization of a monoamine oxidase B selective inhibitor from tobacco smoke. Bioorg Med Chem. 2006;14:3392–8.
32. Lau WK, Chan-Yeung MM, Yip BH, Cheung AH, Ip MS, Mak JC, COPD Study Group of the Hong Kong Thoracic Society. The role of circulating serotonin in the development of chronic obstructive pulmonary disease. PLoS One. 2012;7(2):e31617.

14

Microscopic polyangiitis secondary to *Mycobacterium abscessus* in a patient with bronchiectasis

C. Addy[1,2*], G. Doran[2], A. L. Jones[3], G. Wright[4], S. Caskey[2] and D. G. Downey[1,2]

Abstract

Background: Non-Tuberculous Mycobacterial–pulmonary disease (NTM-PD) is increasing in incidence and prevalence. Mycobacterium abscessus (*M.abscessus*) is a rapid growing multi-resistant NTM associated with severe NTM-PD requiring prolonged antibiotic therapy. Complications of therapy are common but reports on direct complications of active NTM-PD are rare. Vasculitis has been described as a rare complication of NTM-PD, most often in individuals with inherited immune defects. This case is the first to describe an ANCA positive vasculitide (Microscopic Polyangiitis) secondary to *M.abscessus* pulmonary disease.

Case presentation: A 70 year old female with bronchiectasis underwent a clinical decline associated with the growth of *M.abscessus* and was diagnosed with NTM-PD. Before treatment could be initiated she developed small joint arthralgia and a glove and stocking axonal loss sensorimotor neuropathy. Positive Perinuclear Anti-Neutrophil Cytoplasmic Antibodies (P-ANCA) and Myeloperoxidase-ANCA (MPO-ANCA) titres led to a diagnosis of microscopic polyangiitis. Further investigation revealed reduced interferon-gamma production but no other significant immune dysfunction. Dual treatment with immunosuppressive therapy (Corticosteroids/Cyclophosphamide) for vasculitis and antimicrobial therapy for *M.abscessus* NTM-PD was initiated. Clinical stability was difficult to achieve with reductions in immunosuppression triggering vasculitic flares. One flare led to retinal vein occlusion with impending visual loss requiring escalation in immunosuppression to Rituximab infusions. An increase in immunosuppression led to a deterioration in NTM-PD necessitating alterations to antibiotic regimes. Adverse effects including alopecia and Achilles tendonitis have further limited antibiotic choices resulting in a strategy of pulsed intra-venous therapy to stabilise NTM-PD.

Conclusions: This is the first reported case of an ANCA positive vasculitis secondary to *M.abscessus* pulmonary disease. This rare but important complication had a significant impact on the patient adding to the complexity of an already significant disease and treatment burden. The potential role of reduced interferon-gamma production in this case highlights the importance of investigating immune function in those with mycobacterial infection and the intricate relationship between mycobacterial infection and immune dysfunction. Immune dysfunction caused by genetic defects or immunosuppressive therapy is a known risk factor for NTM-PD. Balancing immunosuppressive therapy with prolonged antimicrobial treatment is challenging and likely to become more common as the number of individuals being treated with biologics and immunosuppressive agents increases.

Keywords: Non-tuberculous mycobacteria, Non-tuberculous mycobacterial pulmonary disease Mycobacterium abscessus, Vasculitis, Interferon-gamma, Bronchiectasis

* Correspondence: c.addy@qub.ac.uk
[1]Centre for Experimental Medicine, Queen's University Belfast, 97 Lisburn Road, Belfast BT9 7BL, Northern Ireland
[2]Regional Respiratory Centre, Belfast City Hospital, 51 Lisburn Road, Belfast BT9 7AB, Northern Ireland
Full list of author information is available at the end of the article

Background

The incidence and prevalence of Non-Tuberculous Mycobacterial–pulmonary disease (NTM-PD) is increasing [1, 2]. Understanding the spectrum of disease and pathogenicity of differing Non-Tuberculous Mycobacteria (NTM) has advanced in line with developments in microbiological detection highlighting the need to sub-speciate NTM and alter management accordingly [1]. NTM can cause progressive lung disease or reside within the lungs asymptomatically [1]. Treatment regimens are prolonged, toxic and difficult to tolerate. Decisions to commence treatment are based on a number of factors including disease severity, frequency of positive cultures, progression of radiological appearances, underlying lung disease, co-morbidities and pathogenicity of individual species [1].

Guidance on treating NTM-PD was first published in 2007 [3] with no further guidance published until the 2016 Cystic Fibrosis specific consensus document [4] and 2017 British Thoracic Society guidelines [5]. This is due to lack of evidence in this area and to the complexity of the disease. Increasing incidence and prevalence of NTM-PD highlights the need for further research and guidance [1].

Mycobacterium abscessus *(M.abscessus)* is one of the most pathogenic NTMs, particularly in those with underlying lung disease [5]. It is a multi-resistant organism with limited antibiotic options and is challenging to treat [5]. *M. abscessus* is a rapid growing NTM which can be sub-speciated into *M.a.abscessus*, *M.a.massiliense* and *M.a.bolletii* [5]. The initial treatment aim is eradication, which commonly fails and therefore long-term chronic suppressive therapy becomes necessary. Development of macrolide resistance is associated with reduced rates of culture conversion and increased chronic infection [5]. Evidence on optimal antibiotic regimes and longer-term outcomes of chronic suppressive treatment are limited [3, 5]. Those with the subspecies *M.a.abscessus* have much lower rates of culture conversion [5]. The impact of *M.abscessus* infection on patients should not be underestimated because of prolonged toxic treatment regimens that it requires, the need for stringent infection control precautions and it's relative contra-indication to lung transplantation [4, 5].

Case presentation

A 70-year-old female had been symptomatic with a persistent non-productive cough and recurrent chest infections for 10 years. At presentation to clinic a CT thorax showed right middle lobe bronchiectasis. She was a life-long non-smoker with no childhood history of respiratory disease and normal baseline investigations for immune deficiency. Clinical stability was achieved with long term Azithromycin and regular airway clearance. *Staphyloccocus aureus (S.aureus)* was cultured intermittently from sputum samples with repeatedly negative mycobacterial cultures. A repeat CT 6 years after her initial scan demonstrated progression of disease with bi-apical scarring, right middle lobe atelectasis, right upper lobe cylindrical bronchiectasis and reticulo-nodular densities in both lower lobes. (Fig. 1) Nebulised Tobramycin was trialled to suppress *S.aureus* and stabilise radiological appearances but stopped after 15 months due to worsening cough.

M. abscessus was first isolated from her sputum in November 2013; sub-speciated into *M.a. abscessus.* Commencement of therapy was under consideration when, 3 months from first isolation of *M.abscessus*, paraesthesia developed in her hands and feet with associated small joint arthropathy. A subtle purpuric rash was evident on the lower limbs. Nerve conduction studies confirmed an axonal loss sensorimotor neuropathy. Erythrocyte Sedimentation Ratio was elevated at 49 mm/hr, Perinuclear Anti-Neutrophil Cytoplasmic Antibodies (P-ANCA) titre was highly positive at 80 AI and Myeloperoxidase-ANCA (MPO-ANCA) was >8 AI with Proteinase-3–ANCA (PR3-ANCA) <0.2 AI. Renal function and urine microscopy were normal. A diagnosis of microscopic polyangiitis was made. Treatment with Cyclophosphamide and high dose Prednisolone was commenced with full resolution of her paraesthesia.

Within 4 months of first isolation, all sputum samples ($n = 4$) were culture positive and 66% of those samples were smear positive for *M. abscessus.* C-Reactive Protein was elevated at 86.2 mg/l. A repeat CT thorax showed extensive bronchiectasis with underlying collapse in the right upper and lower lobes. There was extensive tree-in-bud change within the right lower lobe, scattered pulmonary nodules and small areas of ground glass shadowing in both lungs. Deteriorating radiological appearances and commencement of active immunosuppression prompted urgent initiation of *M. abscessus* treatment.

Treatment

Induction phase treatment comprised intravenous (IV) Cefoxitin and Amikacin with oral Clarithromycin and Minocycline and was tolerated for 2 weeks. Long-term nebulised Amikacin was commenced, along with oral Moxifloxacin, Minocycline and Clarithromycin.

A month later she attended the Emergency Department (ED) with rupture of her right Achilles tendon secondary to Moxifloxacin. This was stopped immediately and replaced with Linezolid. Despite dose reduction this was discontinued due to intolerable nausea, diarrhoea and angular stomatitis. She remained on oral Minocycline, Clarithromycin and nebulised Amikacin. Cyclophosphamide was changed to Azathioprine as long-term immunosuppression, but this was poorly tolerated due

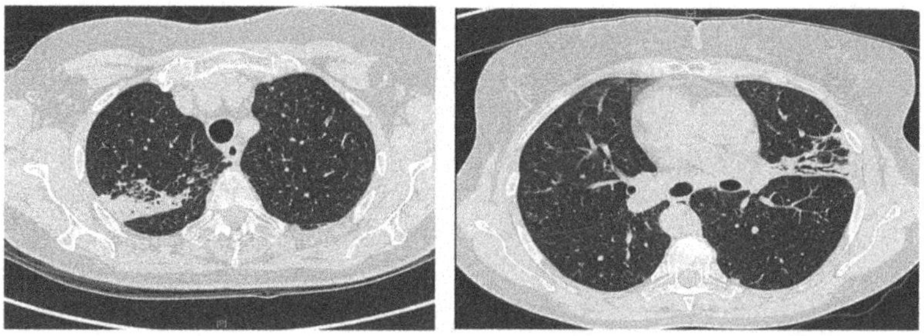

Fig. 1 CT Thorax 2007: CT Thorax from 2007 demonstrating bi-apical scarring, right middle lobe atelectasis, right upper lobe cylindrical bronchiectasis and reticulo-nodular densities in both lower lobes

to nausea. Significant alopecia then developed; attributed to Minocycline, which was also discontinued. Nebulised Meropenem was therefore added to maintain triple antibiotic therapy.

On review 17 months after initiation of treatment her pulmonary disease appeared more stable. A regime of nebulised Meropenem, nebulised Amikacin and oral Clarithromycin was tolerated. Smear and culture negativity was maintained for a further 12 months on this regime. P-ANCA and MPO-ANCA titres remained within normal limits during this period.

Twenty months after starting treatment, cultures again became positive for *M.abscessus*. A month after culture positivity returned, she presented to the ED with visual loss secondary to a right branch retinal vein occlusion. MPO-ANCA had again become highly positive at > 8 AI and P-ANCA titre was 160 AI. Due to active vasculitis with impending visual loss from associated hypercoagulability and thromboembolism higher dose immunosuppression was required. She commenced Rituximab and Methylprednisolone infusions weekly for 4 weeks, followed by 6 monthly Rituximab. Clinical response was achieved with CD19 count reducing from 46% to 0%. Within the following 12 months sputum samples became smear positive again. High resolution CT chest demonstrated extensive airspace opacification, ill-defined nodularity and tree in bud change. (Fig. 2)

Outcome and follow-up

Further assessment of immunological function was carried out, including vaccination response, respiratory oxidative burst, Mannan Binding Lectin, IgG subsets, complement levels, alternative and innate signalling pathways. Specific testing of interferon pathways demonstrated a very low interferon-gamma (IFN-γ) level, with low production of Interleukin-17 (IL-17) but no auto-antibodies to IFN-γ.

No other organisms, including *S.aureus* have been detected by standard sputum culture since 2012. Four years from first isolation she remained *M.abscessus* smear and culture positive. Clarithromycin resistance was now detectable necessitating its cessation. A further 3 weeks of IV Amikacin, Cefoxitin and Tigecycline was commenced. Long-term treatment continued with nebulised Meropenem and Amikacin.

A third oral agent would optimise long-term therapy but intolerances, resistance and risk of visual loss prevent the use of almost all suitable oral agents. Clofazimine was not commenced due to risk of further visual loss. A trial of oral Co-trimoxazole [5] resulted in intolerable nausea and had to be stopped. As no third oral agent could be used, pulsed IV antibiotics have been introduced. The optimal duration between IV courses is unknown and is currently based on recurrence of smear positivity or deteriorating symptoms. The first repeat IV antibiotic course maintained smear negativity for

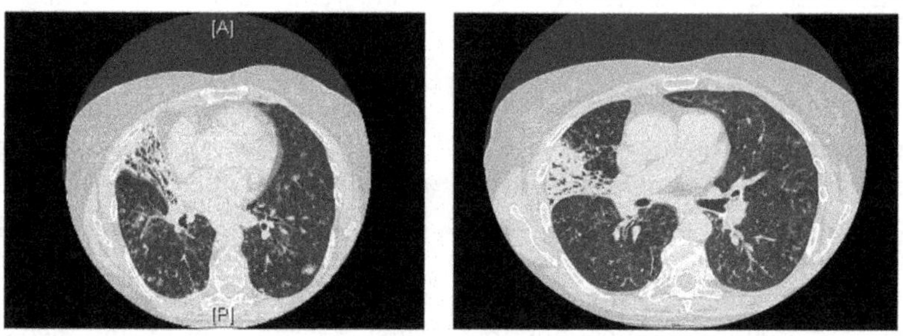

Fig. 2 CT Thorax 2016: High resolution CT Chest from 2016 demonstrating extensive airspace opacification, ill-defined nodularity and tree in bud change

6 months. Recurrence of smear positivity and associated clinical deterioration have required further IV courses (Table 1).

Discussion

This case highlights a rare systemic complication of NTM-PD and is the first reported case of ANCA-positive vasculitis as a consequence of *M. abscessus* infection. It demonstrates the complexity of managing NTM-PD including therapeutic challenges and the relationship between immune function and NTM infection.

NTM-PD is increasing in incidence and prevalence. Determining the clinical relevance of NTM isolates can be difficult [2]. *M. abscessus* is the 3rd most commonly isolated NTM in the USA [5]. It predominantly affects white, female non-smokers over the age of 60 [5]. It can occur in the absence of underlying lung disease where the course can be slow and indolent. In the setting of pre-existing lung disease such as CF or bronchiectasis, it can be fulminant and rapidly progressive [5]. The radiographic picture is of inflammatory nodules, tree-in-bud opacities and cavitation particularly in areas of underlying bronchiectasis [4].

There is wide variation in how patients with *M. abscessus* NTM-PD are treated [4]. An intensive induction phase consisting of three IV antibiotics administered for several weeks in combination with an oral agent is common [4, 5]. This is usually followed by at least two oral antimicrobials in addition to a macrolide antibiotic and inhaled antibiotic(s) [4]. Side effects of antimicrobial therapy are significant and can limit treatment options over a prolonged treatment period. In one study 65% patients stopped at least one antibiotic due to adverse events or toxicity [6]. In this case the additive toxicity of both anti-microbial and immunosuppressive agents further increased the side effect profile (Table 2).

The association between vasculitis and chronic suppurative lung conditions [7, 8] is thought to result from excessive humoral immune responses secondary to circulating immune complexes [8]. Pulmonary infection may trigger vasculitis through induction of ANCA antigen expression on the surface of neutrophils [9]. The temporal relationship between *M.abscessus* growth, ANCA positivity and vasculitic symptoms reduces the chance of the two being unrelated, suggesting *M.abscessus* was a causative trigger for the vasculitides. *S.aureus* had been chronically cultured since presentation with no prior evidence of vasculitis reducing the likelihood of *S.aureus* being a causative factor. Previous case reports have described ANCA-positive vasculitis secondary to *M.avium complex* [10]. Leukocytoclastic vasculitis linked to Salmonella has been reported in children with genetic Interferon-gamma deficiency [11]. Leukocytoclastic vasculitis in an individual with interferon-gamma autoantibodies and disseminated *M. abscessus* has also been reported [12]. Increased susceptibility to mycobacterial disease has been reported in genetic interferon defects but a causal link with associated vasculitides has not been established [13]. It is possible the reduction in IFN-γ seen in this case may have contributed both to development of vasculitis and poor treatment response.

The use of IFN-γ had been considered in this case. IFN-γ production is integral to mycobacterial defence through activation of both innate and adaptive immune systems via the interleukin12-IFN-γ pathway [13, 14]. IFN-γ facilitates mycobacterial killing by enhancing phagocytosis and expression of oxygen free radicals [14]. Administration is associated with a flu like syndrome [15–17]. Intramuscular IFN-γ as adjuvant therapy for *M. avium complex* resulted in clinical benefit over antibiotics alone [5, 15] but of insufficient magnitude to warrant recommending routine use [5]. IFN-γ therapy in management of *M. abscessus* disease is limited to case reports of use in disseminated disease [16, 18].

Rituximab has been successfully used in disseminated *M. abscessus* disease refractory to antibacterial chemotherapy in those with IFN-γ autoantibodies [12, 19]. It can restore IFN-γ signalling in these individuals [12, 19]. Whether this is true in those without autoantibodies, as in this case is unknown, as is any potential interaction between Rituximab and IFN-γ therapy. In this case monitoring Rituximab response first was considered of lowest risk but the addition of IFN-γ could be re-visited.

Treatment regimens for systemic vasculitis comprise high dose induction immunosuppression followed by oral maintenance therapy for 12–18 months [9]. The challenge in this case was balancing adequate immunosuppression with sufficient antimicrobial therapy to maintain clinical stability alongside smear and culture negativity. Reductions in immunosuppression triggered vasculitic flares with sight threatening consequences whilst increases in immunosuppression led to a deterioration in NTM-PD.

This case highlights the complex interplay between immune function and NTM-PD both as a complication and a cause of disease [13, 14, 20]. Defects in IFN-γ pathways, both acquired and genetic are associated with NTM-PD [14, 20]; as are defects in macrophage and dendritic cell function and cytokine signalling [5, 13]. Whole genome sequencing has demonstrated higher rates of genetic variants in immune, Cystic Fibrosis Transmembrane Conductance Regulator, cilial function and connective tissue categories in people with NTM-PD. [21] Screening for immune defects in those with NTM-PD who fail to respond to "standard" treatment is increasingly recommended [5] and may allow better prognostication and management in the future. Equally, those with known immune dysfunction should be screened for NTM.

Table 1 Timeline of Case

Time from Presentation	Relevant Past Medical History and Interventions		
Presentation	First review in Respiratory Clinic- recurrent "chest infections" since 1992 Life-long Non-Smoker No childhood History of Respiratory Illness No significant Past Medical History or Family History of note		
	Summary of progress	Diagnostic Tests	Interventions
Presentation	Initial Diagnosis Bronchiectasis Clinically stable	CT thorax Normal Baseline Investigations for immunodeficiency Sputum Culture and Sensitivity testing Sputum for Acid Fast Bacill (AFB) and NTM culture	Airway Clearance regime initiated Maintenance Azithromycin therapy started
Six years from presentation	Increasing frequency of Exacerbations	HRCT thorax: progression of disease with right middle lobe atelectasis, right upper lobe cylindrical bronchiectasis and reticulo-nodular densities in both lower lobes Serial growth of *S. aureus* in sputum samples	Trial of Nebulised Tobramycin- stopped after 15 months due to cough
Eleven years from presentation	First Isolation of *M.abscessus* from Sputum	Further Sputum Samples for AFB/NTM Culture	Eradication therapy under consideration
Three months from first *M.abscessus* culture	Development of paraesthesia in hands, purpuric rash on limbs and small joint arthropathy	ESR 49 P-ANCA highly positive 80AI MPO-ANCA was > 8 AI; PR3-ANCA < 0.2 AI Nerve conduction studies - axonal loss sensorimotor neuropathy Renal Function and Urine microscopy Normal	Diagnosis of microscopic polyangiitis Commenced on immunosuppression-high dose Prednisolone and Cyclophosphamide
Four months from first *M.abscessus* culture	All sputum samples culture positive for *M.abscessus*, 66% samples smear positive	CRP raised at 86.2 mg/l CT thorax: extensive bronchiectasis with underlying collapse in the right upper and lower lobes.	Induction Phase Treatment for *M.abscessus* initiated (IV Cefoxitin/Amikacin/ Oral Clarithromycin/ Minocycline) Maintenance therapy initiated (Nebulised Amikacin,Oral Moxifloxacin/ Minocycline/Clarithromycin)
Six months from first *M.abscessus* culture	Attended ED with Achilles tendon rupture	Non-surgical management with immobilization	Moxifloxacin stopped Replaced with Linezolid
Seven months from first *M.abscessus* culture	Developed significant Alopecia		Minocycline Discontinued Nebulised Meropenem added
Two years from first *M.abscessus* culture (Seventeen months into treatment)	Sputum became culture positive for *M.abscessus* Presented to ED with right sided visual loss – 1 month later (18 months into treatment)	Right branch retinal vein occlusion secondary to vasculitis confirmed on fluorescein angiography P-ANCA titre = 160; MPO > 8 AI (highly positive)	Higher level of Immunosuppression initiated (IV Methylprednisolone and 6 monthly Rituximab infusions)
Three years from first *M.abscessus* culture	Clinically stable Smear and culture positive for *M.abscessus*	Further assessment of immunological function: • Very low interferon-gamma (IFN-γ) level, with low production of Interleukin-17(IL-17) but no autoantibodies to IFN-γ. • Normal Vaccination response • Normal Respiratory oxidative burst, Mannan Binding Lectin, Alternative and innate signalling pathways Evidence of efficacy of Rituximab • CD19 count reduced from 46 to 0% • P-ANCA and MPO titres suppressed	Remained on maintenance antibiotic regime Ongoing immunosuppression with Rituximab

Table 1 Timeline of Case *(Continued)*

Four years from first *M.abscessus* culture	Persistent *M. abscessus* smear and culture positivity	Clarithromycin resistance detectable on sputum culture	Cessation of Clarithromycin Further 3 weeks IV Amikacin/Cefoxitin/Tigecycline. Maintenance nebulised Meropenem and Amikacin
Current (Five years from first *M.abscessus* culture)	Intermittent *M.abscessus* smear positivity Persistent culture positivity	Sensitivity of *M.abscessus* being monitored No growth of other organisms including *S.aureus* in sputum since 2012	Pulsed IV antibiotics at intervals determined by clinical symptoms and smear positivity

Table 2 Adaption from RA Floto, KN Olivier, L. Saiman et al.US Cystic Fibrosis Foundation and European Cystic Fibrosis Society consensus recommendations for the management of non-tuberculous mycobacteria in individuals with cystic fibrosis. Thorax; 2016:71:i1-i22; Haworth CS, Banks J, Capstick T et al. British Thoracic Society Guidelines for the Diagnosis and Management of Non-Tuberculous Mycobacterial Pulmonary Disease (NTM-PD). Thorax; 2017;72:2; Lallana EC and Fadul CE. Toxicities of Immunosuppressive Treatment of Autoimmune Neurologic Diseases. Curr Neuropharmacol. 2011 Sep; 9 (3):468–477 [24]

Drug	Common Side Effects
Amikacin	Nephrotoxicity, Ototoxicity: irreversible vestibulocochlear nerve damage.
Azithromycin	Nausea, Vomiting, Diarrhoea, Fulminant Hepatitis, Pseudomembranous Colitis Ototoxicity Prolonged QT
Clarithromycin	Hepatitis Taste Disturbance Prolonged QT
Cefoxitin	Fever, Rash Eosinophilia, Anaemia, Leucopenia, Thrombocytopenia
Clofazimine	Pink Brownish-Black Discoloration of Skin, Ichthyosis and dry skin Enteropathy, Nausea and Vomiting Conjunctival pigmentation, Dimness of vision and dry eyes.
Co-Trimoxazole	Nausea, Vomiting, Diarrhoea Anaemia, Leucopenia, Thrombocytopenia Hyponatraemia, Hyperkalaemia Fever, Rash, Steven Johnson Syndrome
Ethambutol	Optic Neuritis Hyperuricaemia Peripheral Neuropathy
Imipenem	Rash and Urticaria Hepatitis, Nausea, Vomiting Diarrhoea
Linezolid	Anaemia, Leucopenia, Thrombocytopenia Peripheral Neuropathy Optic Neuritis
Moxifloxacin	Nausea, Vomiting, Diarrhoea Insomnia, Agitation, Anxiety Tendonitis Photosensitivity Prolonged QT
Minocycline	Photosensitivity Nausea, Vomiting, Diarrhoea, Dysphagia Vertigo, Headache Skin Hyperpigmentation
Rifampicin	Orange discoloration of bodily fluids Hepatitis, Nausea, Vomiting, Diarrhoea Fever, Chills Thrombocytopenia Renal Failure Increased hepatic metabolism of numerous drugs
Streptomycin	Nephrotoxicity Ototoxicity
Tigecycline	Nausea, Vomiting, Diarrhoea, Pancreatitis, Bilirubinaemia Increased risk of infections: sepsis/septic shock Hypoproteinaemia
Corticosteroids	Cataract Increased risk of infection Type 2 Diabetes Mellitus Osteoporosis Gastrointestinal bleeding Altered Mood – rarely psychosis Proximal myopathy Hypertension
Cyclophosphamide	Leucopenia Haemorrhagic Cystitis

Table 2 Adaption from RA Floto, KN Olivier, L. Saiman et al.US Cystic Fibrosis Foundation and European Cystic Fibrosis Society consensus recommendations for the management of non-tuberculous mycobacteria in individuals with cystic fibrosis. Thorax; 2016:71:i1-i22; Haworth CS, Banks J, Capstick T et al. British Thoracic Society Guidelines for the Diagnosis and Management of Non-Tuberculous Mycobacterial Pulmonary Disease (NTM-PD). Thorax; 2017;72:2; Lallana EC and Fadul CE. Toxicities of Immunosuppressive Treatment of Autoimmune Neurologic Diseases. Curr Neuropharmacol. 2011 Sep; 9 (3):468–477 [24] *(Continued)*

Drug	Common Side Effects
	Infertility Long term increase risk of cancer e.g. Bladder Malignancy, Myeloproliferative disorders Nausea, Hair Loss, Skin Irritation
Azathioprine	Hepatotoxicity, Pancreatitis Leucopenia Fatigue, Hair loss Diarrhoea Increased risk of malignancy
Rituximab	Rash GI upset Serious Infection, CNS toxicity

Striking the balance between managing infection and immunosuppression is an increasing issue in clinical medicine with rising numbers of patients receiving biologics, immunosuppressive agents and increasing lifespan post haematological and solid organ transplants [5, 22, 23]. Oral corticosteroid use is up to eight times higher amongst cases of NTM infection [22]. Rates of NTM-PD are five to ten fold higher in patients on anti-TNF alpha therapies [23]. Whilst other biological agents, carry a theoretical increased risk of NTM there is little data on infection rates [15]. Acquisition of NTM infection is likely due to disruption or depletion of cell mediated immunity which is a critical component of host defence against mycobacterium [14]. Adequate screening of high-risk populations for NTM is necessary to further understanding of disease rates and facilitate appropriate intervention [1, 5, 22] (Table 3).

Table 3 Key Learning points and Patient Perspective

Patient Perspective

"When I was diagnosed with bronchiectasis in my late forties, it did not affect me day to day and I continued to work, raise my family and have an active social life. However, since being diagnosed with *Mycobacterium Abscessus* and Vasculitis, I have struggled with tiredness and progressive shortness of breath especially when exerting myself. I am no longer as active as I wish to be, in particular I struggle to keep up with my toddler grand-daughter and make it around the golf course. However, I make the effort to continue to take light exercise every day by meeting friends for coffee, going shopping and short walks when the weather permits."

Learning Points

- NTM Pulmonary disease is increasing in prevalence and should be screened for in in at risk groups. NTM-PD should also be considered if appropriate radiological appearances and /or symptoms develop in these groups.
- Treatment regimens are toxic and difficult to tolerate and therefore timing of treatment and goals of treatment are important as well as clear communication with patients in this regard
- With increases in therapies which impair immunity the rates of NTM-PD in these groups may continue to rise
- Vasculitis triggered by NTM is a rare but significant complication of NTM and this is the first reported case of this being due to M.Abcessus.
- Balancing effective immunosuppression with active treatment for infection is challenging and requires specialist expertise and collaborative working between specialist services.

Conclusion

Effective treatment of NTM-PD requires effective communication and team working between specialities treating this complex group of patients. Balancing immunosuppressive with anti-microbial regimes and their relative toxicities is challenging and requires frequent assessment, monitoring and treatment adjustment. Further research will refine management approaches and improve our understanding of the role of innate, adaptive and auto-immune dysfunction and the incidence of related complications including vasculitis.

Abbreviations

AFB: Acid Fast Bacilli; ANCA: Anti-Neutrophil Cytoplasmic Antibodies; CT: Computed Tomography; ED: Emergency Department; IFN-γ: Interferon – gamma; IL-17: Interleukin-17; IV: Intra-venous; *M.a.abscessus*: Mycobacterium abscessus abscessus; *M.a.bolletii*: Mycobacterium abscessus bolletii; *M.a.massiliense*: Mycobacterium abscessus massiliense; *M.abscessus*: Mycobacterium abscessus; MPO-ANCA: Myeloperoxidase Anti-Neutrophil Cytoplasmic Antibodies; NTM: Non-Tuberculous Mycobacteria; NTM-PD: Non-Tuberculous Mycobacterial Pulmonary disease; P-ANCA: Perinuclear Anti-Neutrophil Cytoplasmic Antibodies; PR3-ANCA: Proteinase – 3-Anti-Neutrophil Cytoplasmic Antibodies; *S.Aureus*: Staphyloccocus aureus; TNF-alpha: Tumour Necrosis Factor - alpha

Acknowledgements

Not applicable.

Funding

Not applicable.

Authors' contributions

CA and GD were major contributors to writing and creating the manuscript. AJ, GW, SC and DGD contributed to writing and editing the manuscript. All authors read and approved the final manuscript.

Authors' information

The authors represent the complexity in managing this case across multiple hospital sites and specialities. Respiratory speciality input has been provided both at Belfast City Hospital, Belfast (CA, GD, SC and DGD) and at Royal Brompton and Harefield Hospital London (AJ) with Rheumatology specialist input provided at Musgrave Hospital, Belfast (GW).

Consent for publication

Written informed consent for publication of their clinical details and/or clinical images was obtained from the patient. A copy of the consent form is available for review by the Editor of this journal.

Competing interests

The authors declare that they have no competing interests.

Author details

[1]Centre for Experimental Medicine, Queen's University Belfast, 97 Lisburn Road, Belfast BT9 7BL, Northern Ireland. [2]Regional Respiratory Centre, Belfast City Hospital, 51 Lisburn Road, Belfast BT9 7AB, Northern Ireland. [3]Department of Respiratory Medicine, Royal Brompton Hospitals, Sydney Street, London SW3 6NP, England. [4]Department of Rheumatology, Musgrave Park Hospital, Stockmans Ln, Belfast BT9 7JB, Northern Ireland.

References

1. Bonaiti G, Pesci A, Marruchella A, et al. Nontuberculous Mycobacteria in Noncystic Fibrosis Bronchiectasis. BioMed Res Int. 2015;2015:197950. https://doi.org/10.1155/2015/197950.
2. Moore J, Kruijsharr M, Ormerod LP, et al. Increasing reports on non-tuberculous mycobacteria in England, Wales and Northern Ireland, 1995–2006. BMC Public Health. 2010;10:612.
3. Griffith DE, Aksamit T, Brown-Elliott BA, et al. An official ATS/IDSA statement: diagnosis, treatment, and prevention of nontuberculous mycobacterial diseases. Am J Respir Crit Care Med. 2007;175(4):367–416.
4. Floto RA, Olivier KN, L. Saiman et al.US Cystic Fibrosis Foundation and European cystic fibrosis society consensus recommendations for the management of non-tuberculous mycobacteria in individuals with cystic fibrosis. Thorax. 2016;71:i1–i22.
5. Haworth CS, Banks J, Capstick T, et al. British Thoracic Society Guidelines for the Diagnosis and Management of Non-Tuberculous Mycobacterial Pulmonary Disease (NTM-PD). Thorax. 2017;72(Suppl.2).
6. Jarand J, Levin A, Zhang L, et al. Clinical and microbiologic outcomes in patients receiving treatment for Mycobacterium abscessus pulmonary disease. Clin Infect Dis. 2011;52:565–71.
7. Tanaka E, Tada K, Amitani R, et al. Systemic hypersensitivity Vasculitis associated bronchiectasis. Chest. 1992;102(2):647–9.
8. Bruce IN, McAteer JA, Gardiner PV, et al. Chronic supprative lung disease with associated vasculitis. Postgrad Med J. 1995;71:24–7.
9. Tagboto SK, Venkatesh AG. Progressive dyspnoea following the treatment of Mycobacterium abscessus infection in an individual with relapsing granulomatosis with polyangiitis (Wegener's), complicated by hearing loss requiring cochlear implantation. BMC Pulm Med. 2012;12:47.
10. Asano S, Mizuno S, Okachiet S, et al. Antineutrophil cytoplasmic antibody-associated Vasculitis superimposed on infection-related glomerulonephritis secondary to pulmonary Mycobacterium avium complex infection. Intern Med. 2016;55:2439–45.
11. Filiz S, Kocacik Uygun DF, Verhard EM, et al. Cutaneous Leukocytoclastic Vasculitis due to Salmonella enteritidis in a child with Interleukin-12 receptor Beta-1 deficiency. Paediatr Dermatol. 2014;31(2):236–40.
12. Czaja CA, Merkel PA, Chan ED, et al. Rituximab as Successful Adjunct Treatment in a Patient With Disseminated Nontuberculous Mycobacterial Infection Due to Acquired Anti–Interferon-γ Autoantibody. Clin Infect Dis. 2014;58(6):115–8.
13. Wu U-I, Holland SM. Host susceptibility to non-tuberculous mycobacterial infections. Lancet Infect Dis. 2015;15:968–80.
14. Haverkamp MH, Van Diesel JT, Holland SM. Human host genetic factors in nontuberculous mycobacterial infection; lessons from single gene disorders affecting innate and adaptive immunity and lessons from molecular defects in interferon-γ-dependent signalling. Microbes Infect. 2006;8:1157–66.
15. Milanés-Virelles MT, García-García I, Santos-Herrera Y, et al. Adjuvant interferon gamma in patients with pulmonary atypical Mycobacteriosis: a randomized, double blind,placebo-controlled study. BMC Infect Dis. 2008;8:17.
16. Colsky A, Hanly A, Elgart G, Kerdel F. Treatment of Refractory Disseminated Mycobacterium abscessus Infection With Interferon Gamma Therapy. Arch Dermatol. 1999;135(2):125–7.
17. Gallin JI, Farber JM, Holland SM. Interferon-y in the Management of Infectious Diseases. Ann Intern Med. 1995;123:216–24.
18. Rivera R, Alrabaa S, List A, Greene J. Successful Treatment of Refractory Disseminated Mycobacterium abscessus Infection Using Interferon Gamma. Infect Dis Clin Prac. 2011;19(2):142–5.
19. Browne SK, Zaman R, Sampaio E, et al. Anti-CD20 (rituximab) therapy for anti–IFN autoantibody–associated nontuberculous mycobacterial infection. Blood. 2012;119(17):3933–9.
20. Lim A, Allison C, Price P, et al. Susceptibility to pulmonary disease due to mycobacterial avium-intracellulare complex may reflect low IL-17 and high IL-10 responses rather than TH1 deficiency. Clin Immunol. 2017;137:296–320.
21. Szymanski E, Leung JM, Fowler CJ, et al. Pulmonary nontuberculous mycobacterial infection: a multisystem, Multigenic Disease. Am J Respir Crit Care Med. 2015;192(5):618–28.
22. Henkle E, Winthrop K. Nontubercuolous mycobacteria infections in immunocompromised hosts. Clin Chest Med. 2015;36(1):91–9.
23. Winthrop KL, Baxter R, Liu L. Mycobacterial diseases and anti-tumour necrosis factor therapy in USA. Ann Rheum Dis. 2013;72:37–42.
24. Lallana EC, Fadul CE. Toxicities of immunosuppressive treatment of autoimmune neurologic diseases. Curr Neuropharmacol. 2011;9(3):468–77.

15

Role of TLR4-p38 MAPK-Hsp27 signal pathway in LPS-induced pulmonary epithelial hyperpermeability

Weiju Wang†, Jie Weng†, Lei Yu, Qiaobing Huang*, Yong Jiang* and Xiaohua Guo*

Abstract

Background: The breakdown of alveolar barrier dysfunction contributes to Lipopolysaccharide stimulated pulmonary edema and acute lung injury. Actin cytoskeleton has been implicated to be critical in regulation of epithelial barrier. Here, we performed in vivo and in vitro study to investigate role of TLR4-p38 MAPK-Hsp27 signal pathway in LPS-induced ALI.

Methods: For in vivo studies, 6–8-week-old C57 mice were used, Bronchoalveolar lavage Fluid /Blood fluorescent ratio, wet-to-dry lung weight ratio, as well as protein concentrations and neutrophil cell counts in BALF were detected as either directly or indirectly indicators of pulmonary alveolar barrier dysfunction. And hematoxylin and eosin staining was performed to estimate pulmonary injury. The in vitro explorations of transepithelial permeability were achieved through transepithelial electrical resistance measurement and testing of FITC-Dextran transepithelial flux in A549. In addition, cytoskeletal rearrangement was tested through F-actin immunostaining. And SB203580 was used to inhibit p38 MAPK activation, while siRNA was administered to genetically knockdown specific protein.

Results: We showed that LPS triggered activation of p38 MAPK, rearrangement of cytoskeleton which resulted in severe epithelial hyperpermeability and lung edema. A549 pretreated with TLR4 siRNA、 p38 MAPK siRNA and its inhibitor SB203580 displayed a lower permeability and fewer stress fibers formation after LPS stimulation, accompanied with lower phosphorylation level of p38 MAPK and Hsp27, which verified the involvement of TLR4-p38 MAPK-Hsp27 in LPS-evoked alveolar epithelial injury. Inhibition of p38 MAPK activity with SB203580 in vivo attenuated pulmonary edema formation and hyperpermeability in response to LPS.

Conclusions: Our study demonstrated that LPS increased alveolar epithelial permeability both in vitro and in vivo and that TLR4- p38 MAPK- Hsp27 signal pathway dependent actin remolding was involved in this process.

Keywords: ALI, Alveolar barrier dysfunction, P38 MAPK, LPS, TLR4, Hsp27, Cytoskeletal rearrangement

Background

Acute lung injury (ALI) is a clinical syndrome that still remains high (30–40%) rates of mortality in spite of the great advances in mechanism research and therapy [1–3]. Among all the causes, Lipopolysaccharide (LPS), the outer layer of the most Gram-negative bacteria, has been wildly studied [4–6]. It has been frequently implicated that exposure to LPS leads to activation of various signal pathways, production of inflammatory mediators, and endothelial barrier dysfunction [7–9]. All these effects facilitate transcelluar permeability and lead to severe edema during ALI. In addition, accumulated evidences point to a role for alveolar epithelial barrier dysfunction during development of ALI [10–12]. However, the precise mechanism responsible for alveolar epithelial injury in LPS-induced ALI remains to be elusive, which is major theme of this study.

Zhijie et al. have performed an in-vivo study to determine the critical role of Toll-like receptor 4 (TLR4) in LPS-induced ALI [13]. Further studies show that binding of LPS and TLR4 triggers induction of NF-κB as well as mitogen-activated protein kinase (MAPK) signal pathways, leading to severe cellular responses [4]. p38 MAPK

* Correspondence: bing@smu.edu.cn; jiang48231@163.com; lanblue@smu.edu.cn
†Weiju Wang and Jie Weng contributed equally to this work.
Department of Pathophysiology, Guangdong Province Key Laboratory for Shock and Microcirculation Research, Guangdong Provincial Key Laboratory of Proteomics, State Key Laboratory of Organ Failure Research, Southern Medical University, Guangzhou 510515, China

belongs to MAPK family that is involved in a signal cascade responsive to stress stimuli [14]. And the activation of p38 MAPK has been implicated as a critical step in the process of pulmonary barrier dysfunction induced by various stimulus, including pertussis toxin, LPS, and H_2O_2. In addition, emerging evidences highlight role of p38 MAPK in pulmonary epithelial injury [15–19]. These data implicated the putative effect of p38 MAPK on LPS-induced epithelial injury. Hsp27 is considered to be an inhibitor of actin polymerization [20]. It has been shown to regulate actin-containing cytoskeletal structure during endothelial barrier dysfunction. Furthermore, S. Hirano et al. has presented that LPS induced endothelial barrier breakdown was associated with the phosphorylation of Hsp27 [21]. Of note, regardless of the endothelium compromised during the development of sepsis, epithelial breakdown is considered to be key mechanism underlying profound pulmonary impairment [22]. Therefore, we seek to uncover the potential role of TLR4-p38MAPK-Hsp27 signal pathway in LPS-induced pulmonary epithelial hyperpermeability.

Methods

Antibodies and reagents

Monoclonal antibody against F-actin was purchased from abcam. Antibodies against p38、p-p38、Hsp27 、β-actin were purchased from ABclonal. Anti-P-Hsp27 antibody was purchased from CST. TLR4 siRNA、p38 siRNA and control siRNA were synthesized by GenePharma (Shanghai, China). The p38 specific inhibitor SB203580 was obtained from MedChem Express. LPS、DAPI were acquired from Sigma.

Cell culture

Adenocarcinomic human alveolar basal epithelial cells (A549) were cultured in 1640 medium (Gibco) supplemented with 10% fetal bovine serum (Gibco) in humidified incubator with 5% CO_2. Experiments were performed after A549 were grown on specific plates, reaching 80%~ 90% confluences and subsequently substitute the culture medium with serum-free one for 12 h to make sure cells in synchronous growth and quiescent state.

Isolation of mouse pulmonary epithelial cells

6–8-week-old male C57 mice, purchased from the Laboratory Animal Center of Southern Medical University, were maintained under controlled temperature (22 ± 1 °C), humidity (60 ± 10%) and light (12 h/day). All the animals were fasted for 8 h with free access to water before the experiment. All the procedures related to mice were approved by the Animal Care Committee of the Southern Medical University of China and were in strict accordance with the Guide for the Care and Use of Laboratory Animals of the National Institutes of Health.

Mice were anesthetized by an intraperitoneal injection of 1.0% pentobarbital sodium (60 mg/kg) and sacrifized through Cervical dislocation and the lungs were collected in PBS, sliced with scissors, aaand then digested with trypsin in 37 °C for 15 min. Collect the supernatant, while the tissue was further digested with 2 mL collagenase in 37 °C for 15 min. Then 70 μm nylon filter was used and the cell suspension was collected in a new tube, followed by 1200 rpm centrifugation for 5 min. Finally, cells was cultured in 37 °C 5% CO_2 incubator.

Cell permeability measurement

The explorations of transepithelial permeability were achieved through Transepithelial electrical resistance (TEER) measurement and testing of FITC-Dextran transepithelial flux. For TEER measurement, A549 cells were seeded on the upper chamber of 0.4 μm-pore-size-transwells (US,Coming Costar), stimulated with 100 ng/mL LPS for corresponding time, and monolayer permeability was measured with $EVOM_2$ (World Precision Instruments, USA). As for FITC-Dextran transepithelial flux, cells were grown on the transwells as mentioned above, and FITC-labeled dextran (1 mg/mL) was administrated for 45 min, followed by determination of FITC-dextran concentration of upper and bottom chamber using HTS 7000 microplate reader. The permeability coefficient of dextran were calculated as follows: $Pd = [A]/t \times 1/A \times V/[L]$,with [A] represents the concentration of bottom chamber, [L] represents the upper ones, t indicates time in seconds, A refers to the membrane area (in cm^2), and V indicates the volume of the bottom chamber.

Western blotting

Cells were cultured in 6-well plates, and treated with 100 ng/mL LPS. Total proteins were prepared in the extraction buffer containing phosphatase and protease inhibitors, and separated by 10% SDS-PAGE followed by transferred to polyvinylidenedifluoride membranes. Then, Membranes were blocked with 5% BSA and incubated with specific primary antibodies overnight at 4 °C. After three times washing, the membranes were incubated with respective second antibodies at room temperature for 1 h, and subsequently detected with chemiluminescence. Finally, analysis of band density was carried out by an imaging station.

siRNA transfection

Cells were cultured in 6-well plates with 50% ~ 70% confluence, and transfected with pre-prepare siRNA- siRNA-Mate™ complex according to GenePharma' s protocol. After 48 h transfection, cells were incubated with or without 100 ng/mL LPS, followed by the corresponding experiment.

Immunofluorescent

A549 cells were seeded on Microporous Petri dish to confluence. After the indicated treatments, they were washed three times with phosphate buffered saline (PBS), fixed with 4% formaldehyde and sequentially permeabilized in 0.5% Triton X-100 at room temperature. Then cells were blocked with 5% BSA after three times wash in PBS and subjected to incubation of rhodamine-phalloidin (2000 U/L) at room temperature for 1 h, following with three times washing in PBS. Finally, DAPI (1:1000) was administrated to lable the nucleus, and Zeiss LSM780 laser confocal scanning microscope (Zeiss, Germany) was used to detect the Immunofluorescent signals.

Animal models

One hundred 6–8-week-old male C57 mice, purchased from the Laboratory Animal Center of Southern Medical University, were used in these experiments. C57 mice were chosen because this strain is wildly used as models of sepsis. They were randomly divided into 4 groups and each group contains 3–4 mice. Afterwards, they were intraperitoneal injected with 200 μL PBS or PBS-diluted LPS (15 mg/kg) for 8 h. For p38 MAPK inhibitor group, SB203580 was administrated intraperitoneally 2 h before PBS or LPS injection. After injection, mice were kept under controlled temperature (22 ± 1 °C), humidity (60 ± 10%) and light (12 h/day). All the animals were fasted for 8 h with free access to water before the experiment.

Measurements of acute lung injury

Mice were euthanized with 13.3% ethyl carbamate plus 0.5% chloralose intraperitoneal injection (0.65 mL/kg) after indicated treatments. The right lobes of the lung were removed and fixed with 4% paraformaldehyde for 48 h, dehydrated in graded alcohol, and embedded in paraffin, subsequently followed by hematoxylin (H) and eosin (E) staining. The total lung injury score was obtained as previously described [23]. The left lobes were removed and immediately stored in – 80 °C prior to protein analysis. Bronchoalveolar lavage Fluid (BALF) was acquired as previously described [24], with which manual cell counts were performed though hemacytometer and total protein concentration was measured using BCA protein assay. As for lung wet-to-dry weight ratio, the lungs were excised and weighted before and after dried to a constant weight at 55 °C for 72 h.

In vivo epithelial permeability assay

Mice were going through carotid veins cannulation after they were anesthetized, and 1 mL APSS-diluted FITC-dextran (100 mg/kg) were injected through carotid veins. 30 min later, apical blood collection was performed with a heparinized syringe and the blood was centrifuged at 3000 rpm for 15 min to obtain the supernatant. BALF was acquired afterwards. BALF/blood fluorescence intensity ratio was measured with fluorospectrophotometer as indicators of epithelial permeability.

Statistical analysis

All data were analyzed by SPSS16.0 software and presented with means ± SD with more than three independent experiments. One-way ANOVA was used in statistical comparisons with significant level set at $P < 0.05$. LSD posthoc analysis was used to compare data among multiple groups.

Results

In vivo study of LPS-induced pulmonary edema and epithelial hyperpermeability

We performed in vivo studies to determine effect of LPS in ALI, specifically in pulmonary epithelial permeability. We found that LPS-injected mice presented higher BALF/Blood fluorescent intensity ratio (Fig. 1a), implicating the breakdown of pulmonary epithelial barrier. The increased wet-to-dry lung weight ratio (Fig. 1b), and higher protein concentrations (Fig. 1c) as well as increased neutrophil cell counts in BALF (Fig. 1d) presented in LPS-treated mice implicated pulmonary edema and inflammation. Hematoxylin (H) and eosin (E) staining were performed to examine the histological changes in lung. Results showed increased lung injury score with irregular alveolar structure with thickened alveolar septa and discontinuous alveoli as well as more neutrophil infiltration in mice injected with LPS (Fig. 1e). These data indicated that alveolar epithelium dysfunction was involved in LPS-induced ALI.

LPS induced epithelial hyperpermeability and cytoskeleton rearrangement

To further confirm the role of LPS in epithelial permeability, A549 cells, which are widely used as an in vitro model for a type II pulmonary epithelial cells, were stimulated by LPS, and TEER value and permeability coefficient for dextran (Pd) in dextran trans-epithelial flux were evaluated. Data show that TEER was decreased (Fig. 2a) and Pd was gradually increased with significant differences at 12 h (Fig. 2b). When different concentrations of LPS were administrated, cells showing gradually decline trend of TEER (Fig. 2c) and incline trend of Pd (Fig. 2d) with significant differences at 100 ng/mL and 200 ng/mL. These data well confirmed that LPS could induce pulmonary epithelial hyperpermeability. Since cytoskeletal network was considered to be a key component to alveolar barrier integrity, we then monitored F-actin morphological changes to investigate whether LPS induced A549 cytoskeleton rearrangement. We found that after LPS stimulation, the periphery-located F-actin was substituted with centralized stress fibers, and the regular shaped cells with continuous intercellular connections become irregular (Fig. 2e). And

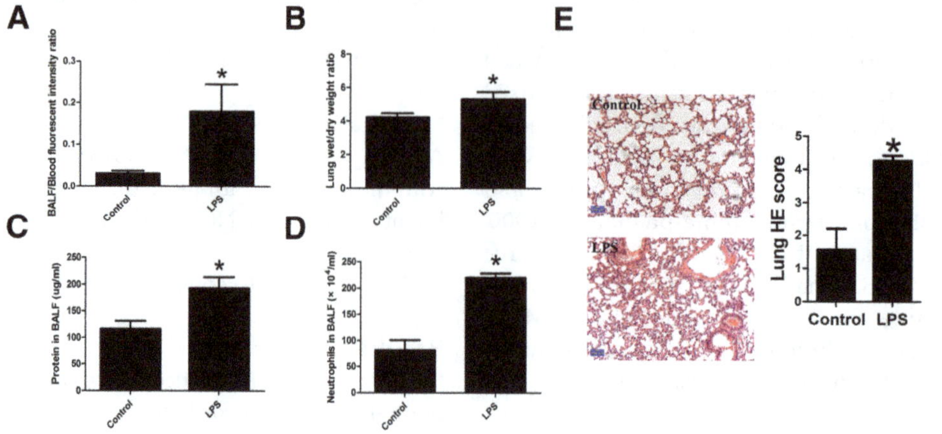

Fig. 1 LPS induce pulmonary edema and alveolar epithelial hyperpermeability in vivo. C57 mice were intraperitoneal injected with PBS or PBS-diluted LPS (15 mg/kg) for 8 h. (**a**) BALF/blood fluorescence intensity ratio and (**b**) Wet-to-dry lung weight ratio were measured; (**c**) protein concentration and (**d**) neutrophil cell counts in BALF were obtained; $n = 3$, $^*P < 0.05$ versus control. (**e**) Lung Hematoxylin and eosin staining were obtained and lung injury score was calculated. $n = 5$, $^*P < 0.05$

the fluorescense intensity was increased after LPS administration in a time dependent manner (Fig. 2f). These data showed that cytoskeletal rearrangement was involved in LPS-induced epithelial barrier dysfunction.

LPS induced p38 MAPK phosphorylation

Due to the pivotal role of p38 MAPK in epithelial injury, we verified whether it is involved in LPS-induced epithelial hyperpermeability. The phosphorylation of p38 MAPK was measured after cells incubated with LPS for different time courses or at different concentrations. Results showed LPS stimulation increased p38 MAPK phosphorylation in a time-dependent manner, with reaching a peak at 30 min (Fig. 3a). Also dose-dependently enhanced p38 MAPK phosphorylation was observed. These results suggested activation of p38 MAPK was involved in LPS-mediated epithelial injury (Fig. 3b).

Role of TLR4 in LPS-induced epithelial hyperpermeability

We next explored whether TLR4 was required for p38 MAPK activation in LPS-induced epithelial hyperpermeability. We First examined that knockdown of TLR4 with siRNA significantly abolished LPS-mediated A549 hyperpermeability, rescued TEER and Pd to normal

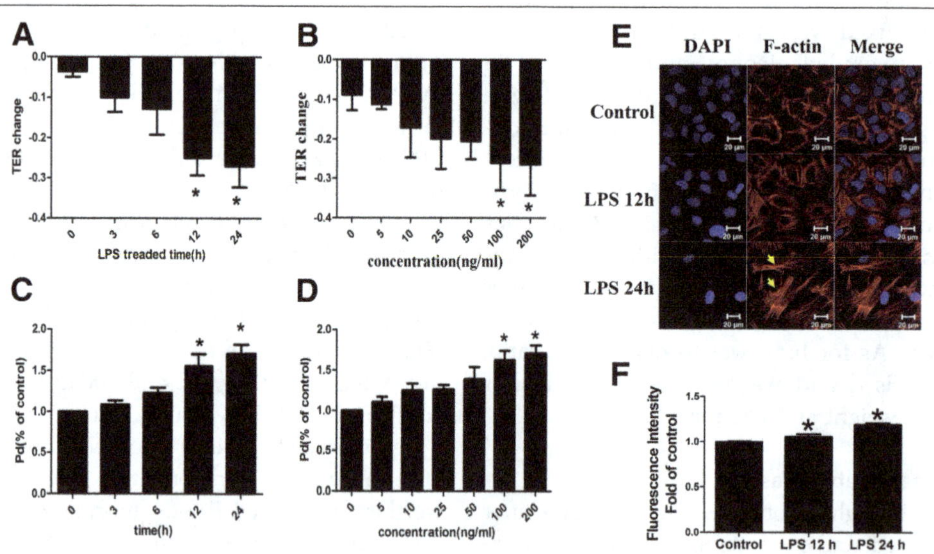

Fig. 2 LPS induce A549 hyperpermeability and cytoskeleton rearrangement. A549 cells were stimulated by LPS in (**a**, **c**) time- or (**b**, **d**) dose-dependent manner, and (**a**, **b**) TER value and (**c**, **d**) permeability coefficient for dextran (Pd) in dextran trans-epithelial flux were evaluated. (**e**) A549 were treated with or without 100 ng/mL LPS and the image of rhodamine-phalloidin stained F-actin was obtained through a laser confocal microscopy; (**f**) Fluorescence intensity of F-actin was qualified. $n = 3$, $^*P < 0.05$ versus control

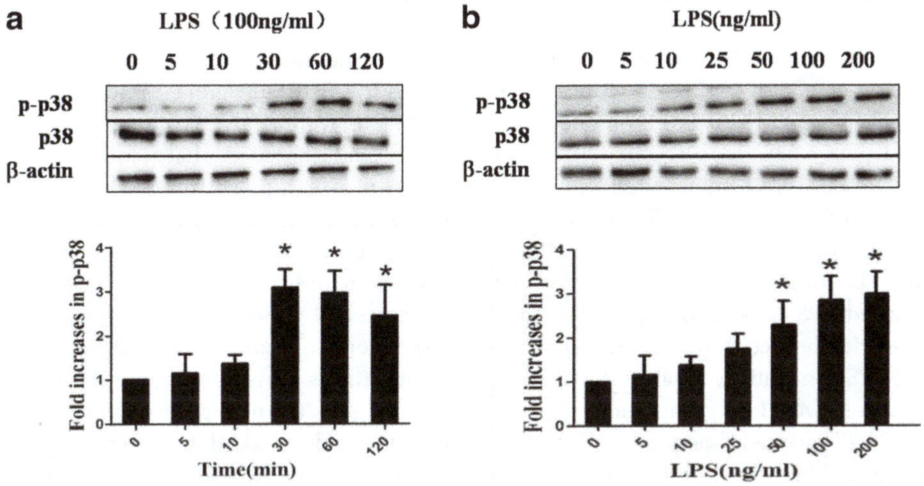

Fig. 3 Effect of LPS on p38 MAPK phosphorylation. A549 cells were stimulated by LPS in (**a**) time- or (**b**) dose-dependent manner. p-p38 was detected by western blotting. $n = 3$, $^{*}P < 0.05$ versus control

level (Fig. 4a, b). As well as the phosphorylation of p38 MAPK induced by LPS was also inhibited by TLR4 siRNA (Fig. 4c). Since Hsp27 was considered to be a downstream signal molecule of p38 MAPK, and the phosphorylation of Hsp27 was reported to be a key factor to regulate cytoskeletal alteration, we therefore investigated whether Hsp27 activation was involved in this process. Predictably, we found that LPS-mediated Hsp27 phosphorylation and F-actin rearrangement were blocked by TLR4 siRNA pretreatment (Fig. 4c, d). Fluorescence intensity of F-actin was qualified (Fig 4e).These data suggested that LPS-evoked p38MAPK-Hsp27 activation via TLR4.

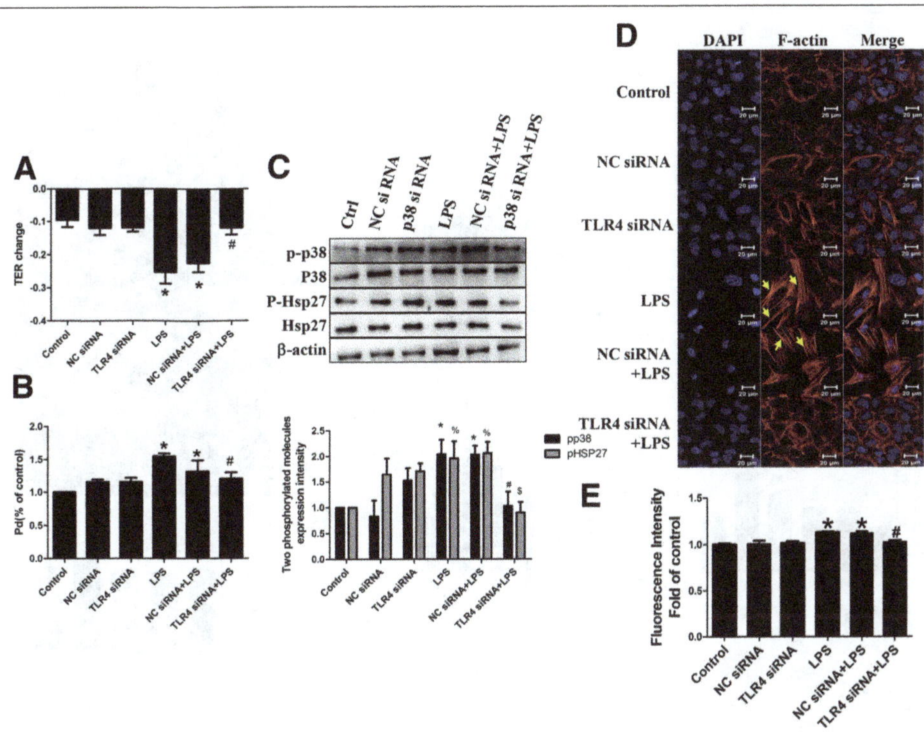

Fig. 4 Role of TLR4 in LPS-induced A549 hyperpermeability. A549 was pretreated with TLR4 siRNA followed by LPS exposure. (**a**) TER value and (**b**) permeability coefficient for dextran (Pd) in dextran trans-epithelial flux were measured; (**c**) P-p38 and P-Hsp27 were detected by western blotting; (**d**) The image of rhodamine-phalloidin stained F-actin was obtained through a laser confocal microscopy; (**e**) Fluorescence intensity of F-actin was qualified. $n = 3$, $^{*}P < 0.05$ versus control, $^{\#}P < 0.05$ versus LPS

Role of p38 MAPK in LPS-induced epithelial hyperpermeability

So far, we have identified that p38 MAPK was activated in response to combination of LPS and TLR4 in vitro. To further understand the role of p38 MAPK in LPS-induced epithelial barrier dysfunction, p38 MAPK siRNA or the selective inhibitor SB203580 were administrated before LPS stimulation. Results showed that p38 MAPK siRNA significantly reversed LPS-induced epithelial hyperpermeability (Fig. 5a, b). Western blotting analysis showed that p38 MAPK siRNA attenuated LPS- mediated Hsp27 phosphorylation (Fig. 5c). In addition, cells pretreated with p38 MAPK siRNA before LPS stimulation, exhibited fewer stress fibers formation compared with LPS group, indicating that p38 siRNA prevented LPS-induced F-actin remolding (Fig. 5d). Fluorescence intensity of F-actin was qualified (Fig. 5e). Accordingly, inhibition of p38 MAPK with SB203580 blocked Hsp27 phosphorylation induced by LPS (Fig. 6c), reversed LPS-mediated cytoskeleton rearrangement (Fig. 6d, e) and thus attenuated LPS-evoked A549 hyperpermeability (Fig. 6a, b). We also examined the F-actin rearrangement induced by LPS in primary mice pulmonary epithelial cells, and got the same effects (Fig. 6f).

In vivo study of effects of p38 MAPK in LPS-induced ALI

To further verify involvement of p38 MAPK activation in LPS-mediated ALI in vivo, p38 inhibitor SB203580 was administered before LPS injection, and the severity of ALI as well as alveolar barrier dysfunction was evaluated. Data showed that, compared with LPS group, mice pretreated with SB 203580 followed by LPS injection presented decreased wet-to-dry lung weight ratio (Fig. 7b), lower protein concentration (Fig. 7c) and less neutrophil cell counts (Fig. 7d) in BALF, and decreased BALF/blood fluorescence intensity ratio (Fig. 7a) when compared with LPS counterparts. All these observations implicated that inhibition of p38 MAPK activity significantly reversed LPS-mediated pulmonary edema and epithelial hyperpermeability. Results of Hematoxylin (H) and eosin (E) staining showed that SB203580 attenuated LPS-mediated alveolar structure disruption and neutrophil infiltration, indicated by decreased lung injury score with ameliorated irregulation of alveolar structure as well as decreased neutrophil infiltration when compared with LPS, suggesting that activation of p38 MAPK was involved in LPS-mediated ALI (Fig. 7e).

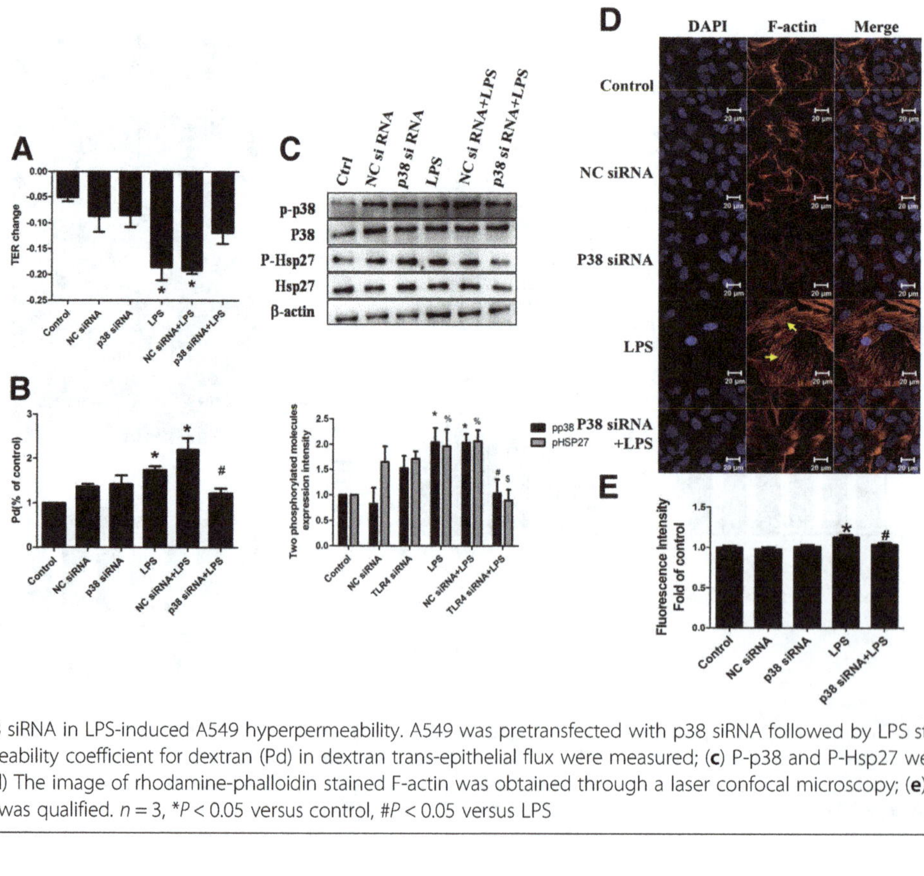

Fig. 5 Effect of p38 siRNA in LPS-induced A549 hyperpermeability. A549 was pretransfected with p38 siRNA followed by LPS stimulation. (**a**) TER value and (**b**) permeability coefficient for dextran (Pd) in dextran trans-epithelial flux were measured; (**c**) P-p38 and P-Hsp27 were detected by western blotting; (**d**) The image of rhodamine-phalloidin stained F-actin was obtained through a laser confocal microscopy; (**e**) Fluorescence intensity of F-actin was qualified. $n = 3$, $^*P < 0.05$ versus control, $\#P < 0.05$ versus LPS

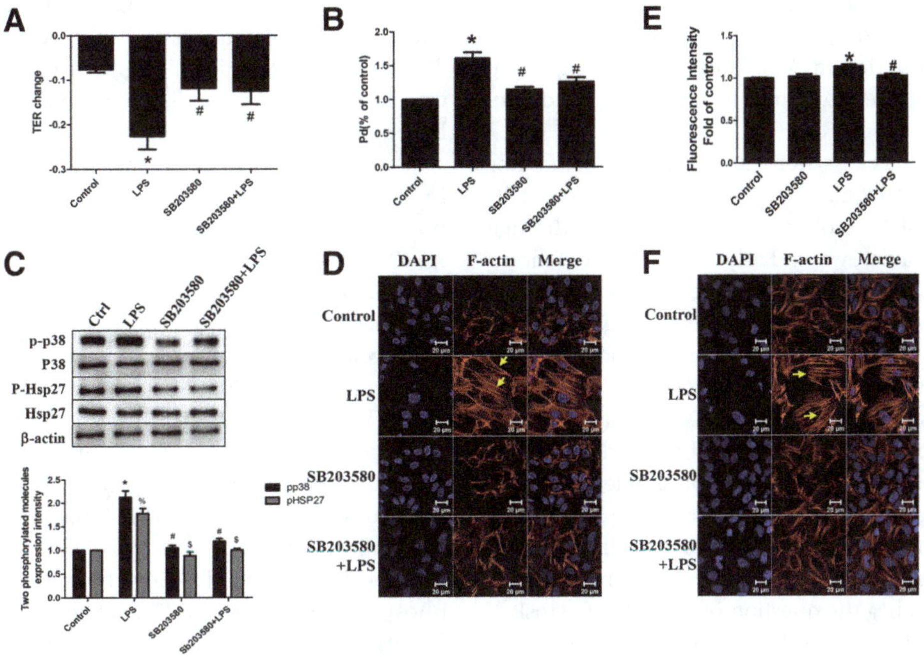

Fig. 6 Role of p38 inhibitor SB203580 in LPS-induced A549 hyperpermeability. A549 was pretreated with SB203580 followed by LPS exposure. (**a**) TER value and (**b**) permeability coefficient for dextran (Pd) in dextran trans-epithelial flux were measured; (**c**) P-p38 and P-Hsp27 were detected by western blotting; (**d**) The image of rhodamine-phalloidin stained F-actin was obtained through a laser confocal microscopy; (**e**) Fluorescence intensity of F-actin was qualified; (**f**) The image of rhodamine-phalloidin stained F-actin was obtained through a laser confocal microscopy by using primary mice pulmonary epithelial cells. $n = 3$, $^*P < 0.05$ versus control, $\#P < 0.05$ versus LPS

Discussion

LPS-mediated ALI has been primarily characterized by severe edema that is caused by alveolar-capillary barrier dysfunction [25], with numerous available evidences support the critical role of pulmonary epithelium in this syndrome of respiratory failure [10, 26]. Gorin AB et al. had performed a precise study demonstrating that pulmonary epithelium accounted for more than 92% of resistance effect to albumin transit across the barrier, and that epithelial injury alone are sufficient in pulmonary edema formation

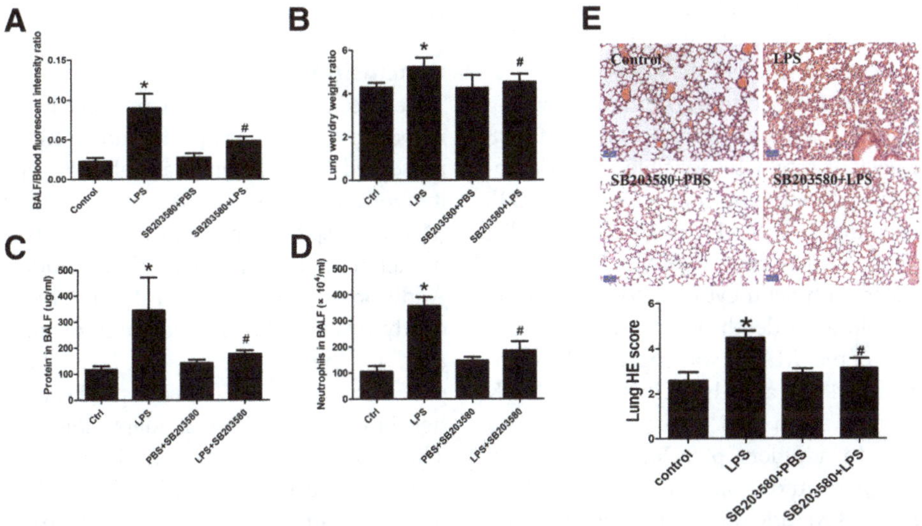

Fig. 7 In vivo study of effect of p38 MAPK in LPS-induced ALI. C57 mice were pretreated with SB203580 before LPS (15 mg/kg) injection. (**a**) BALF/blood fluorescence intensity ratio and (**b**) Wet-to-dry lung weight ratio were measured; (**c**) protein concentration and (**d**) neutrophil cell counts in BALF were obtained; $n = 3{\sim}4$, $^*P < 0.05$ versus control. (**e**) Lung Hematoxylin and eosin staining were obtained and lung injury score was calculated. $n = 5$, $^*P < 0.05$

[27]. This data, accompanying with other emerging evidences [11, 28] strongly spotlight pulmonary epithelium barrier dysfunction in ALI. Therefore, we highlight effect of alveolar epithelium in current study of LPS-induced ALI.

Epithelium serves as a barrier between the air-containing and the aqueous interstitial compartment. It is structurally optimized to regulate molecular transportation through trans- and paracellular ways. Early investigations shown that cytochalasin D and B, the actin altering agents, can increase epithelial permeability [29, 30], indicating the potential relationship between actin dynamics and epithelial barrier dysfunction. In addition, it has been well recognized that intracellular stress fiber formation is strongly related to cellular hyperpermeability. As reviewed by Rodgers, stress fibers resulted from actin polymerization is one of the primary elements that comprises the contractile machinery in cells and has been suggested with increased cell contractility, which is responsible for intracellular gap formation [28]. These observations beg the question of the role of cytoskeleton rearrangement in LPS-induced epithelial hyperpermeability, which remains the major theme of this study [31].

Firstly, in vivo studies were performed to investigate whether alveolar-capillary permeability was increased after mice exposure to LPS. Results presented increased wet-to-dry lung weight ratio, higher protein concentration as well as more neutrophil cell counts in BALF, higher score of total lung injury, and enhanced BALF/blood fluorescence intensity ratio, all of which indirectly or directly indicated that LPS induce breakdown of alveolar barrier integrity. This impairment was confirmed by decline of TEER and incline of Pd in dextran trans-epithelial flux in LPS-stimulated A549 cells. Afterwards, our postulation, cytoskeleton remodeling is involved in this process, was certified by morphological alteration of A549 compatible with the enhancement of stress fibers.

Sequentially, we sought to shed light on the underlying mechanism. It has been frequently implicated that p38 MAPK is either partially or totally responsible for endothelial actin polymerization during lung injury [5, 15, 32, 33]. It could also be shown that p38 MAPK mediated epithelial hyperpermeability [34]. In other cases, p38 MAPK was suggested to be cooperated with actin cytoskeleton alternation in epithelium [33]. More in-depth mechanism analysis suggest that activation of p38 MAPK was triggered by combination of LPS and TRL4 [4], and that TLR4-p38 MAPK signal pathway was involved in LPS mediated pulmonary edema formation [6]. In addition, p38 MAPK has been considered to be the upstream of Hsp27. And Hsp27 phosphrylation induced by p38 MAPK was associated with actin filament dependent endothelial hyperpermeability caused by LPS [17]. Further work showed that unphosphorylated Hsp27 binds to actin, while phosphorylated Hsp27 dissociates from actin, which facilitates actin polymerization and stress fiber formation [35]. Given those information, we naturally postulated that LPS-mediated activation of TLR4-p38 MAPK-Hsp27 signal pathway is involved in cytoskeleton rearrangement dependent alveolar epithelial hyperpermeability.

To this end, we testified that p38 was activated by LPS in A549 cells in a time- and concentration-dependent manner. Then, role of TLR4 in LPS in LPS-mediated A549 hyperpermeability was investigated by using TLR4 siRNA. Data showed that knockdown of TLR4 abolished LPS-mediated p38 and Hsp27 phosphrylation, attenuated LPS-evoked A549 hyperpermeability, and suppressed LPS-triggered cytoskeleton rearrangement, suggesting that TLR4 is involved in LPS induced pulmonary epithelial barrier dysfunction and act upstream of p38 and Hsp27. Subsequently, we testified that either genetically knockdown of p38 with siRNA or pharmacologically inhibit p38 activation with SB203580 would significantly reverse LPS-induced A549 hyperpermeability, reduce phosphorylation of Hsp27 evoked by LPS, and suppress LPS-triggered cytoskeleton rearrangement, suggesting that priming activation of p38 MAPK leads to subsequent phosphorylation of Hsp27 which in turn triggers rearrangement of actin filament and breakdown of pulmonary epithelial barrier. Afterwards, SB203580 were used in C57 mice to further confirm the pivotal role of p38 MAPK in LPS-induced ALI. Data presented decreased wet-to-dry lung weight ratio, lower protein concentration and less neutrophil cell counts in BALF, lower score of total lung injury, and decreased BALF/blood fluorescence intensity aratio, suggesting that inactivation of p38 MAPK significantly reverses LPS-induced ALI and alveolar epithelial hyperpermeability.

Conclusion

Taken together, in the current study, we highlighted the response of alveolar epithelium to LPS-induced ALI, and presented that LPS increase alveolar epithelial permeability both in vitro and in vivo. Furthermore, TLR4- p38 MAPK- Hsp27 signal pathway was studied in an in vitro model to better understand the underlying mechanism. Additionally, we presented that inhibit p38 MAPK significantly reverse LPS-induced pulmonary epithelial dysfunction, and hence release ALI. These findings add to other promising endothelial based studies advance our comprehension of multicellular adaptation to LPS-induced ALI. The dysregulation of epithelial function during sepsis contributes to leakage of fluid and even inflammatory mediators into air-containing alveolar space, which leads to severe edema and may favor the development secondary infection. Therefore, septic alveolar epithelium should be considered either therapeutic or diagnostic targets to improve outcomes in patients.

Abbreviations

ALI: Acute lung injury; BALF: Bronchoalveolar lavage fluid; HE: Hematoxylin and eosin; LPS: Lipopolysaccharide; PBS: Phosphate buffered saline; TEER: Transepithelial electrical resistance

Acknowledgements

We thank Biying zhou for providing technical support in mice experiment.

Funding

This work was supported by National Natural Science Foundation of China (81670076, 31871183, 81372030); Guangdong Natural Science Foundation (2014A030313301, 2017A030313462); General Program from Natural Science Foundation of China (81370226,81170297); The Team-project of Natural Science Foundation of Guangdong, China (S2013030013217); Grant of NSFC-Guangdong Joint Foundation of China (U1601225); Key Scientific and Technological Program of Guangzhou City (201607020016); Special Funds for the Cultivation of Guangdong College Students' Scientific and Technological Innovation [pdjh2017a0095]. The funding bodies had no role in the design of the study and collection, analysis, and interpretation of data and in writing the manuscript.

Authors' contributions

QH, YJ and XG conceived the study, arranged the collaboration, edited and compiled the final version for submission. JW initiated the manuscript and participated in its design. WW, JW, and LY performed laboratory and studied design. All authors reviewed and approved the final manuscript.

Consent for publication

Not applicable.

Competing interests

The authors declare that they have no competing interests.

References

1. Dossow-Hanfstingl W. Advances in therapy for acute lung injury[J]. Anesthesiol Clin. 2012;30(4):629–39.
2. Bosmann M, Ward PA. Protein-based therapies for acute lung injury: targeting neutrophil extracellular traps.[J]. Expert Opin Ther Targets. 2014;18(6):703–14.
3. Leng YX, Yang SG, Song YH, et al. Ulinastatin for acute lung injury and acute respiratory distress syndrome: a systematic review and meta-analysis[J]. World J Crit Care Med. 2014;3(1):34.
4. Lu YC, Yeh WC, Ohashi PS. LPS/TLR4 signal transduction pathway[J]. Cytokine. 2008;42(2):145–51.
5. Reiss LK, Uhlig U, Uhlig S. Models and mechanisms of acute lung injury caused by direct insults[J]. Eur J Cell Biol. 2012;91(6–7):590–601.
6. Liu H, Yu X, Yu S, et al. Molecular mechanisms in lipopolysaccharide-induced pulmonary endothelial barrier dysfunction[J]. Int Immunopharmacol. 2015;29(2):937–46.
7. Lipke AB, Matutebello G, Herrero R, et al. Death receptors mediate the adverse effects of febrile-range hyperthermia on the outcome of lipopolysaccharide-induced lung injury.[J]. Am J Physiol Lung Cell Mol Physiol. 2011;301(1):L60.
8. Herold S, Tabar TS, Janssen H, et al. Exudate macrophages attenuate lung injury by the release of IL-1 receptor antagonist in gram-negative pneumonia[J]. Am J Respir Crit Care Med. 2011;183(10):1380.
9. Hou YC, Chiu WC, Yeh CL, et al. Glutamine modulates lipopolysaccharide-induced activation of NF-κB via the Akt/mTOR pathway in lung epithelial cells.[J]. Am J Physiol Lung Cell Mol Physiol. 2012;302(1):L174.
10. Sartori C, Matthay MA. Alveolar epithelial fluid transport in acute lung injury: new insights[J]. Eur Respir J. 2002;20(5):1299–313.
11. Zhou G, Dada LA, Sznajder JI. Regulation of alveolar epithelial function by hypoxia[J]. Eur Respir J. 2008;31(5):1107–13.
12. Rezaee F, DeSando SA, Ivanov AI, et al. Sustained protein kinase D activation mediates respiratory syncytial virus-induced airway barrier disruption[J]. J Virol. 2013;87(20):11088–95.
13. He Z, Chen X, Wang S, et al. Toll-like receptor 4 monoclonal antibody attenuates lipopolysaccharide-induced acute lung injury in mice[J]. Exp Ther Med. 2014;8(3):871–6.
14. Qian F, Deng J, Wang G, et al. Pivotal role of mitogen-activated protein kinase-activated protein kinase 2 in inflammatory pulmonary diseases[J]. Curr Protein Pept Sci. 2016;17(4):332–42.
15. Garcia JGN, Wang P, Schaphorst KL, et al. Critical involvement of p38 MAP kinase in pertussis toxin-induced cytoskeletal reorganization and lung permeability[J]. Faseb J Off Publ Fed Am Soc Exp Biol. 2002; 16(9):1064.
16. Chen P, Cai Y, Yang ZG, et al. Involvement of PKC, p38 MAPK and AP-2 in IL-1beta-induced expression of cyclooxygenase-2 in human pulmonary epithelial cells[J]. Respirology. 2006;11(1):18–23.
17. Liu T, Guevara OE, Warburton RR, et al. Modulation of hsp27 alters hypoxia-induced endothelial permeability and related signaling pathways[j]. J Cell Physiol. 2009;220(3):600–10.
18. Kolosova I, Nethery D, Kern JA. Role of Smad2/3 and p38 MAP kinase in TGF-β1-induced epithelial–mesenchymal transition of pulmonary epithelial cells[J]. J Cell Physiol. 2011;226(5):1248–54.
19. Ning W, Song R, Li C, et al. TGF-beta1 stimulates HO-1 via the p38 mitogen-activated protein kinase in A549 pulmonary epithelial cells[J]. Am J Physiol Lung Cell Mol Physiol. 2002;283(5):L1094.
20. Mounier N, Arrigo AP. Actin cytoskeleton and small heat shock proteins: how do they interact?[J]. Cell Stress Chaperones. 2002;7(2):167–76.
21. Hirano S, Rees RS, Yancy SL, et al. Endothelial barrier dysfunction caused by LPS correlates with phosphorylation of HSP27 in vivo[J]. Cell Biol Toxicol. 2004;20(1):1–14.
22. Chawla LS, Fink M, Goldstein SL, et al. The epithelium as a Target in Sepsis[J]. Shock. 2016;45(3):249–58.
23. Bastarache JA, Sebag SC, Clune JK, et al. Low levels of tissue factor lead to alveolar haemorrhage, potentiating murine acute lung injury and oxidative stress[J]. Thorax. 2012;67(12):1032–9.
24. Su X, Song Y, Jiang J, et al. The role of aquaporin-1 (AQP1) expression in a murine model of lipopolysaccharide-induced acute lung injury[J]. Respir Physiol Neurobiol. 2004;142(1):1–11.
25. Herold S, Gabrielli NM, Vadasz I. Novel concepts of acute lung injury and alveolar-capillary barrier dysfunction[J]. Am J Physiol Lung Cell Mol Physiol. 2013;305(10):L665–81.
26. Frank JA. Claudins and alveolar epithelial barrier function in the lung[J]. Ann N Y Acad Sci. 2012;1257:175–83.
27. Gorin AB, Stewart PA. Differential permeability of endothelial and epithelial barriers to albumin flux.[J]. J Appl Physiol Respir Environ Exerc Physiol. 1980; 47(6):1315–24.
28. Rodgers LS, Fanning AS. Regulation of epithelial permeability by the actin cytoskeleton[J]. Cytoskeleton (Hoboken). 2011;68(12):653–60.
29. Ma TY, Hollander D, Le TT, et al. Cytoskeletal regulation of Caco-2 intestinal monolayer paracellular permeability[J]. J Cell Physiol. 1995; 164(3):533–45.
30. Madara JL, Barenberg D, Carlson S. Effects of cytochalasin D on occluding junctions of intestinal absorptive cells: further evidence that the cytoskeleton may influence paracellular permeability and junctional charge selectivity.[J]. J Cell Biol. 1986;102(6):2125.
31. Wu JT, Tu MC, Zhung P. Advanced glycation end product (AGE): characterization of the products from the reaction between D-glucose and serum albumin[J]. J Clin Lab Anal. 1996;10(1):21–34.
32. Chu ZG, Zhang JP, Song HP, et al. p38 MAP kinase mediates burn serum-induced endothelial barrier dysfunction: involvement of F-actin rearrangement and L-caldesmon phosphorylation[J]. Shock. 2010;34(3):222.

33. Ng CT, Fong LY, Sulaiman MR, et al. Interferon-gamma increases endothelial permeability by causing activation of p38 MAP kinase and actin cytoskeleton alteration[J]. J Interf Cytokine Res. 2015;35(7):513.
34. Wang Q, Guo XL, Wells-Byrum D, et al. Cytokine-induced epithelial permeability changes are regulated by the activation of the p38 mitogen-activated protein kinase pathway in cultured Caco-2 cells.[J]. Shock. 2008;29(4):531–7.
35. Sun HB, Ren X, Liu J, et al. HSP27 phosphorylation protects against endothelial barrier dysfunction under burn serum challenge[J]. Biochem Biophys Res Commun. 2015;463(3):377–83.

The usefulness of pleural fluid presepsin, C-reactive protein, and procalcitonin in distinguishing different causes of pleural effusions

Naoki Watanabe[1*], Tomoya Ishii[1], Nobuyuki Kita[1], Nobuhiro Kanaji[1], Hiroyuki Nakamura[2], Nobuki Nanki[3], Yutaka Ueda[4], Yasunori Tojo[5], Norimitsu Kadowaki[1] and Shuji Bandoh[1]

Abstract

Background: We aimed to determine the presepsin concentration in pleural fluid from patients with pleural effusions of different aetiologies and to compare its diagnostic value with that of pleural fluid C-reactive protein (CRP) and procalcitonin (PCT).

Methods: We enrolled 132 patients with pleural effusion who underwent diagnostic evaluation, and we classified them into six categories: empyema, parapneumonic effusion, tuberculous effusion, malignant effusion, paramalignant effusion, and transudate effusion. Additionally, all pleural effusions were categorised as infectious or non-infectious effusions.

Results: Receiver operating characteristic analysis was used to evaluate diagnostic performance. When diagnosing empyema, the marker with the highest sensitivity was pleural fluid presepsin (cut-off: 754 pg/mL; sensitivity: 90.9%, specificity: 74.4%) and that with the highest specificity was pleural fluid CRP (cut-off: 4.91 mg/dL; sensitivity: 63.6%, specificity: 89.3%). Pleural fluid PCT tended to be lower in patients with empyema than in those with parapneumonic effusion, but this was not useful for the diagnosis of empyema. When diagnosing infectious pleural effusion, a combination of pleural fluid CRP (cut-off: 2.59 mg/dL) and presepsin (cut-off: 680 pg/mL) produced the highest diagnostic accuracy (83.3%).

Conclusions: Pleural fluid presepsin was found at high levels in patients with empyema and parapneumonic effusion. This pattern closely resembles the previously reported pattern of pleural fluid CRP. Some combinations of pleural fluid inflammatory markers may be more clinically useful than these markers in isolation.

Keywords: Presepsin, C-reactive protein, Procalcitonin, Empyema, Pleural effusion

Background

To investigate the aetiology of pleural effusion, a variety of examinations are typically performed, including pleural fluid cell and differential white blood cell counts, cytological examination, and bacterial culture following Light's criteria [1]. However, the information obtained by these methods is limited, and delays in the diagnosis and the initiation of appropriate therapy for infectious effusions can increase the rate of complications. Therefore, rapid diagnosis and determination of whether the cause of pleural effusion is infection are beneficial in the treatment of this condition.

Although clinical microbiology testing can confirm the presence of infection, a positive culture is observed in only about 60% of parapneumonic effusions, and the time required to obtain a positive culture can be prolonged [2]. Various pleural biomarkers have therefore been investigated as methods for differentiating infectious pleural effusion [3–5].

* Correspondence: naoki-w@med.kagawa-u.ac.jp
[1]Department of Internal Medicine, Hematology, Rheumatology and Respiratory Medicine, Faculty of Medicine, Kagawa University, 1750-1 Ikenobe, Miki-cho, Kita-gun, Kagawa 761-0793, Japan
Full list of author information is available at the end of the article

Presepsin, also known as soluble CD14 subtype, is a protein reported to be increased specifically in the blood of patients with sepsis [6] and is therefore used to predict sepsis in patients in emergency or intensive care units [7]. Following stimulation by pathogens, presepsin is released via shedding from the surface of various types of immune cells, including macrophages, monocytes, and neutrophils, which are implicated in phagocytosis and the cleavage of membrane CD14 by lysosomal enzymes from granulocytes in response to bacterial infection [8]. Several studies have confirmed that presepsin is a more specific and sensitive marker for the diagnosis of sepsis compared with C-reactive protein (CRP), interleukin-6 (IL-6), or procalcitonin (PCT) [7], [9–11]. However, few studies have investigated the diagnostic value of presepsin levels in body fluids.

The aim of the present study was to evaluate the pleural fluid concentrations of presepsin, CRP, and PCT in patients with pleural effusions of various causes and to explore the usefulness of these markers in predicting an infectious aetiology.

Methods

Study design

In this cross-sectional study, we set the target number of cases based on feasibility. An average of 30 thoracentesis procedures are performed at the participating institutions annually. Allowing for ineligible patients and a consent rate of 90%, the target number of cases was set at 135. This study protocol was approved by the institutional review boards of Kagawa University Hospital and all other participating institutions. All patients provided written informed consent prior to participation.

Between November 2015 and March 2017, 145 patients aged ≥18 years with pleural effusion and planned thoracentesis for diagnosis were initially enrolled in the study. Among these, seven patients with chronic maintenance dialysis or continuous hemodiafiltration and six patients with severe renal failure (GFR of < 15 mL/min/1.73 m^2) were excluded from further participation.

Diagnostic criteria

Pleural fluid samples were collected from 132 patients. Each diagnosis was made according to the diagnostic criteria described below. The cases were also categorised as infectious or non-infectious effusions.

We classified the aetiology of pleural effusion into seven categories. 1) Empyema was defined as a grossly purulent pleural effusion accompanied by bacteria detected by Gram staining or a positive culture for bacteria. 2) Parapneumonic effusion was defined as pleural effusion associated with bacterial pneumonia. 3) Tuberculous pleural effusion was based on the presence of a caseous granuloma in the pleural biopsy and/or a positive culture for *Mycobacterium tuberculosis* in the pleural fluid or biopsy material or a positive sputum culture with an exudative pleural effusion and both a clinical and radiological response to anti-tuberculous treatment. 4) Malignant effusion was diagnosed when malignant cells were found in the pleural fluid or in a biopsy specimen. 5) Paramalignant effusion was diagnosed in patients with a known malignancy or subsequent diagnosis of malignancy but with negative cytology and no obvious alternative diagnosis. 6) Transudate effusion was diagnosed by the attending physician based on Light's criteria as well as the general condition of the patient. 7) Any pleural effusion not meeting one of the above diagnostic criteria was categorised as an unclassifiable pleural effusion.

Notably, the cases of unclassifiable pleural effusion were divided into infectious or non-infectious effusions, based on the judgment of the attending physician and the reactivity of the condition to antimicrobial drugs. Therefore, the infectious pleural effusion cases in this study included all the patients with empyema, parapneumonic effusion, and tuberculous pleural effusion as well as those with unclassifiable pleural effusion who were clinically diagnosed as having infectious pleural effusion.

Procedures

Thoracentesis was performed under local anaesthesia. Samples of pleural fluid were immediately subjected to routine examinations for analysis (e.g. pH, total protein, glucose, and lactate dehydrogenase), total and differential cell counts, and cytological and microbiological examination. Pleural fluid was collected in a serum-separating tube for CRP measurement and in a tube containing EDTA for presepsin and PCT measurement. Samples were centrifuged at 1200×*g* for 5 min at 4 °C, and the resulting supernatants were stored at − 30 °C until they were assayed. Simultaneously, venous blood was obtained and analysed for white blood cell count and for lactate dehydrogenase, total protein, blood urea nitrogen, creatinine, and CRP content in addition to any other appropriate assessments ordered by the attending physician. Aliquots of blood plasma were stored at − 30 °C prior to the assessment of presepsin and PCT levels.

Biomarker assays

Assays for the three inflammatory markers, presepsin, CRP, and PCT, were performed on the cell-free supernatants of pleural fluid and blood plasma samples. All samples were tested in random order by technicians blinded to the clinical diagnosis.

Pleural fluid CRP measurement was performed by a latex-enhanced immunoturbidimetric assay at an external clinical laboratory testing facility (SRL Inc., Tokyo, Japan). PCT concentrations in pleural fluid and blood plasma were measured using the Wako i30 micro-total analysis system (μTAS) and Wako–BRAHMS PCT assay (Wako Pure Chemical Industries, Ltd., Osaka, Japan), respectively. Presepsin concentrations in pleural fluid and blood plasma were determined using a compact automated immunoanalyser based on a chemiluminescent enzyme immunoassay (PATHFAST; Mitsubishi Chemical Medience Corporation, Tokyo, Japan).

Statistical analysis

Data are presented as means ± standard deviation (SD) for data with a normal distribution and as medians with interquartile ranges in parentheses for skewed data. Normality of distribution was ascertained using the Shapiro–Wilk test. For comparing categorical data, a chi-squared test was performed. For the evaluation of diagnostic performance, receiver operating characteristic (ROC) analysis was performed, ROC curves were generated by plotting sensitivity against 1-specificity, and the area under the curve (AUC) with 95% confidence intervals (CI) was calculated. The Youden index was used to identify the cut-off values with potential diagnostic significance. All statistical analyses were performed using JMP software version 12.2.0 (SAS institute Inc., Cary, NC, USA), and p-values of < 0.05 were considered statistically significant.

Results

General characteristics of pleural effusions

Of the 132 patients classified as having pleural effusions, 122 (92.4%) were diagnosed with exudative effusion and 10 (7.6%) were diagnosed with transudate effusion. Additionally, 38 (28.8%) patients were diagnosed with infectious pleural effusions, while 94 (71.2%) were diagnosed with non-infectious pleural effusions.

The exudative effusion group was further divided into the following six subgroups according to the diagnosis: empyema, 11 (9.0%); parapneumonic effusion, 16 (13.1%); tuberculous pleural effusion, 9 (7.4%); malignant effusion, 46 (37.7%); paramalignant effusion, 13 (10.7%); and unclassified effusion, 27 (22.1%). Although the attending physician investigated thoroughly to determine the cause of pleural effusion, the cause remained unknown in 17 cases. Among the other 10 cases of unclassified effusion, there were 2 cases associated with pneumothorax, 2 cases of chronic empyema, 1 case associated with collagen disease, 1 case associated with trauma, 1 case associated with interstitial pneumonia, 1 case associated with asbestos, 1 case of chylous pleural effusion, and 1 case of reactive pleural effusion due to *Clonorchis sinensis*. The chronic empyema cases categorised as unclassified effusions did not meet the diagnostic criteria of empyema for this study. Of the 27 unclassifiable pleural effusion cases, only the two chronic empyema cases were judged as being infectious pleural effusion. The demographic data and the pleural fluid characteristics of the 132 patients included in the present study are shown in Table 1.

Pleural fluid levels of presepsin, CRP, and PCT

Presepsin measurements

Pleural fluid presepsin levels were significantly higher in patients with empyema or parapneumonic effusion compared with patients who had other types of effusions. However, no difference in the pleural fluid presepsin level was observed between these two types of effusions (Table 2, Fig. 1a). Presepsin levels were significantly higher in pleural fluid than in blood for all types of effusions.

The diagnostic performance of pleural fluid presepsin values as determined from a ROC analysis is presented in Table 3. Pleural fluid presepsin may represent a useful marker for the differentiation of empyema from other types of effusions. Using a cut-off point of 754 pg/mL, pleural presepsin presented 90.9% sensitivity and 74.4% specificity for the diagnosis of empyema.

A similar cut-off point was observed in another pair comparison. In distinguishing parapneumonic effusion from other types of effusions (excluding empyema) with a cut-off point of 680 pg/mL, the sensitivity was 81.3% and the specificity was 74.3%.

CRP measurements

Pleural fluid CRP levels were significantly higher in patients with empyema, parapneumonic effusion, and tuberculous effusion compared with patients who had malignant or transudate effusions. There was no difference in pleural fluid CRP levels between empyema and parapneumonic effusion cases. Additionally, no difference in pleural fluid CRP levels was observed between malignant effusion, paramalignant effusion, and transudate effusion cases. CRP levels were significantly lower in pleural fluid than in blood for all types of effusions (Table 2, Fig. 1b).

The CRP diagnostic performance based on a ROC analysis of pleural fluid CRP values is presented in Table 4. Pleural fluid CRP was found to represent a useful marker for the diagnosis of empyema; using a cut-off point of 4.91 mg/dL, pleural fluid CRP presented 63.6% sensitivity and 89.3% specificity for the diagnosis of empyema. In distinguishing between infectious effusions and non-infectious effusions, the sensitivity was 65.8% and the specificity was 90.4% when using a pleural fluid CRP cut-off point of 2.59 mg/dL. Pleural fluid CRP showed the highest accuracy compared with pleural fluid presepsin and PCT.

PCT measurements

Pleural fluid PCT levels were significantly higher in patients with parapneumonic effusion compared with patients who had tuberculous effusion, malignant effusion, paramalignant effusion, or transudate effusion. No difference in pleural

Table 1 Demographic data and pleural fluid characteristics ($n = 132$)

	Empyema ($n = 11$)	Parapneumonic ($n = 16$)	Tuberculous ($n = 9$)	Malignant ($n = 46$)	Paramalignant (n = 13)	Transudates ($n = 10$)	Unclassified ($n = 27$)
Age (years)	74.3 ± 11.1	76.7 ± 10.1	76.1 ± 17.4	74.5 (67, 82.3)	77.2 ± 10.9	80.7 ± 9.5	79 (73, 88)
Sex (male/female)	9/2	13/3	4/5	25/21	9/4	9/1	20/7
Pleural fluid white blood cell count	6355 (2160, 23,693)	1870 (963, 6338)	931 (782, 1325)	1290 (890, 2355)	1532 ± 999	658 ± 356	1045 (613, 4029)
Pleural fluid lymphocytes (%)	22.3 ± 22.4	33.3 ± 26.5	81.1 ± 11.3	36.5 (17.3, 63.5)	57.3 ± 28.9	54.9 ± 16.1	73 (35.5, 86.5)
Pleural fluid neutrophils (%)	67.7 ± 31.1	45.5 (8.9, 77.1)	5.2 ± 5.2	5.0 (1.4, 20)	10.0 (4.5, 16.5)	16.1 ± 16.1	8.0 (1.1, 15)
Pleural fluid glucose (mg/dL)	10 (1, 107)	160 ± 62	104 ± 28	106 (74, 123)	104 ± 33	117 (110, 141)	93 ± 43
Total protein in pleural fluid (g/L)	3.8 ± 1.1	3.9 ± 0.6	4.2 ± 0.9	4.6 (3.8, 5.1)	3.9 (3.5, 4.8)	2.7 ± 1.0	4.5 ± 1.1
Total protein in serum (g/L)	6.0 ± 1.1	6.3 (5.8, 6.6)	6.5 ± 0.6	6.8 ± 0.7	6.9 ± 0.7	6.0 (5.3, 6.4)	7.1 ± 1.2
Total protein in pleural fluid/ serum ratio	0.65 ± 0.19	0.67 (0.54, 0.71)	0.64 ± 0.11	0.67 (0.58, 0.72)	0.62 ± 0.10	0.44 ± 0.14	0.63 ± 0.14
Pleural fluid LDH (U/L)	1076 (474, 2522)	496 ± 247	396 ± 250	410 (267, 775)	234 (164, 392)	117 (94, 128)	232 (171, 543)
Serum LDH (U/L)	189 ± 71	254 (194, 325)	205 (186, 245)	269 (237, 395)	240 ± 68	250 (209, 363)	191 (152, 238)
LDH pleural fluid/serum ratio	6.22 (1.41, 29.67)	1.45 (0.90, 3.41)	1.77 ± 1.02	1.25 (0.97, 2.92)	0.88 (0.76, 1.77)	0.42 ± 0.17	1.24 (0.85, 2.45)

LDH, lactate dehydrogenase; Data are presented as the mean ± SD for normally distributed data or as the median (interquartile ranges) for skewed data

fluid PCT levels was observed between empyema and parapneumonic effusion cases. Interestingly, pleural fluid PCT levels tended to be lower in empyema cases than in parapneumonic effusion cases. Pleural fluid PCT levels did not differ from blood PCT levels, except in patients with empyema (Table 2, Fig. 1c).

The PCT diagnostic performance based on a ROC analysis of pleural fluid PCT values is presented in Table 5. This analysis revealed that pleural fluid PCT is unsuitable as a marker for the differentiation of empyema because its AUC was < 0.5. However, pleural fluid PCT may be a useful marker in differentiating parapneumonic effusion from other type of effusions (excluding empyema); when using a cut-off point of 0.11 ng/mL, the sensitivity was 75.0% and the specificity was 79.0%.

The diagnostic accuracy of different marker combinations

The diagnostic accuracy of combined cut-off values for the three inflammatory markers obtained in each ROC analysis is shown in Table 6. To distinguish between empyema and other type of effusions, a pleural fluid presepsin level of > 754 pg/mL and a pleural fluid CRP level of > 4.91 mg/dL yielded the highest accuracy rate (90.9%). Similarly, when distinguishing between infectious pleural

Table 2 Levels of presepsin, CRP, and PCT in the pleural fluid and blood ($n = 105$)

	Empyema ($n = 11$)	Parapneumonic ($n = 16$)	Tuberculous ($n = 9$)	Malignant ($n = 46$)	Paramalignant ($n = 13$)	Transudates ($n = 10$)
Presepsin (pg/mL)						
PF	1496 ± 971	854 (682, 1423)	548 ± 188	463 (347, 609)	438 (319, 812)	531 ± 172
Blood	776 ± 362	395 (251, 851)	392 ± 183	258 (162, 318)	259 (200, 322)	402 ± 144
p-value	0.0139	0.0330	0.0019	< 0.0001	0.0111	0.0125
CRP (mg/dL)						
PF	5.57 ± 4.40	3.67 (2.28, 7.59)	3.29 ± 2.22	0.55 (0.21, 1.48)	0.90 (0.53, 2.46)	0.41 ± 0.43
Blood	19.11 ± 9.88	8.04 (2.97, 19.35)	8.06 ± 6.18	1.62 (0.49, 5.80)	3.12 (1.37, 10.66)	1.00 (0.25, 2.18)
p-value	0.0001	0.0114	0.0047	< 0.0001	0.0069	0.0130
PCT (ng/mL)						
PF	0.30 (0.11, 0.77)	0.28 (0.07, 2.72)	0.08 ± 0.06	0.05 (0.03, 0.10)	0.10 (0.04, 0.50)	0.12 ± 0.08
Blood	1.43 (0.25, 3.26)	0.30 (0.13, 2.13)	0.08 ± 0.05	0.06 (0.03, 0.12)	0.06 (0.04, 0.23)	0.12 ± 0.10
p-value	0.0272	ns	ns	ns	ns	ns

Data are presented as the mean ± SD for normally distributed data or median (interquartile ranges) for skewed data. PF: pleural fluid

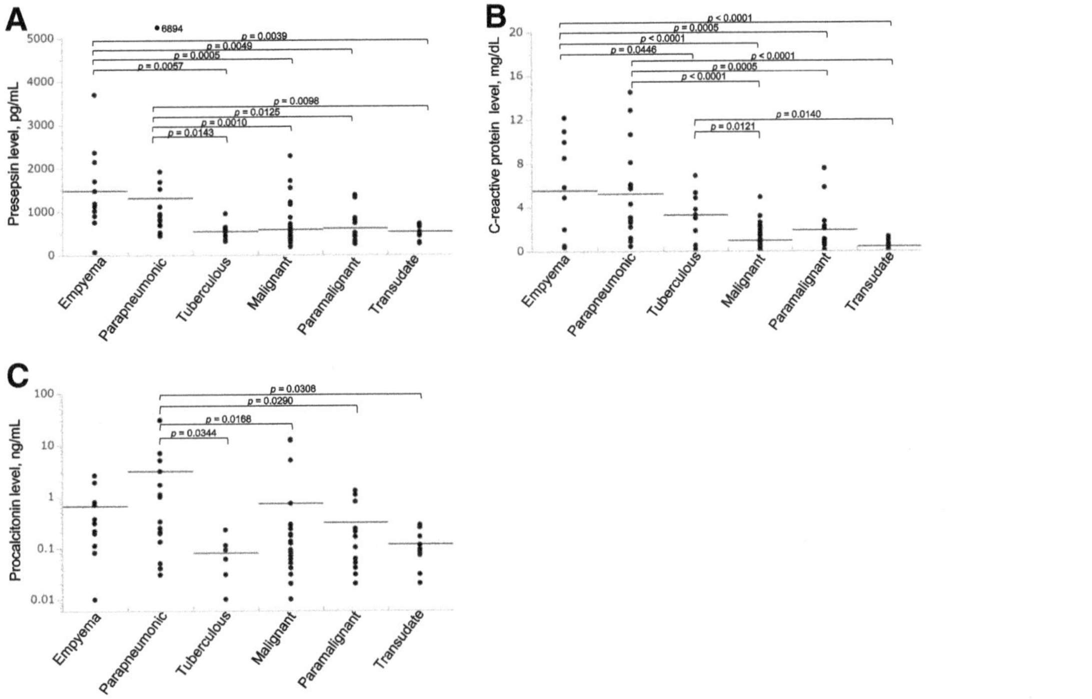

Fig. 1 Pleural fluid presepsin, CRP, and PCT levels. (**a–c**) Pleural fluid presepsin (**a**), CRP (**b**), and PCT (**c**) levels in the different diagnostic subgroups. Individual values are plotted. Bars represent the means of the values, and *p*-values are shown between only groups with statistically significant differences

effusion and non-infectious pleural effusion, the accuracy rate peaked at 83.3% for pleural fluid presepsin levels of > 680 pg/mL and pleural fluid CRP levels of > 2.59 mg/dL. Furthermore, when distinguishing between parapneumonic pleural effusion and other types of effusions (excluding empyema in both groups), pleural fluid presepsin levels of > 680 pg/mL and pleural fluid CRP levels of > 2.18 mg/dL yielded the highest accuracy rate (90.1%). The combination of pleural fluid PCT levels of < 2.57 ng/mL and pleural fluid CRP levels of > 4.91 mg/dL yielded the second highest accuracy rate (87.9%) in the differentiation of empyema. The combination of PCT and CRP also showed better accuracy than the combination of PCT and presepsin in distinguishing between infectious and non-infectious pleural effusion, parapneumonic pleural effusion, and other types of effusions (excluding empyema in both groups).

Discussion

We hypothesised that pleural fluid presepsin, CRP, and/or PCT concentration(s) may be of value in the differentiation between several causes of pleural effusions. Thus, this study investigated the diagnostic performance of these three inflammatory markers in the blood and pleural fluid of a well-characterised population of patients with several types of effusions. We found that pleural fluid presepsin levels were significantly higher in cases of empyema and parapneumonic effusion compared with other types of effusions, as well as in cases with infectious pleural effusions compared with non-infectious effusions, although the pleural fluid presepsin level was not elevated in tuberculous effusion cases. Furthermore, pleural fluid presepsin was found to be the most sensitive of the three tested markers for distinguishing between infectious and non-infectious pleural effusions.

Table 3 Diagnostic performance of pleural fluid presepsin based on the ROC analysis ($n = 132$)

	Optimal cut-off point (pg/mL)	Sensitivity (%)	Specificity (%)	+LR	−LR	PPV (%)	NPV (%)	AUC	Accuracy (%)
Emp vs. other	≥754	90.9	74.4	1.39	0.12	24.4	98.9	0.809	75.8
Emp and PE vs. other	≥680	85.2	74.3	3.31	0.20	46.0	95.1	0.803	76.5
Emp, PE, and TB vs. other	≥680	66.7	72.9	2.46	0.46	48.0	85.4	0.728	71.2
PE vs. other (excluding Emp)	≥680	81.3	74.3	3.16	0.25	32.5	96.3	0.785	75.2
Infectious vs. non-infectious	≥680	68.4	74.5	2.68	0.42	52.0	85.4	0.746	72.7

Emp empyema, *PE* parapneumonic effusions, *TB* tuberculosis, *+LR* positive likelihood ratio, *−LR* negative likelihood ratio *PPV* positive predictive value, *NPV* negative predictive value, *AUC* area under the curve

Table 4 Diagnostic performance of pleural fluid CRP based on the ROC analysis ($n = 132$)

	Optimal cut-off point (mg/dL)	Sensitivity (%)	Specificity (%)	+LR	−LR	PPV (%)	NPV (%)	AUC	Accuracy (%)
Emp vs. other	≥4.91	63.6	89.3	5.93	0.41	35.0	96.4	0.757	87.1
Emp and PE vs. other	≥2.59	70.4	85.7	4.92	0.35	55.9	91.8	0.834	82.6
Emp, PE and TB vs. other	≥2.59	69.4	90.6	7.40	0.34	73.5	88.8	0.840	84.9
PE vs. other (excluding Emp)	≥2.18	81.3	81.0	4.27	0.23	39.4	96.6	0.859	81.0
Infectious vs. non-infectious	≥2.59	65.8	90.4	6.87	0.38	73.5	86.7	0.820	83.3

Emp empyema, *PE* parapneumonic effusions, *TB* tuberculosis, *+LR* positive likelihood ratio *−LR* negative likelihood ratio, *PPV* positive predictive value, *NPV* negative predictive value, *AUC* area under the curve

Our findings on pleural fluid presepsin may support a pathophysiological mechanism of the acute phase response during the development of infection. Kiropoulos et al. [12] investigated the levels of CRP, IL-6, and TNF-α in various types of pleural effusions and reported that pleural fluid CRP was likely to reflect the systemic inflammation induced by the local production of IL-6 and TNF-α in the pleural cavity. Notably, although IL-6 and TNF-α levels were higher in the pleural fluid than in the serum, we found that pleural fluid CRP levels were significantly lower than serum CRP levels. Similarly, pleural fluid presepsin levels may reflect local production in the pleural cavity as well as the production mechanism of pleural fluid IL-6 and TNF-α.

Although the biological function of presepsin remains unclear, studies in rabbits [13] showed that its release mechanism is likely to be associated with the phagocytosis and cleavage of microorganisms by lysosomes. This finding supports the high levels of pleural fluid presepsin observed in empyema cases in this study. We suggest that locally increased pleural fluid presepsin levels may be attributed to bacterial phagocytosis in pleural effusion. Furthermore, this connection may be one of the reasons that pleural fluid presepsin does not increase in tuberculous effusion compared with empyema or parapneumonic effusion. As confirmed in the present study (Table 1), the proportion of lymphocytes is relatively high in tuberculous pleural effusion [14]. Thus, there are relatively few macrophages and neutrophils in this condition, and the low numbers of these phagocytes may lead to low presepsin production. Presepsin is produced in the pleural space; therefore, measuring presepsin in the pleural fluid may provide a more accurate marker for distinguishing the cause of pleural effusion than measuring presepsin in the blood.

We found that pleural fluid CRP levels were higher in infectious effusions compared with non-infectious effusions. This result supports the value of pleural fluid CRP measurement in diagnosing infectious effusions. Furthermore, it confirms and extends the findings of previous investigations, in which pleural CRP levels were found to be higher in parapneumonic effusions than in other types of exudates. Izhakian et al. [15] reported that pleural CRP levels were higher in parapneumonic effusion than in other effusion types, with a cut-off value of > 1.38 mg/dL. Pleural CRP had a low positive predicted value (37.6%) but a very high negative predicted value (96.7%), which suggests that it could be a powerful tool for excluding parapneumonic effusion as a diagnosis. Several other studies have investigated the relationship between pleural fluid CRP and the cause of pleural effusions, with similar findings [16, 17]. Although the exact cut-off value varies among studies, pleural fluid CRP levels appear capable of differentiating between infectious effusions and non-infectious effusions. Porcel et al. [4] found that pleural fluid CRP levels of > 10 mg/dL were associated with complicated parapneumonic effusion and with the need for pleural effusion drainage. Here, we examined whether the marker distribution differed between patients treated with antibiotics alone ($n = 5$) and those treated with drainage or surgical treatment ($n = 11$). No difference in PCT or presepsin levels was found between these groups, but CRP levels trended higher in the group with drainage or surgical treatment.

Table 5 Diagnostic performance of pleural fluid PCT based on the ROC analysis ($n = 132$)

	Optimal cut-off point (ng/mL)	Sensitivity (%)	Specificity (%)	+LR	−LR	PPV (%)	NPV (%)	AUC	Accuracy (%)
Emp vs. other	≤2.57	100.0	5.8	1.06	0.00	8.8	100.0	0.244	13.6
Emp and PE vs. other	≥0.19	70.4	83.8	4.35	0.35	52.8	91.7	0.791	81.1
Emp, PE and TB vs. other	≥0.11	66.7	75.0	2.67	0.44	50.0	85.7	0.718	72.7
PE vs. other (excluding Emp)	≥0.13	75.0	79.0	3.58	0.32	35.3	95.4	0.783	78.5
Infectious vs. non-infectious	≥0.11	63.2	74.5	2.47	0.49	50.0	83.3	0.696	71.2

Emp empyema, *PE* parapneumonic effusion, *TB* tuberculosis, *+LR* positive likelihood ratio, *−LR* negative likelihood ratio, *PPV* positive predictive value, *NPV* negative predictive value, *AUC* area under the curve

Table 6 Diagnostic performance of different marker combinations ($n = 132$)

Cut-off value	Sensitivity (%)	Specificity (%)	+LR	−LR	PPV (%)	NPV (%)	Accuracy (%)
Emp vs. other							
Presepsin, 754 pg/mL + CRP, 4.91 mg/dL	63.6	93.4	9.63	0.39	46.7	96.6	90.9
Presepsin, 754 pg/mL + PCT, ≤ 2.57 ng/mL	90.9	78.5	4.23	0.12	27.8	99.0	79.6
CRP, 4.91 mg/dL + PCT, ≤ 2.57 ng/mL	63.6	90.1	6.42	0.40	36.8	96.5	87.9
PE vs. other (excluding Emp)							
Presepsin, 680 pg/mL + CRP, 2.18 mg/dL	68.8	93.3	10.31	0.33	61.1	95.1	90.1
Presepsin, 680 pg/mL + PCT, 0.13 ng/mL	68.8	90.5	7.22	0.35	52.4	95.0	87.6
CRP, 2.18 mg/dL + PCT, 0.13 ng/mL	68.8	92.4	9.02	0.34	57.9	95.1	89.3
Infectious vs. non-infectious							
Presepsin, 680 pg/mL + CRP, 2.59 mg/dL	65.8	90.4	6.87	0.38	73.5	86.7	83.3
Presepsin, 680 pg/mL + PCT, 0.11 ng/mL	55.3	89.4	5.19	0.50	67.7	83.2	79.6
CRP, 2.59 mg/dL + PCT, 0.11 ng/mL	50.0	92.6	6.71	0.54	73.1	82.1	80.3

Emp empyema, *PE* parapneumonic effusions, *+LR* positive likelihood ratio, *−LR* negative likelihood ratio, *PPV* positive predictive value, *NPV* negative predictive value

Thus, although the number of cases in the present study was small, its results also suggest that pleural fluid CRP levels vary depending on the treatment.

We examined the relationship between pleural fluid PCT levels and different causes of pleural effusions, which has also been investigated by several previous studies. Among those studies, some reported that pleural fluid PCT measurement is useful in differentiating between parapneumonic and other types of effusions, while others have found that it is not useful for this purpose. Wang et al. [18] reported that PCT levels could differentiate empyema and parapneumonic effusion from non-parapneumonic effusion at a cut-off point of 0.18 ng/mL and an AUC of 0.776 (sensitivity, 69.7%; specificity, 72.1%). Lin et al. [19] also reported that PCT could differentiate parapneumonic effusion from non-parapneumonic effusion at a cut-off point of 0.18 ng/mL and an AUC of 0.752 (sensitivity, 66.7%; specificity, 77.4%). However, Porcel et al. [3] determined that PCT levels in pleural fluid were of little value. Our results show that pleural fluid PCT levels tended to be higher in cases of parapneumonic effusion than in other pleural effusions, supporting its potential use as a tool for diagnosing parapneumonic effusion. Although the small number of cases in this study makes it impossible to make definitive conclusions, pleural fluid PCT levels do not necessarily increase in empyema.

A novel finding of our study is that combinations of pleural fluid markers can distinguish pleural fluid from certain causes with a higher accuracy rate than that of any single pleural fluid marker. In the differentiation of empyema, a combination of pleural fluid presepsin and CRP yielded the highest accuracy rate. In clinical practice, simple cut-off values are easier to remember and apply. Notably, we found that changing the cut-off value of presepsin from 754 pg/mL to 750 pg/mL and the CRP cut-off value from 4.91 mg/dL to 4.9 mg/dL, did not affect the diagnostic performance. Although PCT alone was not useful for the differentiation of empyema, it was found that this marker can be a useful tool when combined with CRP or presepsin. However, for distinguishing between infectious effusion and non-infectious effusion, the accuracy rate of combined markers was not improved over that of pleural fluid CRP alone. Further research on the clinical applicability of various marker combinations is required.

This study should be interpreted in the context of certain limitations. First, the sample size was small, and there was a large variation in case accumulation; although multiple study centres participated, patients were enrolled from both respiratory medicine and outpatient wards. This may have limited the power of its findings. Second, diagnosis based on the physician's judgment may have resulted in the misclassification of some patients, thus compromising the assessment of diagnostic accuracy of the pleural fluid markers. However, as the diagnoses of pleural effusions were performed by board-certified members of the Japanese Respiratory Society at each institution and were made following the same diagnostic criteria, we consider the diagnosis method to have been relatively standardised. Third, dialysis patients and patients with severe renal failure were not included in this study; thus, the findings of this study may not be applicable to patients with severe renal failure. Because presepsin is mainly excreted in the urine, patients with chronic renal failure [20], especially chronic maintenance dialysis patients, tend to have high levels of presepsin. Fourth, the effect of patient background (e.g. underlying disease or the administration of chemotherapy, steroids, or antibiotics) was not analysed in detail; neither was the effect of the type, duration, or dose of antibiotic treatment or the tumour burden [21]. These parameters may have affected the levels of acute inflammatory markers. Finally, because the decision to initiate thoracentesis was based on the judgement of the pulmonary physician, a sampling bias may have been present, which could explain the very low number of cases of congestive pleural effusion representative of transudate effusion that were registered during the study period.

Conclusions

In summary, this study showed that pleural fluid presepsin, CRP, and PCT levels may be of value as additional tools in the assessment of pleural effusions to support the differential diagnosis. High levels of pleural fluid presepsin were found in cases of empyema and parapneumonic effusion; this closely resembles the previously reported pattern of pleural fluid CRP levels. Some combinations of these pleural fluid inflammatory marker may be more likely to be clinically useful compared with these markers in isolation.

Abbreviations

95% CI: 95% confidence interval; AUC: area under the curve; CRP: C-reactive protein; IL-6: interleukin-6; PCT: procalcitonin; ROC: receiver operator characteristics; SD: standard deviation

Acknowledgements

We thank Dr. Masahiro Yamaguch and Dr. Akira Tadokoro of the Department of Respiratory Medicine, National Hospital Organization Takamatsu Medical Center; Dr. Takuya Inoue of the Department of Respiratory Medicine, Sakaide City Hospital; and Dr. Hiroshi Miyawaki and Dr. Kenichiro Sakai of the Department of Respiratory Medicine, Kagawa Prefectural Central Hospital for their help in data acquisition. We also thank Katie Oakley, PhD, from Edanz Group for proofreading this manuscript in English.

Funding

This research did not receive any specific grant from funding agencies in the public, commercial, or not-for-profit sectors.

Authors' contributions

NW contributed to the study design, data acquisition, interpretation of the results and statistical analysis, drafting of the manuscript, and critical revisions of the manuscript for its intellectual content. IT, NK1, NK2, and SB participated in the study design, data acquisition, interpretation of the results, and literature review. HN, NN, YU, and YT were involved in data acquisition and interpretation of the results. NK3 supervised manuscript drafting. All authors have read and approved the final version of the manuscript.

Consent for publication

Not applicable.

Competing interests

The authors declare that they have no competing interests.

Author details

[1]Department of Internal Medicine, Hematology, Rheumatology and Respiratory Medicine, Faculty of Medicine, Kagawa University, 1750-1 Ikenobe, Miki-cho, Kita-gun, Kagawa 761-0793, Japan. [2]Department of Respiratory Medicine, Sakaide City Hospital, 3-1-2, Kotobuki-cho, Sakaide, Kagawa 762-8550, Japan. [3]Department of Respiratory Medicine, Sanuki Municipal Hospital, 387-1, Ishidahigashi-kou, Sangawa-cho, Sanuki, Kagawa 769-2393, Japan. [4]Department of Respiratory Medicine, Kagawa Prefectural Central Hospital, 1-2-1, Asahimachi, Takamatsu, Kagawa 760-8557, Japan. [5]Department of Respiratory Medicine, National Hospital Organization Takamatsu Medical Center, 8, Shindencho-otsu, Takamatsu, Kagawa 761-0193, Japan.

References

1. Light RW, Macgregor MI, Luchsinger PC, Ball WC Jr. Pleural effusions: the diagnostic separation of transudates and exudates. Ann Intern Med. 1972; 77(4):507–13.
2. Maskell NA, Davies CW, Nunn AJ, Hedley EL, Gleeson FV, Miller R, Gabe R, Rees GL, Peto TE, Woodhead MA, et al. U.K. controlled trial of intrapleural streptokinase for pleural infection. N Engl J Med. 2005;352(9):865–74.
3. Porcel JM, Vives M, Cao G, Bielsa S, Ruiz-Gonzalez A, Martinez-Iribarren A, Esquerda A. Biomarkers of infection for the differential diagnosis of pleural effusions. Eur Respir J. 2009;34(6):1383–9.
4. Porcel JM, Bielsa S, Esquerda A, Ruiz-Gonzalez A, Falguera M. Pleural fluid C-reactive protein contributes to the diagnosis and assessment of severity of parapneumonic effusions. Eur J Intern Med. 2012;23(5):447–50.
5. Daniil ZD, Zintzaras E, Kiropoulos T, Papaioannou AI, Koutsokera A, Kastanis A, Gourgoulianis KI. Discrimination of exudative pleural effusions based on multiple biological parameters. Eur Respir J. 2007;30(5):957–64.
6. Yaegashi Y, Shirakawa K, Sato N, Suzuki Y, Kojika M, Imai S, Takahashi G, Miyata M, Furusako S, Endo S. Evaluation of a newly identified soluble CD14 subtype as a marker for sepsis. J Infect Chemother. 2005;11(5):234–8.
7. Endo S, Suzuki Y, Takahashi G, Shozushima T, Ishikura H, Murai A, Nishida T, Irie Y, Miura M, Iguchi H, et al. Presepsin as a powerful monitoring tool for the prognosis and treatment of sepsis: a multicenter prospective study. J Infect Chemother. 2014;20(1):30–4.
8. Mussap M, Noto A, Fravega M, Fanos V. Soluble CD14 subtype presepsin (sCD14-ST) and lipopolysaccharide binding protein (LBP) in neonatal sepsis: new clinical and analytical perspectives for two old biomarkers. J Matern Fetal Neonatal Med. 2011;24(Suppl 2):12–4.
9. Shozushima T, Takahashi G, Matsumoto N, Kojika M, Okamura Y, Endo S. Usefulness of presepsin (sCD14-ST) measurements as a marker for the diagnosis and severity of sepsis that satisfied diagnostic criteria of systemic inflammatory response syndrome. J Infect Chemother. 2011;17(6):764–9.
10. Endo S, Suzuki Y, Takahashi G, Shozushima T, Ishikura H, Murai A, Nishida T, Irie Y, Miura M, Iguchi H, et al. Usefulness of presepsin in the diagnosis of sepsis in a multicenter prospective study. J Infect Chemother. 2012;18(6):891–7.
11. Klouche K, Cristol JP, Devin J, Gilles V, Kuster N, Larcher R, Amigues L, Corne P, Jonquet O, Dupuy AM. Diagnostic and prognostic value of soluble CD14 subtype (Presepsin) for sepsis and community-acquired pneumonia in ICU patients. Ann Intensive Care. 2016;6(1):59.
12. Kiropoulos TS, Kostikas K, Oikonomidi S, Tsilioni I, Nikoulis D, Germenis A, Gourgoulianis KI. Acute phase markers for the differentiation of infectious and malignant pleural effusions. Respir Med. 2007;101(5):910–8.
13. Shirakawa K, Naitou K, Hirose J, Nakamura M, Takeuchi T, Hosaka Y, Furusako S. The new sepsis marker, sCD14-ST, induction mechanism in the rabbit sepsis models. Crit Care. 2010;14(Supple 2).
14. Epstein DM, Kline LR, Albelda SM, Miller WT. Tuberculous Pleural Effusions. Chest. 1987;91(1):106–9.
15. Izhakian S, Wasser WG, Fox BD, Vainshelboim B, Kramer MR. The diagnostic value of the pleural fluid C-reactive protein in Parapneumonic effusions. Dis Markers. 2016;2016:7539780.
16. Skouras V, Boultadakis E, Nikoulis D, Polychronopoulos V, Daniil Z, Kalomenidis I, Gourgoulianis KI. Prognostic value of C-reactive protein in parapneumonic effusions. Respirology. 2012;17(2):308–14.

17. Yilmaz Turay U, Yildirim Z, Turkoz Y, Biber C, Erdogan Y, Keyf AI, Ugurman F, Ayaz A, Ergun P, Harputluoglu M. Use of pleural fluid C-reactive protein in diagnosis of pleural effusions. Respir Med. 2000;94(5):432–5.
18. Wang CY, Hsiao YC, Jerng JS, Ho CC, Lai CC, Yu CJ, Hsueh PR, Yang PC. Diagnostic value of procalcitonin in pleural effusions. Eur J Clin Microbiol Infect Dis. 2011;30(3):313–8.
19. Lin MC, Chen YC, Wu JT, Ko YC, Wang CC. Diagnostic and prognostic values of pleural fluid procalcitonin in parapneumonic pleural effusions. Chest. 2009;136(1):205–11.
20. Kotera A, Sagishima K, Tashiro T, Niimori D, Kamohara H, Kinoshita Y. A validation of presepsin levels in kidney dysfunction patients: four case reports. J Intensive Care. 2014;2(1):63.
21. Heikkila K, Ebrahim S, Lawlor DA. A systematic review of the association between circulating concentrations of C reactive protein and cancer. J Epidemiol Community Health. 2007;61(9):824–33.

17

Initiation of LPS-induced pulmonary dysfunction and its recovery occur independent of T cells

Eva Verjans[1,2*], Stephanie Kanzler[2], Kim Ohl[1], Annette D. Rieg[2,3], Nadine Ruske[2], Angela Schippers[1], Norbert Wagner[1], Klaus Tenbrock[1], Stefan Uhlig[2] and Christian Martin[2]

Abstract

Background: The acute respiratory distress syndrome (ARDS) is a serious disease in critically ill patients that is characterized by pulmonary dysfunctions, hypoxemia and significant mortality. Patients with immunodeficiency (e.g. SCID with T and B cell deficiency) are particularly susceptible to the development of severe ARDS. However, the role of T cells on pulmonary dysfunctions in immune-competent patients with ARDS is only incompletely understood.

Methods: Wild-type (wt) and RAG2$^{-/-}$ mice (lymphocyte deficient) received intratracheal instillations of LPS (4 mg/kg) or saline. On day 1, 4 and 10 lung mechanics and bronchial hyperresponsiveness towards acetylcholine were measured with the flexiVent ventilation set-up. The bronchoalveolar lavage fluid (BALF) was examined for leukocytes (FACS analysis) and pro-inflammatory cytokines (ELISA).

Results: In wt mice, lung mechanics, body weight and body temperature deteriorated in the LPS-group during the early phase (up to d4); these alterations were accompanied by increased leukocyte numbers and inflammatory cytokine levels in the BALF. During the late phase (day 10), both lung mechanics and the cell/cytokine homeostasis recovered in LPS-treated wt mice. RAG2$^{-/-}$ mice experienced changes in body weight, lung mechanics, BAL neutrophil numbers, BAL inflammatory cytokines levels that were comparable to wt mice.

Conclusion: Following LPS instillation, lung mechanics deteriorate within the first 4 days and recover towards day 10. This response is not altered by the lack of T lymphocytes suggesting that T cells play only a minor role for the initiation, propagation or recovery of LPS-induced lung dysfunctions or function of T lymphocytes can be compensated by other immune cells, such as alveolar macrophages.

Keywords: ARDS, Acute lung injury, T cell deficiency, Lung function, Lung mechanics, Lung inflammation

Background

The acute respiratory distress syndrome (ARDS) is a life-threatening disease that is characterized by the rapid onset of severe respiratory failure with decreased pulmonary compliance, pulmonary inflammation and hypoxemia [1, 2]. It is frequently associated with sepsis, pneumonia and polytrauma [3] and the incidence of ARDS in the United States is 79 per 100,000 with a mortality of 40% [1]. Up to now, no pharmacological therapy is available that mitigates disease severity and/or mortality. The treatment remains largely supportive and the use of mechanical ventilation (MV) is mandatory [4–6].

ARDS commences with an inflammatory phase that is followed after 4–10 days by a fibroproliferative phase [7]. With respect to this paradigm, at least two important yet unsolved questions need to answered: (1) Because not all pulmonary inflammation leads to a measurable decline in physiological lung functions, the relationship between inflammation and lung functions deserves further study. (2) It remains unclear why some patients recover after the first phase while others enter the fibroproliferative phase [7]. The present paper addresses

* Correspondence: everjans@ukaachen.de
Eva Verjans and Stephanie Kanzler are considered as co-authors.
Eva Verjans and Stephanie Kanzler contributed equally to this project.
[1]Department of Pediatrics, Medical Faculty, RWTH Aachen, Aachen, Germany
[2]Institute of Pharmacology and Toxicology, RWTH Aachen, Aachen, Germany
Full list of author information is available at the end of the article

both questions by examining the role of T lymphocytes for LPS-induced lung dysfunction for 10 days.

During acute lung injury neutrophils are recruited well before lymphocytes [8, 9]. Based on these and other observations, it is thought that neutrophils are responsible for many of the pathophysiological alterations in the first phase, while T lymphocytes may be involved in the second-line defense and/or the recovery and resolution of inflammation. A recent study of BALF obtained from ARDS patients within 48 h of disease onset reported unchanged proportions of CD4 and CD8 lymphocytes and no increase in regulatory T cells (Treg), but found that T cells were activated (HLA-DR expression), proliferated (KI-67) and produced IL-17 [10]. A possible role of T cells in ARDS is further highlighted by patients with primary immunodeficiency (PID) with T cell dysregulation or absence. They show an enhanced susceptibility to pulmonary infections [11–13] that might be related to the overexpression of CREMα in the lymphocytes of these patients/mice [14].

A common way to study the role of lymphocytes in disease is the use of lymphocyte deficient mice. In LPS-induced lung injury at day 2 or later such studies have yielded conflicting results, i.e. fewer [8], similar [15] or higher numbers [16] of neutrophils in the BALF; similar inconsistencies were observed for lung injury scores, that were found to be either higher [16] or similar [17]. An important question in such models is the severity of the organ injury that can be assessed in a clinically relevant manner by lung function measurements. Up to date, such measurements had never been performed in lymphocyte-deficient mice.

Therefore, we first characterized lung mechanics and the associated inflammatory changes in LPS-induced lung injury for 10 days, i.e. for a time span long enough to observe the possible effects of lymphoyctes. Subsequently, we used RAG2$^{-/-}$ mice to examine the impact of T cell deficiency on lung function parameters and disease activity during early and late phase of ARDS.

Materials and methods

Animals

Experiments were performed with 8 to 12 weeks old wild-type C57Bl/6 J mice (wt) and RAG2$^{-/-}$ littermates, weighing 20 to 25 g. All mice were bred in our animal facility and kept under specific pathogen-free conditions. Room conditions were controlled for humidity (40–70%) and temperature (21–23 °C) with a 12-h light/dark cycle. Wild type and transgenic mice were age-matched for all experiments. The study was approved by regional governmental authorities and animal procedures were performed according to the German animal protection law and approved by regional governmental authorities (Landesamt für Natur, Umwelt und Verbraucherschutz Nordrhein-Westfalen, permission number: AZ 84-02.04.2016.A290).

Experimental design and lung function measurements

Anesthetized mice (pentobarbital 70 mg/kg) were instilled intratracheally with an LPS (E.coli O111.B4, Sigma-Aldrich, Germany) aerosol (4 mg/kg) via a microsprayer (PennCentury, USA). Control animals received NaCl 0.9% and physiological parameters (body weight, behavior and temperature) were monitored in both groups during sleeping time of 20-30 min and the following 24-240 h. After 1, 4 or 10 days mice were tracheotomized with a 20G cannula and directly connected to the ventilator. All mice were initially anaesthetized with pentobarbital sodium (70 mg/kg) and fentanyl (0.1 mg/kg). Anaesthesia was maintained with pentobarbital sodium (20 mg/kg) after 30 min. All mice were mechanically ventilated with a tidal volume (Vt) of 10 ml/kg and a positive end-expiratory pressure (PEEP) of 2 cm H_2O using the flexiVent (SCIREQ, Canada) ventilation setup. Body temperature was rectally controlled and adjusted between 36.5 and 37.5 ° C during the whole ventilation period. Continuous data recording of heart rate and ECG was performed to monitor the function of the cardiovascular system.

Dynamic lung mechanics were measured by applying a sinusoidal standardized breath and analyzed with forced oscillation technique. We used a 1.2 s, 2.5 Hz single-frequency forced oscillation manoeuvre (SnapShot perturbation) and a 3 s, broadband low frequency forced oscillation manoeuvre containing 13 mutually prime frequencies between 1 and 20.5 Hz (Quick Prime perturbation). Total lung resistance (Rrs) and elastance (Ers) were calculated by the *flexiVent* software (flexiWare 7.0.1, SCIREQ, Canada) by fitting measured SnapShot values to the linear single compartment model using multiple linear regressions. Respiratory system input impedance was calculated from the QuickPrime data and tissue resistance (tissue damping, G) and tissue elastance (H) were assessed by iteratively fitting the constant-phase model to input impedance.

During the first 25 min of ventilation time baseline values were recorded using a standardized script with measurements every 30 s. Every 5 min short volume controlled recruitment maneuvers (deep inspirations over 3 s) were used to avoid atelectasis [18]. The data are presented as the maximum value obtained during these 25 min.

Following basal ventilation, airway hyperresponsiveness was provoked with nebulized acetylcholine (Ach). For each concentration lung function was measured 12 times (SnapShot and QuickPrime) during a period of 3 min.

After provocation of bronchial hyperresponsiveness, mice were sacrified by exsanguination via the carotid artery.

Bronchoalveolar lavage and cytokine measurements

Following ventilation, lungs were removed. To obtain single lung cell suspensions, lungs were perfused with

5 ml sterile PBS through the right ventricle and the pulmonary artery at a constant hydrostatic pressure (15 cmH_2O). The entire right lung was used for bronchoalveolar lavage fluid (BALF) by instilling 700 µL ice-cold PBS. Murine IL-6, TNF-α and KC were analyzed in supernatants of BALF samples with sandwich ELISAs according to manufacturer's protocols (R&D Systems/eBioscience, Germany).

FACS analysis

30 µL of BALF and 170 µL PBS/0.5% BSA were taken without staining to calculate absolute numbers of BALF cells with the BD LSR Fortessa analyzer (BD Bioscience, Germans). The remaining BALF was centrifuged for 10 min at 1250 × g and the pellet was resolved in 1 ml of PBS/0.5% BSA to wash the cells for a second time. After red blood cell lysis with lysis buffer, cells were stained with antibodies diluted in PBS/0.5% BSA for 20 min at 4 °C. For detection of T cells and the T cell subsets CD3-APC (eBioscience, Germany), CD4-PE (eBioscience, Germany), CD8-Pacific Blue and CD25-APC (eBioscience, Germany) were used. Neutrophil granulocytes were stained with Gr-1-FITC (Immuno Tools, Germany) and CD11b-Pacific Blue (eBioscience, San Diego). To identify alveolar macrophages, CD11c-APC-Cy7 (BD Bioscience, NJ, USA) and F4/80-PE (eBioscience, San Diego) were used. A minimum of 10,000 events were collected for evaluation.

Statistical analysis

Time dependent data of body weight and temperature are shown as mean ± standard deviation (SD) and the area under the curve (AUC) was used for univariate analysis. All other data were presented as mean ± standard error (SEM). For all data, the Brown Forsythe test was used to check for equal variances and the BoxCox transformation was performed to achieve homoscedasticity if suitable. The ShapiroWilk test was used to verify normal distributions. For parametric data, differences between groups were tested using unpaired two-sided Student's t-tests or ANOVA corrected by the Tukey post-test. Non-parametric data were analysed by Kruskall-Wallis test followed by Dunn's post test. Graph generation and statistical analysis were performed by using Graph Pad Prism version 5.0 (GraphPad Software) or JMP 7.0.1 (SAS Institute). * $p < 0.05$, ** $p < 0.01$, *** $p < 0.001$.

Results

Wild-type animals

Body weight and rectal temperature

Body weight and rectal temperature were followed for10 days. LPS-treated animals showed a continuous weight loss until day 3 and reached their initial body weight on day 9 to 10 (Fig. 1a). The NaCl-treated group developed normally (Fig. 1a). LPS treated mice showed a temperature drop on day 1, but not thereafter (Fig. 1b).

Lung mechanics

LPS-treated mice showed higher resistance (Rrs) and elastance (Ers) on day 1 and 4 after instillation and returned to baseline on day 10 (Fig. 1c–d). The resistance of the smaller airways (G) showed only slight differences between LPS-treated and control animals, whereas tissue elastance (H) was significantly increased on day 1 and 4 in the LPS-treated mice (Fig. 1e–f). Figure 1g–h exemplary presents lung mechanics over a ventilation time of 25 min on day 1 in comparison to control animals (Rrs and tissue elastance, H). Higher tissue elastance represents stronger stiffness of the smaller airways and therefore deteriorated lung function. Frequent increases in these graphs result from TLC manoeuvres every 5 min to avoid atelectasis [18]. As lung function parameters of saline-treated controls did not differ significantly at several time points after NaCl-instillation, these mice were summarized as control group in these time-dependent graphs for reason of clarity (Fig. 1c–d).

To study the occurrence of bronchial hyperresponsiveness (AHR), animals were provoked by 0.4 mg/kg Ach (Additional file 1: Figure S1A-D). Control animals responded only marginally to Ach, while ARDS mice showed a small increase in airway responsiveness towards methacholine (compare to Fig. 1c–f without acetylcholine).

BALF inflammatory mediators and cell counts

Levels of IL-6 and KC peaked on day 1 after LPS-instillation and dropped during the following days (Fig. 2a–b). The amounts of TNF in BALF tended to be higher in ARDS-mice on all days, but its upregulation was not as high compared to the other cytokines (Fig. 2c).

As expected, levels of total cells in the BALF were much higher in LPS-treated animals than in control mice, but there were no significant differences in total cell counts (without lysis of erythrocytes) in different stages of disease (Fig. 2d). Therefore, we determined cell subpopulations in the LPS-treated groups. $CD11b^+$ / $GR\text{-}1^+$ positive cells were considered as neutropils; their levels were highest on day 1 after LPS-instillation and then continuously dropped until day 10 (Fig. 2e). In contrast, the amounts of T lymphocytes determined by total $CD3^+$ cells as well as $CD3^+/CD4^+$, $CD3^+/CD4^+/CD25^+$ and $CD3^+/CD8^+$ cells, increased over time. The ratio of $CD4^+/CD8^+$ cells clearly decreased from early to late stages of ARDS (Fig. 2f–j).

LPS-instillation in $RAG^{-/-}$ mice

Our study demonstrated a strong increase of T cells during different phases of ARDS (Fig. 2f–i). To study the

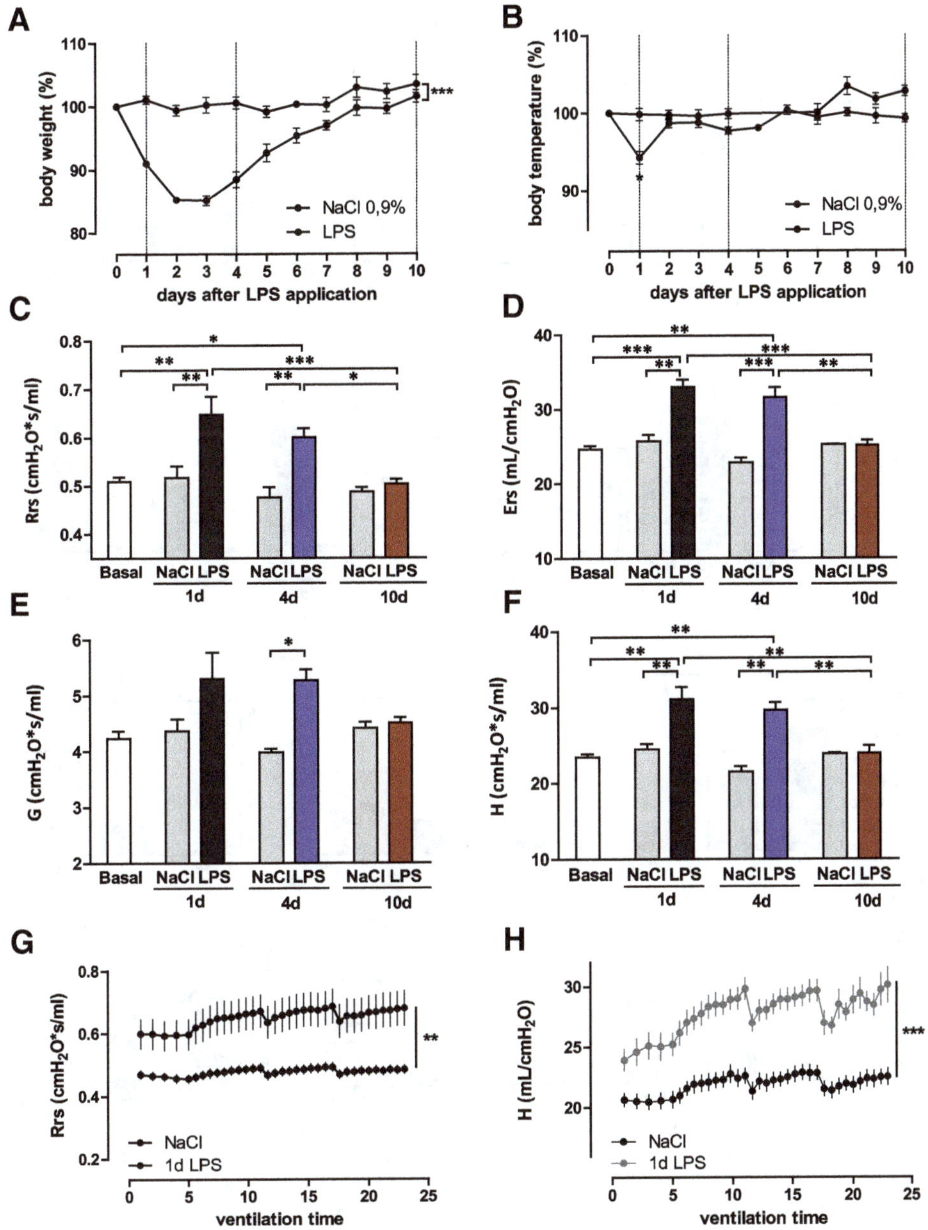

Fig. 1 Characteristics of LPS-induced acute lung injury in C57BL6 mice. Mice were instilled with 50 µL of LPS (4 mg/kg) or saline (controls) on day 0 and were mechanically ventilated 1, 4 or 10 days after ARDS induction. Control mice were mechanical ventilated without prior i.t. instillation. ARDS disease activity was determined via body weight (**a**) and temperature (**b**) over the time (controls $n = 4$ and ARDS group $n = 8$ per time point, means ± SEM). **c**–**f** Lung function parameters resistance (Rrs), elastance (Ers), tissue damping (**g**) and tissue elastance (**h**) on day 1, 4 and 10 after ARDS-induction. (controls $n = 4$, ARDS group $n = 6$ per time point, means ± SEM). Lung function parameters over a ventilation time of 25 min, exemplary resistance (Rrs) and tissue elastance (H) of treated ARDS-animals and controls on day 1 are depicted in (**g**) and (**h**) (controls $n = 12$, summarized from all time points, ARDS group $n = 8$, means ± SEM). * $p \leq 0.05$, ** $p \leq 0.01$, *** $p \leq 0.001$

role of T cells in our model, we used RAG2$^{-/-}$ mice that lack mature lymphocytes.

Body weight and rectal temperature

Weight loss and the following weight gain as well as the temperature drop after LPS instillation were nearly the same in LPS-treated wt- and RAG2$^{-/-}$ mice (Fig. 3a–b).

Lung mechanics

The lack of T lymphocytes in RAG2$^{-/-}$ mice did not alter resistance and elastance of central and smaller airways on day 1, 4 or 10 after LPS instillation (basal ventilation) (Fig. 3c–h, g–h exemplary time courses on day 1). Further, there were no relevant differences in lung function parameters of RAG2$^{-/-}$ and wt mice after provocation of bronchial

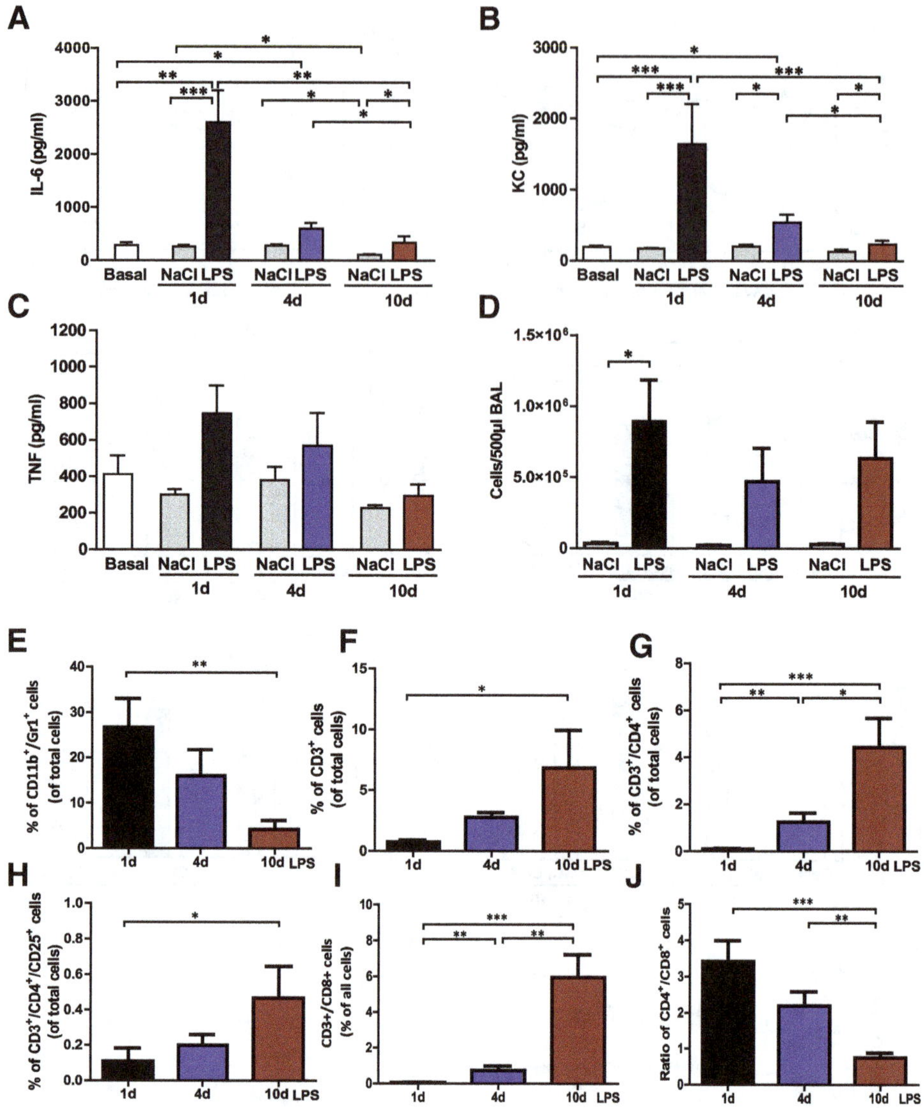

Fig. 2 LPS induced inflammatory response in C57BL/6 mice. Proinflammatory cytokines IL-6 (**a**) and TNF-α (**c**) as well as the chemokine KC (**b**) were quantified in BALF supernatants on day 1, 4 and 10 after ARDS induction by ELISA. **d** Total cell numbers in BALF of LPS-treated animals and saline-instilled controls were calculated by FACS analysis. **e–j** Several cell subpopulations in ARDS mice were differentiated by specific antibodies, neutrophil granulocytes (**e**), T cell subpopulations (**f–i**) and $CD4^+/CD8^+$ ratio (F). Data are shown as means ± SEM. **a–j** Controls n = 4, ARDS groups $n = 6$. * $p \leq 0.05$, ** $p \leq 0.01$, *** $p \leq 0.001$

hyperresponsiveness with acetylcholine (Additional file 2: Figure S2A-D).

BALF inflammatory mediators and cell counts

BALF Levels of IL-6, KC and TNF declined after day 1, both in wt and in $RAG2^{-/-}$ mice. The total BALF cell counts were the same in wt and $RAG2^{-/-}$ mice on day 1, 4 and 10 (Fig. 4a). Flow cytometric measurements demonstrated that all of the $RAG2^{-/-}$ mice were lacking T lymphocytes: nearly no cells were counted in LPS-treated $RAG2^{-/-}$ mice in the $CD3^+$, $CD3^+/CD4^+$ and $CD3^+/CD8^+$ gates, whereas their wt littermates showed increasing numbers of different subpopulations of T lymphocytes over the time (Fig. 4b–d). Numbers of neutrophils (characterized by $CD11b^+/Gr1^+$) were not significantly different between wt and $RAG2^{-/-}$ mice (Fig. 4e). Notably, the amount of $CD11b^{low+}/CD11c^{high+}/F4\text{–}80^+$ cells (alveolar macrophages) was the same in both groups on day 1 and 4 but clearly differed on day 10 with 22% of total cells (wt) versus 57% ($RAG2^{-/-}$) (Fig. 4f).

Discussion

In a murine ARDS model lasting for 10 days we found that the major pathophysiological alterations – from inflammation to recovery – can occur independent of lymphocytes. In wt mice we observed the expected alterations

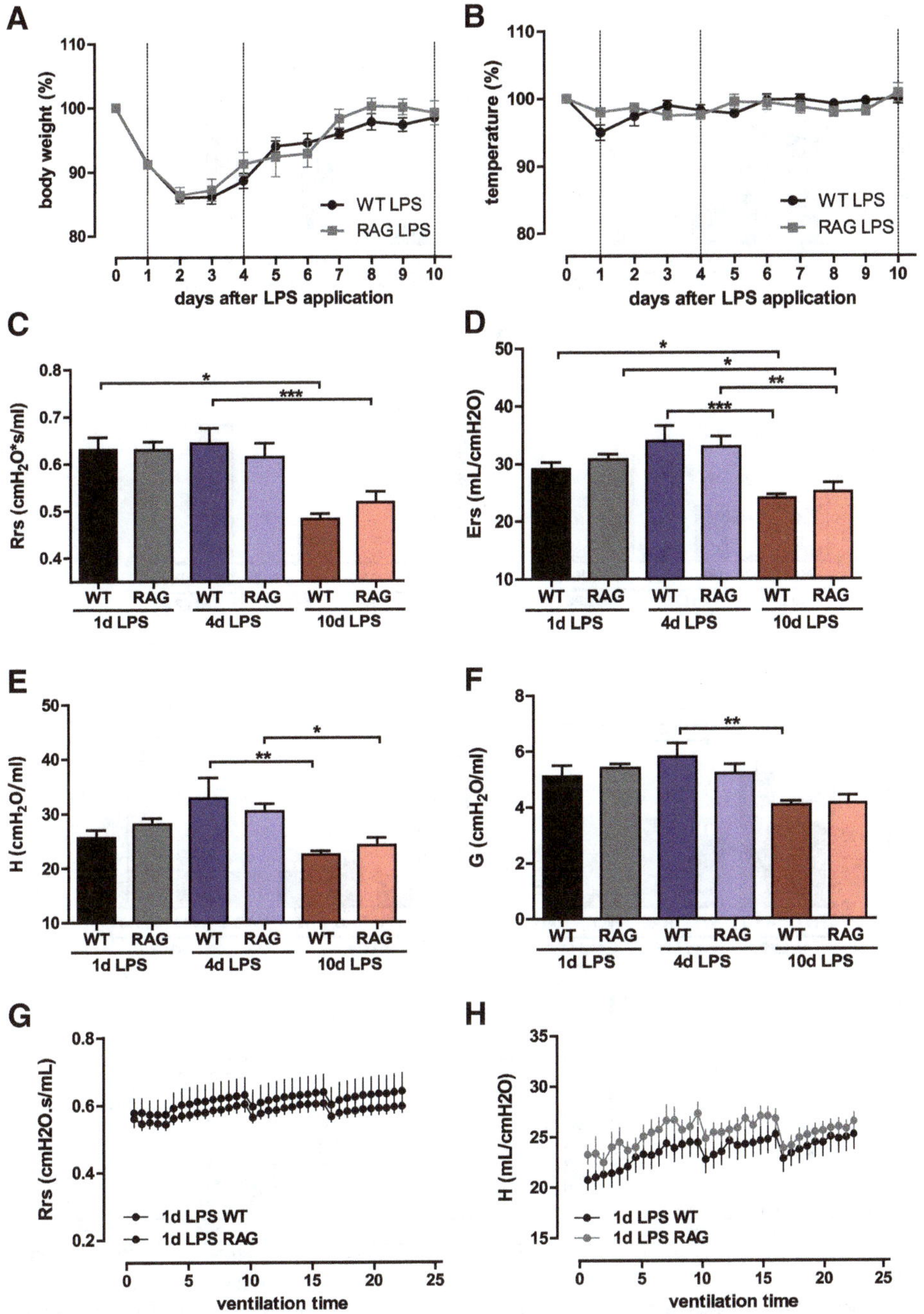

Fig. 3 Characteristics of LPS-induced acute lung injury in $RAG2^{-/-}$ and wildtype mice. ARDS was induced as described before in wildtype (WT) and $RAG2^{-/-}$ (RAG) mice and animals were mechanically ventilated on day 1, 4 and 10 after ARDS induction. ARDS disease activity was determined via body weight and temperature over the time (**a**, **b**). **c**–**f** Lung function parameters resistance (Rrs), elastance (Ers), tissue damping (**g**) and tissue elastance (**h**) on day 1, 4 and 10 after ARDS-induction. Lung function parameters over a ventilation time of 25 min, exemplary resistance (Rrs) and tissue elastance (**h**) of treated ARDS-animals and controls on day 1 are depicted in (**g**) and (h). **a**–**h** ($n = 8$ in each group at each time point, means ± SEM). * $p \leq 0.05$, ** $p \leq 0.01$, *** $p \leq 0.001$

in lung functions and inflammation during the early phase (up to day 4), and their recovery until day 10. Although pulmonary lymphocyte counts increased over the observational period of 10 days, mice lacking B and T lymphocytes ($RAG2^{-/-}$), showed no relevant alterations in body weight, body temperature, lung functions, BALF cytokines or neutrophil counts compared to immune-competent wt littermates. Only the number of alveolar macrophages ($CD11b^+/CD11c^{high +}/F4–80^+$) were higher in LPS-treated $RAG2^{-/-}$ mice on day 10 and it may be speculated that

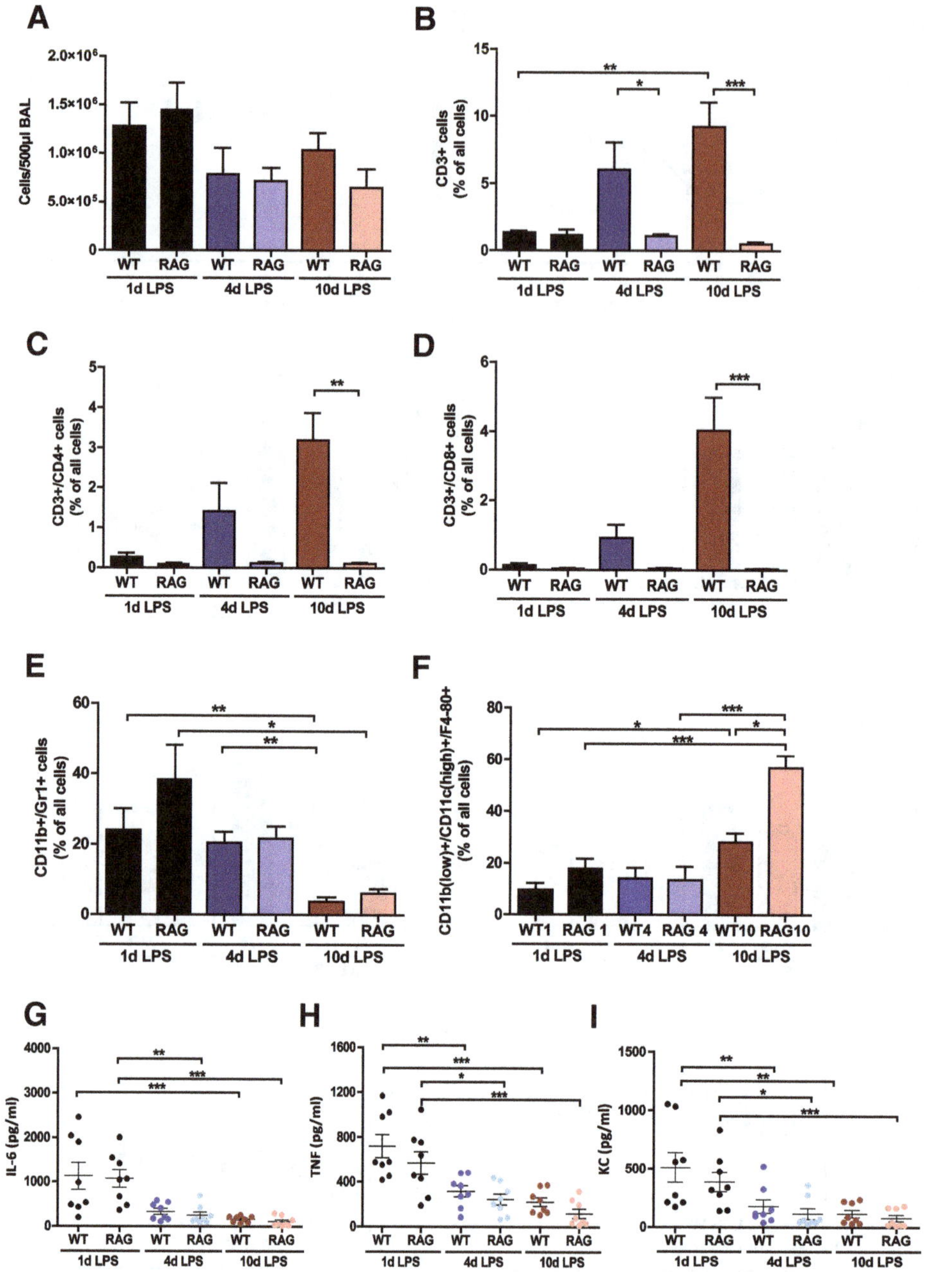

Fig. 4 LPS induced inflammatory response in $RAG2^{-/-}$ and wildtype mice. **a** Total cell numbers in BALF of LPS-treated $RAG2^{-/-}$ animals and wildtype mice were calculated by FACS analysis. **b–f** Several cell subpopulations in ARDS mice were differentiated by specific antibodies. Proinflammatory cytokines IL-6 (**g**) and TNF-α (**h**) as well as the chemokine KC (**i**) were quantified in BALF supernatants on day 1, 4 and 10 after ARDS induction by ELISA. Data are shown as means ± SEM. **a–i** n = 8 per group, means ± SEM. * $p \leq 0.05$, ** $p \leq 0.01$, *** $p \leq 0.001$

these cells can compensate for the lack of lymphocytes during the recovery phase.

The instillation of LPS showed the expected time course with all changes being maximal between d1-d3, and recovery thereafter. The use of the constant phase model of lung mechanics allows to partition lung mechanics into a central airway component (R_N) and a peripheral tissue component (G and H). The increase of G and H in LPS-treated mice therefore indicate increased stiffness and heterogeneity of the distal lung compartment including the small airways. We believe that lung function measurements are a highly useful readout in ARDS models, because they do not change in case of mild inflammation [18, 19] and because they provide an absolute measure that allows to compare the severity of lung injury across studies and with that of human ARDS.

For instance, the loss of compliance in ARDS patients may typically be about 50% (e.g. 1.25 $mL/cmH_2O/kg$ BW [20] in anaesthetized healthy individuals vs 0.55 mL/cmH2O/kg BW in ARDS patients [21]), whereas in the present work it was roughly 30%, indicating that our lung injury was less severe than in ARDS patients. Based on these considerations we cannot exclude that lymphocytes play a role for the recovery or resolution in more severe ARDS.

The fact that all previous studies with lymphocyte deficient animals were lacking such measurements of compliance or other features of ARDS, makes it difficult to compare our studies to the previous ones.

According to the Berlin definition, there is no use of the term Acute Lung Injury (ALI) anymore. The committee felt that this term was used inappropriately in many contexts and hence was not helpful. In the Berlin definition, ARDS was classified as mild, moderate and severe according to the value of PaO_2/FiO_2 ratio. In our study, we do not reach ARDS according to this definition or we did not measure all necessary parameters according to PaO_2/FiO_2 ratio or chest radiation. However, our animals showed typical features of acute lung inflammation and a relevant tachypnoea. In human models, we would have assessed CPAP to our patients but this is not possible in our mouse model. Therefore, following the definition, we would classify our disease as milde ARDS or ARDS-typical acute lung inflammation.

ARDS is typically divided into at least two phases, where the acute phase is thought to be governed by the innate immune system, and later phases at least in part also by the adaptive immune system. As confirmed in the present work, the influx of T cells is usually low in the early phase, and rises until and during the recovery phase. According to our findings, however, this increase in lymphocyte has no bearing on the development or the recovery of the LPS-induced lung inflammation. Our findings in lymphocyte deficient RAG-$2^{-/-}$ are in line with other studies showing unaltered lung injury in WT, nude and RAG-$1^{-/-}$ mice [15, 17], but are in contrast to observations in RAG-$1^{-/-}$ mice where inflammation was either less [8] or stronger [22, 23] and are also in conflict to the observation that pulmonary inflammation was increased in the absence of γδ T cells [24].

At present it is difficult to reconcile these contrasting findings for several reasons: (i) All these models used a similar model (LPS-administration via the airways), yet T-cell deficiency resulted in all possible outcomes, i.e. reduced, similar or increased lung injury; (ii) RAG$1^{-/-}$ and RAG$2^{-/-}$ are thought to possess nearly identical phenotypes [25]; (iii) T-cell dependent changes in TNF levels that have been proposed to explain the increased inflammation seen in γδ-knockout mice, were nearly the same in wt and RAG$2^{-/-}$mice in the present study [24]. (iv) Treg cells that have been made responsible for the resolution of the LPS-induced inflammation, behaved as described [22, 23]: they increased towards d10 in wt mice and were lacking in the RAG2−/− mice. Thus, our findings seem to indicate that the recovery of inflammation is possible in the absence of γδ T cells and of regulatory T cells (which are not increased in human ARDS) [10]. Of course, these finding do not rule out the possibility that dysfunctional lymphocytes, such as those that overexpress CREMa, can exacerbate ARDS in both the acute and the recovery phase [14]. In general, the diversity of the published findings suggests that the role of lymphocytes during ARDS is highly context-dependent.

The only difference that we observed between wt- and RAG$2^{-/-}$ mice was the number of alveolar macrophages ($CD11b^+/CD11c^{high\ +}/F4{-}80^+$) that were increased in the lymphocyte-deficient mice on d10. It may be speculated that these cells could perhaps compensate T cell function [26], possibly through NOS expression [27]. Other cells that may organize the recovery and resolution of inflammation are M2 macrophages [28, 29] or even alveolar epithelial cells [30].

Conclusion

In our model of LPS-induced lung injury, inflammation increased strongly while lung functions dropped by 30% within the first 3 days. Both inflammation and lung functions recovered until day 10 independent of the absence or presence of lymphocytes. These findings indicate that T cells play only a minor role for the initiation, propagation or recovery of LPS-induced lung dysfunctions. The many discrepant findings on the role of lymphocytes in ARDS suggest that their role is highly context-dependent and that further research in well defined and comparable models is required to improve our understanding of the role of the innate immune system in ARDS.

Additional files

Additional file 1: Figure S1. Bronchial hyperresponsiveness in C57BL6 mice in LPS-induced acute lung injury. Mice were instilled with 50 μL of LPS (4 mg/kg) or saline (controls) on day 0 and were mechanically ventilated 1, 4 or 10 days after ARDS induction. Mice of basal group were mechanical ventilated without prior i.t. instillation. (A-D) Lung function parameters resistance (Rrs), elastance (Ers), tissue damping (G) and tissue elastance (H) on day 1, 4 and 10 after ARDS-induction following acetylcholine stimulation (controls $n = 4$, ARDS group $n = 6$ per time point, means ± SEM). * $p \leq 0.05$, ** $p \leq 0.01$, *** $p \leq 0.001$.

Additional file 2: Figure S2. Bronchial hyperresponsiveness in RAG$2^{-/-}$ and wildtype mice in LPS-induced acute lung injury. Mice were instilled with 50 μL of LPS (4 mg/kg) on day 0 and were mechanically ventilated 1, 4 or 10 days after ARDS induction. (A-D) Lung function parameters resistance (Rrs), elastance (Ers), tissue damping (G) and tissue elastance (H) on day 1, 4 and 10 after ARDS-induction following acetylcholine stimulation) ($n = 8$ in each group at each time point, means ± SEM). * $p \leq 0.05$, ** $p \leq 0.01$, *** $p \leq 0.001$.

Abbreviations

Ach: Acetylcholine; AHR: Airway hyperresponsiveness; ARDS: Acute respiratory distress syndrome; AUC: Area under the curve; BALF: Bronchoalveolar lavage fluid; CREM: CAMP-response element modulator; *E. coli*: *Eschericia coli*; ECG: Electrocardiography; ELISA: Enzyme-linked immunosorbent assay; FACS: Fluorescence-activated cell sorting; FoxP3: Forkhead box protein P3; IL-6: Interleukin 6; iNOS: Inducible nitric oxide synthase; KC: Keratinocyte chemoattractant; LPS: Lipopolysaccharide; MV: Mechanical ventilation; PBS: Phosphate buffered saline; PEEP: Positive end-expiratory pressure; PID: Primary immunodeficiency; RAG: Recombination-activating gene; SCID: Severe combined immunodeficiency; SD: Standard deviation; SEM: Standard error of the mean; TNF: Tumor necrosis factor; Vt: Tidal volume; WT: Wildtype

Acknowledgements

Not applicable.

Funding

This project was supported by a grant of the German respiratory society (new translation of the German term), paying part of the animal costs. This organization finances new and innovative projects in the field of lung research, especially young researchers. The society did neither influence study design, data collection, analyses of data nor interpretation of the data.

Authors' contributions

EV, SK and NR performed the mouse experiments and performed several data analysis. EV, AR, AS, KO, NW, SU, KT, CM planned the study design and participated in data analysis. EV, SK, CM, SU performed statistical analysis. EV, SU, SK and CM were major contributors in writing the manuscript. All authors read and approved the final manuscript.

Consent for publication

Not applicable.

Competing interests

The authors declare that they have no competing interests.

Author details

[1]Department of Pediatrics, Medical Faculty, RWTH Aachen, Aachen, Germany. [2]Institute of Pharmacology and Toxicology, RWTH Aachen, Aachen, Germany. [3]Department of Anaesthesiology, Medical Faculty, RWTH Aachen, Aachen, Germany.

References

1. Rubenfeld GD, Caldwell E, Peabody E, Weaver J, Martin DP, Neff M, Stern EJ, Hudson LD. Incidence and outcomes of acute lung injury. N Engl J Med. 2005;353:1685–93.
2. Vadasz I, Sznajder JI. Update in acute lung injury and critical care 2010. Am J Respir Crit Care Med. 2011;183:1147–52.
3. Tsushima K, King LS, Aggarwal NR, De Gorordo A, D'Alessio FR, Kubo K. Acute lung injury review. Intern Med. 2009;48:621–30.
4. Fan E, Needham DM, Stewart TE. Ventilatory management of acute lung injury and acute respiratory distress syndrome. JAMA. 2005;294:2889–96.
5. Yasuda H, Nishimura T, Kamo T, Sanui M, Nango E, Abe T, Takebayashi T, Lefor AK, Hashimoto S. Optimal plateau pressure for patients with acute respiratory distress syndrome: a protocol for a systematic review and meta-analysis with meta-regression. BMJ Open. 2017;7:e015091.
6. Theerawit P, Sutherasan Y, Ball L, Pelosi P. Respiratory monitoring in adult intensive care unit. Expert Rev Respir Med. 2017;11:453–68.
7. Wheeler AP, Bernard GR. Acute lung injury and the acute respiratory distress syndrome: a clinical review. Lancet. 2007;369:1553–64.
8. Nakajima T, Suarez CJ, Lin KW, Jen KY, Schnitzer JE, Makani SS, Parker N, Perkins DL, Finn PW. T cell pathways involving CTLA4 contribute to a model of acute lung injury. J Immunol. 2010;184:5835–41.
9. Abraham E. Neutrophils and acute lung injury. Crit Care Med. 2003;31:S195–9.
10. Risso K, Kumar G, Ticchioni M, Sanfiorenzo C, Dellamonica J, Guillouet-de Salvador F, Bernardin G, Marquette CH, Roger PM. Early infectious acute respiratory distress syndrome is characterized by activation and proliferation of alveolar T-cells. Eur J Clin Microbiol Infect Dis. 2015;34:1111–8.
11. Allenspach E, Rawlings DJ, Scharenberg AM. X-Linked Severe Combined Immunodeficiency. In: Pagon RA, Adam MP, Ardinger HH, Wallace SE, Amemiya A, LJH B, Bird TD, Ledbetter N, Mefford HC, RJH S, Stephens K, editors. GeneReviews(R). Seattle; 1993. PMID: 20301584
12. Fazlollahi MR, Pourpak Z, Hamidieh AA, Movahedi M, Houshmand M, Badalzadeh M, Nourizadeh M, Mahloujirad M, Arshi S, Nabavi AM, et al. Clinical, laboratory and molecular findings of 63 patients with severe combined immunodeficiency: a decade's experience. J Investig Allergol Clin Immunol. 2017;27(5):299-304.
13. Reisi M, Azizi G, Kiaee F, Masiha F, Shirzadi R, Momen T, Rafiemanesh H, Tavakolinia N, Modaresi M, Aghamohammadi A. Evaluation of pulmonary complications in patients with primary immunodeficiency disorders. Eur Ann Allergy Clin Immunol. 2017;49:122–8.
14. Verjans E, Ohl K, Yu Y, Lippe R, Schippers A, Wiener A, Roth J, Wagner N, Uhlig S, Tenbrock K, Martin C. Overexpression of CREMalpha in T cells aggravates lipopolysaccharide-induced acute lung injury. J Immunol. 2013;191:1316–23.
15. Morris PE, Glass J, Cross R, Cohen DA. Role of T-lymphocytes in the resolution of endotoxin-induced lung injury. Inflammation. 1997;21:269–78.
16. D'Alessio FR, Tsushima K, Aggarwal NR, West EE, Willett MH, Britos MF, Pipeling MR, Brower RG, Tuder RM, McDyer JF, King LS. CD4+CD25+Foxp3+ Tregs resolve experimental lung injury in mice and are present in humans with acute lung injury. J Clin Invest. 2009;119:2898–913.
17. Clark JG, Madtes DK, Hackman RC, Chen W, Cheever MA, Martin PJ. Lung injury induced by alloreactive Th1 cells is characterized by host-derived mononuclear cell inflammation and activation of alveolar macrophages. J Immunol. 1998;161:1913–20.
18. Reiss LK, Kowallik A, Uhlig S. Recurrent recruitment manoeuvres improve lung mechanics and minimize lung injury during mechanical ventilation of healthy mice. PLoS One. 2011;6:e24527.
19. Reiss LK, Uhlig U, Uhlig S. Models and mechanisms of acute lung injury caused by direct insults. Eur J Cell Biol. 2012;91:590–601.
20. Gold MI, Helrich M. Pulmonary compliance during anesthesia. Anesthesiology. 1965;26:281–8.
21. Thompson BT, Hayden D, Matthay MA, Brower R, Parsons PE. Clinicians' approaches to mechanical ventilation in acute lung injury and ARDS. Chest. 2001;120:1622–7.
22. Aggarwal NR, D'Alessio FR, Tsushima K, Sidhaye VK, Cheadle C, Grigoryev DN, Barnes KC, King LS. Regulatory T cell-mediated resolution of lung injury: identification of potential target genes via expression profiling. Physiol Genomics. 2010;41:109–19.
23. Pietropaoli A, Georas SN. Resolving lung injury: a new role for Tregs in controlling the innate immune response. J Clin Invest. 2009;119:2891–4.
24. Wehrmann F, Lavelle JC, Collins CB, Tinega AN, Thurman JM, Burnham EL, Simonian PL. gammadelta T cells protect against LPS-induced lung injury. J Leukoc Biol. 2016;99:373–86.
25. Jones JM, Gellert M. The taming of a transposon: V(D)J recombination and the immune system. Immunol Rev. 2004;200:233–48.
26. Zaynagetdinov R, Sherrill TP, Kendall PL, Segal BH, Weller KP, Tighe RM, Blackwell TS. Identification of myeloid cell subsets in murine lungs using flow cytometry. Am J Respir Cell Mol Biol. 2013;49:180–9.
27. Rentsendorj O, D'Alessio FR, Pearse DB. Phosphodiesterase 2A is a major negative regulator of iNOS expression in lipopolysaccharide-treated mouse alveolar macrophages. J Leukoc Biol. 2014;96:907–15.
28. Johnston LK, Rims CR, Gill SE, McGuire JK, Manicone AM. Pulmonary macrophage subpopulations in the induction and resolution of acute lung injury. Am J Respir Cell Mol Biol. 2012;47:417–26.
29. Hume DA. The many alternative faces of macrophage activation. Front Immunol. 2015;6:370.
30. Fehrenbach H. Alveolar epithelial type II cell: defender of the alveolus revisited. Respir Res. 2001;2:33–46.

18

Recurrence of allergic bronchopulmonary aspergillosis after adjunctive surgery for aspergilloma

Kohei Horiuchi[1*], Takanori Asakura[1,2,3], Naoki Hasegawa[4] and Fumitake Saito[1]

Abstract

Background: Coexistence of aspergilloma and allergic bronchopulmonary aspergillosis (ABPA) has rarely been reported. Although the treatment for ABPA includes administration of corticosteroids and antifungal agents, little is known about the treatment for coexisting aspergilloma and ABPA. Furthermore, the impact of surgical resection for aspergilloma on ABPA is not fully understood. Here, we present an interesting case of recurrent ABPA with long-term follow-up after surgical resection of aspergilloma.

Case presentation: A 53-year-old man with a medical history of tuberculosis was referred to our hospital with cough and dyspnea. Imaging revealed multiple cavitary lesions in the right upper lobe of the lung, with a fungus ball and mucoid impaction. The eosinophil count, total serum immunoglobulin E (IgE), and *Aspergillus*-specific IgE levels were elevated. Specimens collected on bronchoscopy revealed fungal filaments compatible with *Aspergillus* species. Based on these findings, a diagnosis of ABPA with concomitant aspergilloma was made. Although treatment with corticosteroids and antifungal agents was administered, the patient's respiratory symptoms persisted. Therefore, he underwent lobectomy of the right upper lobe, which resulted in a stable condition without the need for medication. Twenty-three months after discontinuation of medical treatment, his respiratory symptoms gradually worsened with a recurrence of elevated eosinophil count and total serum IgE. Imaging revealed recurrent bronchiectasis and cavities with mucoid impaction in the right lower lobe, suggesting relapse of aspergilloma and ABPA. Corticosteroids and antifungal agents were re-administered; aspergilloma improved slightly over a 5-year period, and ABPA remained well controlled with low-dose prednisolone (5 mg/day).

Conclusions: We describe the long-term follow-up outcomes of a patient with concomitant ABPA and aspergilloma, who underwent surgical resection for aspergilloma. Physicians should carefully monitor patients with coexisting ABPA and aspergilloma, as the condition may relapse after remission, even despite surgical resection for aspergilloma. Additionally, surgical resection for aspergilloma could result in resolution of ABPA.

Keywords: Allergic bronchopulmonary aspergillosis, *Aspergillus*, Pulmonary *Aspergillus* overlap syndrome, Relapse

* Correspondence: kohei.horiuchi17@gmail.com
[1]Department of Pulmonary Medicine, Eiju General Hospital, 2-23-16 Higashi Ueno, Taito-ku, Tokyo 110-8645, Japan
Full list of author information is available at the end of the article

Background

Aspergillus is a ubiquitous fungus isolated from both outdoor and indoor environments, including hospitals. Although *Aspergillus* spores are inhaled daily, only a minority of the population consequently develops pulmonary disease. Depending on the interaction between the fungal burden and host's immune status or immune hyperactivity, pulmonary aspergillosis has a wide spectrum of disease presentations, including chronic pulmonary aspergillosis such as aspergilloma and chronic necrotizing aspergillosis, invasive pulmonary aspergillosis, and allergic bronchopulmonary aspergillosis (ABPA) [1]. Aspergilloma is the most common form of the infection, and mostly occurs secondary to pre-existing cavitary conditions, such as previous pulmonary tuberculosis, bronchiectasis, and bronchial cysts [2], while ABPA, a hypersensitivity reaction to *Aspergillus* spp. that have colonized the lung, occurs almost exclusively in patients with asthma, cystic fibrosis, or chronic obstructive pulmonary disease [3].

The coexistence of ABPA and aspergilloma has infrequently been reported. A previous case series reported that eight of 179 (4%) ABPA patients had aspergilloma, which was associated with severe disease and relapse [4]. In terms of the treatment for aspergilloma, symptomatic patients, especially those with hemoptysis, are candidates for surgical resection, while observation is recommended for asymptomatic patients who do not demonstrate progression [5]. For ABPA, corticosteroids and anti-fungal agents are used to control inflammation and reduce fungal burden, respectively [5, 6]. However, little is known about the treatment for coexisting aspergilloma and ABPA [1]. Furthermore, the impact of surgical resection for aspergilloma on ABPA is not fully understood. Here, we present an interesting case of recurrent ABPA with long-term follow-up after surgical resection for aspergilloma.

Case presentation

A 53-year-old man was referred to our hospital with purulent cough and progressive dyspnea of a few months' duration. He had a history of tuberculosis at 31 years of age and had no other pulmonary diseases. He had never smoked cigarettes.

Upon physical examination, chest auscultation detected coarse crackles from the right lung and slight wheezes, bilaterally. Chest radiography showed cavitary lesions in the right upper lung field and consolidation in the right lower lung field (Fig. 1a). Chest computed tomography (CT) revealed bronchiectasis and cavitary

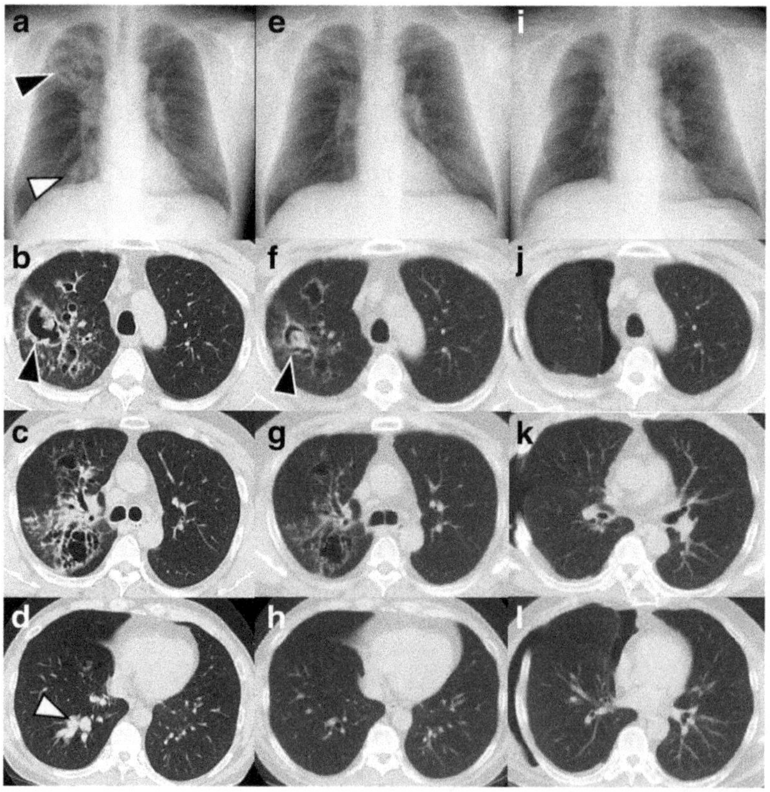

Fig. 1 (**a-d**) Chest imaging on admission showed cavitary lesions in the right upper lobe (black arrowhead) and mucoid impaction in the right lower lobe bronchi (white arrowhead). (**e-h**) Improvement was seen on chest imaging after administration of prednisolone and antifungal therapy; multiple cavities with fungus in the right upper lobe persisted (black arrowhead). (**i-l**) All the lesions improved after right upper lobe resection

lesions with a fungus ball in the right upper lobe and mucoid impaction in the bronchi of the right lower lobe (Fig. 1b–d).

Laboratory examination revealed a total leukocyte count of 14,000 cells/μL (reference range 3500–8500 cells/μL) with 45.1% eosinophils (reference range 1–6%), elevated serum total IgE levels of 19,100 IU/ml (reference range < 173 IU/ml), elevated *Aspergillus*-specific IgE of 46.3 kUA/L (reference range < 0.35 kUA/L) by fluorescence-enzyme immunoassay, as determined at a commercial laboratory (SRL Inc., Tokyo, Japan).

Pathological examination of transbronchial lung biopsy specimens from the right B3 revealed fungal filaments compatible with *Aspergillus* species. Examination of bronchoalveolar lavage fluid (BALF) showed 3056 cells/μL with 70.5% eosinophils, 17.5% neutrophils, 10.5% macrophages, and 1.5% lymphocytes. Culture of sputum and BALF did not grow any fungus. Head and neck examination by fiberscope and magnetic resonance imaging revealed no evidence of sinusitis. Thus, ABPA with concomitant aspergilloma was diagnosed based on the International Society for Human and Animal Mycology criteria [7].

One month after referral, prednisolone (0.5 mg/kg/day) and itraconazole (ITC, 200 mg/day) were administered for ABPA. ITC was switched to voriconazole (VRC, 400 mg/day) 1 month later, as the patient's symptoms and radiographic findings showed no improvement. Although the imaging findings revealed improvement of the cavitary lesions and mucoid impaction after 1 month (Fig. 1e–h), he still had cough and productive sputum. At the time, VRC was decreased to 200 mg/day due to liver dysfunction. To control the disease further, lobectomy of the right upper lobe was performed without any complication, 4 months after initiation of treatment. Pathological examination of the resected lobe revealed fungal filaments compatible with *Aspergillus* species without evidence of malignancy. The surgery resulted in gradual improvement of the patient's symptoms, imaging findings (Fig. 1i–l), and serum total IgE levels. Due to his stable course, prednisolone and VRC were discontinued 5 and 7 months after surgery, respectively.

Twenty-three months after discontinuation of the medical treatment, the patient complained of gradually worsening cough and dyspnea. Additionally, the patient's eosinophil count and serum total IgE had been steadily increasing throughout the previous year. CT showed recurrent bronchiectasis and cavities with mucoid impaction in the right lower lobe (Fig. 2a). Bronchoscopy was performed and culture results of bronchial washings from the right lower lobe revealed no evidence of bacteria, mycobacteria, or fungus. Despite the lack of evidence of *Aspergillus* infection, prednisolone (0.5 mg/kg/day) was prescribed for relapsed ABPA, based on the elevated serum IgE and pathological CT findings. Two months after treatment was initiated, the patient remained symptomatic, and CT showed a cavitary lesion with fungus in the right lower lobe (Fig. 2b). Additional treatment with VRC (400 mg/day) for 3 months resulted in improvement of his symptoms and CT findings (Fig. 2c).

Due to the markedly elevated serum total IgE, CT imaging was repeated 18 months after the re-treatment,

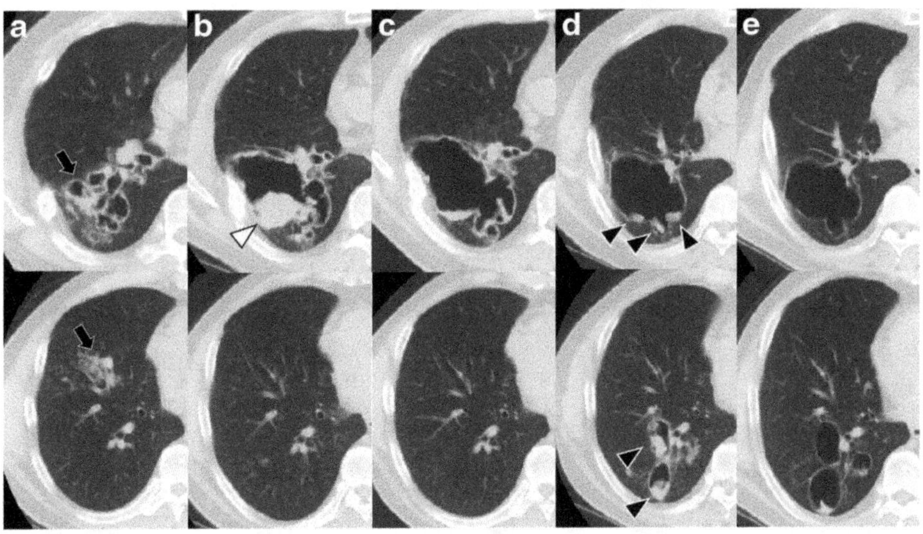

Fig. 2 Chest computed tomography (CT) at the time of relapse (**a**), 2 months (**b**), 3 months (**c**), 22 months (**d**), and 6 years after the relapse (**e**). (**a**) Recurrence of bronchiectasis and cavities with mucoid impaction (black arrow) in the right lower lobe. (**b**) A cavitary lesion with a fungus ball (white arrowhead) was observed in the right lower lobe. (**c**) Improvement seen on CT after additional treatment with voriconazole. (**d**) CT scan showing advancement of fungus balls inside the large cavity in the right lower lobe (black arrowhead). (**e**) No fungus balls seen on CT 6 years after the relapse

although the patient's symptoms had remained stable. CT revealed progression of the fungus balls inside the large cavity in the right lower lobe (Fig. 2d). The addition of VRC (400 mg/day) resulted in a decrease in the serum total IgE. VRC was discontinued after 20 months as the patient's condition had become stable by that time. The aspergilloma improved slightly over a 5-year period (Fig. 2e), and ABPA remained well-controlled with low-dose prednisolone (5 mg/day). The summary of the treatment course is shown in Fig. 3.

Discussion and conclusions

This case describes a recurrence of ABPA, with long-term follow-up after surgical resection for aspergilloma. The surgery resulted in ABPA remission without the use of corticosteroids and anti-fungal agents for about 2 years. However, the patient had recurrence of ABPA with aspergilloma in the residual lung. Eventually, re-administration of corticosteroids and adjunctive anti-fungal therapy achieved long-term remission of ABPA. This case highlights the need for careful monitoring of patients with coexistent ABPA and aspergilloma, as the condition may relapse after remission, even despite surgical resection for aspergilloma. The formation of aspergilloma may also be observed at the recurrence of ABPA. Additionally, surgical resection for aspergilloma could result in resolution of ABPA.

In our case, adjunctive surgery resulted in ABPA remission for 2 years. Previous studies have reported the outcome of surgical resection for aspergilloma in ABPA patients, due to pneumothorax [8] and hemoptysis [9, 10]. However, only one case involved a report of surgical resection for aspergilloma that contributed to disease control of ABPA; the patient was followed up without ABPA treatment for 6 months after receiving surgical resection for aspergilloma with antifungal therapy [11], whereas our case was followed up for a number of years.

Several pathogenic mechanisms have been suggested to be responsible for the overlap between ABPA and aspergilloma. On the one hand, in terms of aspergilloma development in cases of ABPA, in the early phase, bronchiectatic lesions affected by ABPA may enlarge to form cavities that become colonized with *Aspergillus* to create fungus balls [12, 13]. In the late phase, aspergilloma may form in patients with fibrosis and cavitation associated with long-standing or poorly treated ABPA. On the other hand, ABPA may develop due to a hypersensitivity reaction to an increased fungal burden in a patient with aspergilloma with pre-existing fibrocavitary disease, such as tuberculosis [14]. Thus, ABPA and aspergilloma have a synergistic relationship, which can result in a severe disease and recurrent relapse [4]. Furthermore, corticosteroids administered for the treatment of ABPA might accelerate the formation of aspergilloma [12] and lead to hemoptysis. Thus, adjunctive surgery for aspergilloma might be beneficial in ABPA patients as it reduces the fungal burden and allows the use of corticosteroid.

Although the patient had long-term remission after surgery, ABPA and aspergilloma relapsed concurrently, suggesting an overlap in the pathogenesis of these conditions in this patient. CT imaging (Fig. 2) showed severe bronchiectatic lesions with mucoid impaction, leading to the formation of cavities with aspergilloma. Previous

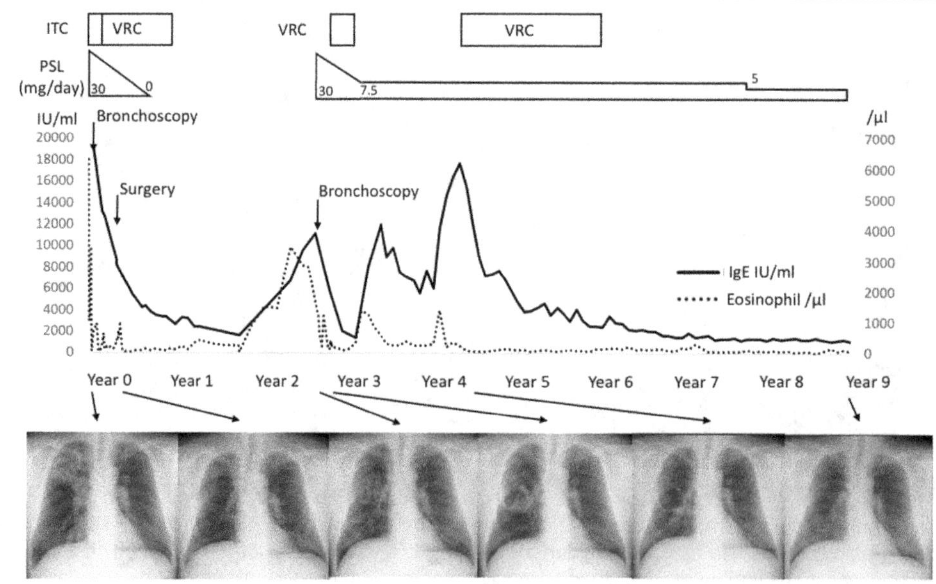

Fig. 3 Clinical course of our case, including the changes in eosinophil counts (dotted line) and IgE levels (solid line). IgE; immunoglobulin E, ITC; itraconazole, VRC; voriconazole, PSL; prednisolone

studies in ABPA have reported a range of radiological features associated with recurrence or relapse, including extensive bronchiectasis, aspergilloma, and high-attenuation mucus [4, 15–17]. Notably, our patient relapsed even though the treatment, including surgery, resulted in initial improvement of all the pulmonary lesions caused by ABPA and aspergilloma (Fig. 1i–l). Therefore, maintenance therapy with corticosteroid or antifungal therapy might be needed to prevent relapse in high-risk patients, even after surgical resection of aspergilloma.

The treatment options for ABPA have included corticosteroid, anti-fungal therapy, and biologic agents, such as omalizumab and mepolizumab. In the acute phase, recent studies have suggested that medium-dose oral corticosteroid are as effective as and safer than high doses for the treatment of ABPA [18], and that ITC was also effective in a significant number of patients, with fewer side effects than prednisolone [19]. In our case, corticosteroids and ITC were simultaneously administered for concomitant aspergilloma, and we decided on surgical resection due to persistent symptoms, resulting in ABPA remission for 2 years. Although we could control ABPA by corticosteroid and anti-fungal therapy at the post-surgical relapse, other new therapies could be options for refractory cases. Recent studies have shown that omalizumab, a humanized anti-IgE monoclonal antibody, can be used safely for ABPA [20], and addition of mepolizumab, an anti-interleukin 5 monoclonal antibody, was also effective for refractory ABPA [21]. Furthermore, nebulized amphotericin could be beneficial for decreasing the frequency of exacerbations [22]. Since steroid therapy might deteriorate the formation of aspergilloma and further surgical resection may be limited, these treatments will be options in case of relapse.

The limitation of our case is that we were unable to detect the precise species of *Aspergillus* by culture of sputum, bronchial wash, or BALF. Additionally, molecular identification of fungal species was not available at our clinical site. Knowing the exact species and the resistance profile may have enabled us to provide better patient care in terms of the choice of antifungal agents. Although infrequent, *Aspergillus terreus* shows resistance to amphotericin B [23, 24]; is has been reported to cause ABPA and may form aspergilloma [25], which is reminiscent of our case. Another concern is that azole-resistant *Aspergillus fumigatus* is becoming a global health problem due to treatment failure and high mortality [26]. Regarding the treatment for azole-resistant *Aspergillus fumigatus*, most experts recommend a change from VRC monotherapy to liposomal amphotericin B or an azole–echinocandin combination [27]. These therapies are also considered in hospitals or wards where a 10% resistance threshold is exceeded [27].

In conclusion, we describe the long-term follow-up outcomes of a case with concomitant ABPA and aspergilloma, who underwent surgical resection for aspergilloma. This case emphasizes that physicians should carefully monitor patients with coexistent ABPA and aspergilloma, as the condition may relapse after remission, even after surgical resection for aspergilloma. Additionally, the case illustrates that surgical resection for aspergilloma could result in resolution of ABPA.

Abbreviations

ABPA: Allergic bronchopulmonary aspergillosis; BALF: bronchoalveolar lavage fluid; CT: computed tomography; IgE: immunoglobulin E; ITC: itraconazole; VRC: voriconazole

Acknowledgements

Not applicable.

Funding

Not applicable.

Authors' contributions

KH provided patient care and drafted the manuscript. TA, NH, and FS supervised the manuscript revision. All authors read and approved the final manuscript.

Consent for publication

Written informed consent was obtained from the patient for publication of this case report.

Competing interests

The authors declare that they have no competing interests.

Author details

[1]Department of Pulmonary Medicine, Eiju General Hospital, 2-23-16 Higashi Ueno, Taito-ku, Tokyo 110-8645, Japan. [2]Division of Pulmonary Medicine, Department of Medicine, Keio University School of Medicine, Tokyo, Japan. [3]Department of Mycobacteriology, National Institute of Infectious Diseases, Tokyo, Japan. [4]Center for Infectious Diseases and Infection Control, Keio University School of Medicine, Tokyo, Japan.

References

1. Kousha M, Tadi R, Soubani AO. Pulmonary aspergillosis: a clinical review. Eur Respir Rev. 2011;20(121):156–74.
2. Kauffman CA. Quandary about treatment of aspergillomas persists. Lancet. 1996;347(9016):1640.
3. Agarwal R, Hazarika B, Gupta D, Aggarwal AN, Chakrabarti A, Jindal SK. *Aspergillus* hypersensitivity in patients with chronic obstructive pulmonary disease: COPD as a risk factor for ABPA? Med Mycol. 2010;48(7):988–94.
4. Agarwal R, Aggarwal AN, Garg M, Saikia B, Gupta D, Chakrabarti A. Allergic bronchopulmonary aspergillosis with aspergilloma: an immunologically severe disease with poor outcome. Mycopathologia. 2012;174(3):193–201.
5. Patterson TF, Thompson GR 3rd, Denning DW, Fishman JA, Hadley S, Herbrecht R, Kontoyiannis DP, Marr KA, Morrison VA, Nguyen MH, et al. Practice guidelines for the diagnosis and Management of Aspergillosis: 2016

update by the Infectious Diseases Society of America. Clin Infect Dis. 2016; 63(4):e1–e60.

6. Muldoon EG, Strek ME, Patterson KC. Allergic and noninvasive infectious pulmonary aspergillosis syndromes. Clin Chest Med. 2017;38(3):521–34.
7. Agarwal R, Chakrabarti A, Shah A, Gupta D, Meis JF, Guleria R, Moss R, Denning DW. Allergic bronchopulmonary aspergillosis: review of literature and proposal of new diagnostic and classification criteria. Clin Exp Allergy. 2013;43(8):850–73.
8. Reich JM. Pneumothorax due to pleural perforation of a pseudocavity containing aspergillomas in a patient with allergic bronchopulmonary aspergillosis. Chest. 1992;102(2):652–3.
9. Bhagat R, Shah A, Jaggi OP, Khan ZU. Concomitant allergic bronchopulmonary aspergillosis and allergic *Aspergillus* sinusitis with an operated aspergilloma. J Allergy Clin Immunol. 1993;91(5):1094–6.
10. Dogra V, Sinha AK, Saxena R, Talwar D. *Aspergillus* march: from ABPA to aspergilloma to subacute invasive aspergillosis. Allergy Asthma Clin Immunol. 2016;12:64.
11. Montani D, Zendah I, Achouh L, Dorfmuller P, Mercier O, Garcia G, Humbert M. Association of pulmonary aspergilloma and allergic bronchopulmonary aspergillosis. Eur Respir Rev. 2010;19(118):349–51.
12. Safirstein BH, D'Souza MF, Simon G, Tai EH, Pepys J. Five-year follow-up of allergic bronchopulmonary aspergillosis. Am Rev Respir Dis. 1973;108(3):450–9.
13. Israel RH, Poe RH, Bomba PA, Gross RA. The rapid development of an aspergilloma secondary to allergic bronchopulmonary aspergillosis. Am J Med Sci. 1980;280(1):41–4.
14. Ein ME, Wallace RJ Jr, Williams TW Jr. Allergic bronchopulmonary aspergillosis-like syndrome consequent to aspergilloma. Am Rev Respir Dis. 1979;119(5):811–20.
15. Agarwal R, Gupta D, Aggarwal AN, Saxena AK, Chakrabarti A, Jindal SK. Clinical significance of hyperattenuating mucoid impaction in allergic bronchopulmonary aspergillosis: an analysis of 155 patients. Chest. 2007;132(4):1183–90.
16. Agarwal R, Gupta D, Aggarwal AN, Saxena AK, Saikia B, Chakrabarti A, Jindal SK. Clinical significance of decline in serum IgE levels in allergic bronchopulmonary aspergillosis. Respir Med. 2010;104(2):204–10.
17. Agarwal R, Khan A, Gupta D, Aggarwal AN, Saxena AK, Chakrabarti A. An alternate method of classifying allergic bronchopulmonary aspergillosis based on high-attenuation mucus. PLoS One. 2010;5(12):e15346.
18. Agarwal R, Aggarwal AN, Dhooria S, Singh Sehgal I, Garg M, Saikia B, Behera D, Chakrabarti A. A randomised trial of glucocorticoids in acute-stage allergic bronchopulmonary aspergillosis complicating asthma. Eur Respir J. 2016;47(2):490–8.
19. Agarwal R, Dhooria S, Singh Sehgal I, Aggarwal AN, Garg M, Saikia B, Behera D, Chakrabarti A. A randomized trial of itraconazole vs prednisolone in acute-stage allergic bronchopulmonary aspergillosis complicating asthma. Chest. 2018;153(3):656–64.
20. Voskamp AL, Gillman A, Symons K, Sandrini A, Rolland JM, O'Hehir RE, Douglass JA. Clinical efficacy and immunologic effects of omalizumab in allergic bronchopulmonary aspergillosis. J Allergy Clin Immunol Pract. 2015;3(2):192–9.
21. Altman MC, Lenington J, Bronson S, Ayars AG. Combination omalizumab and mepolizumab therapy for refractory allergic bronchopulmonary aspergillosis. J Allergy Clin Immunol Pract. 2017;5(4):1137–9.
22. Ram B, Aggarwal AN, Dhooria S, Sehgal IS, Garg M, Behera D, Chakrabarti A, Agarwal R. A pilot randomized trial of nebulized amphotericin in patients with allergic bronchopulmonary aspergillosis. J Asthma. 2016;53(5):517–24.
23. Steinbach WJ, Benjamin DK Jr, Kontoyiannis DP, Perfect JR, Lutsar I, Marr KA, Lionakis MS, Torres HA, Jafri H, Walsh TJ. Infections due to *Aspergillus terreus*: a multicenter retrospective analysis of 83 cases. Clin Infect Dis. 2004;39(2):192–8.
24. Won EJ, Choi MJ, Shin JH, Park YJ, Byun SA, Jung JS, Kim SH, Shin MG, Suh SP. Diversity of clinical isolates of *Aspergillus terreus* in antifungal susceptibilities, genotypes and virulence in *Galleria mellonella* model: comparison between respiratory and ear isolates. PLoS One. 2017;12(10):e0186086.
25. Laham MN, Carpenter JL. *Aspergillus terreus*, a pathogen capable of causing infective endocarditis, pulmonary mycetoma, and allergic bronchopulmonary aspergillosis. *Am Rev Respir Dis*. 1982;125(6):769–72.
26. Verweij PE, Chowdhary A, Melchers WJ, Meis JF. Azole resistance in *Aspergillus fumigatus*: can we retain the clinical use of mold-active antifungal azoles? Clin Infect Dis. 2016;62(3):362–8.
27. Chowdhary A, Sharma C, Meis JF. Azole-resistant aspergillosis: epidemiology, molecular mechanisms, and treatment. J Infect Dis. 2017; 216(Suppl 3):S436–s444.

19

WISP1 mediates lung injury following hepatic ischemia reperfusion dependent on TLR4 in mice

Yao Tong[†], Zhuang Yu[†], Renlingzi Zhang[†], Xibing Ding, Zhixia Chen and Quan Li[*]

Abstract

Background: Hepatic ischemia-reperfusion injury (IRI) is a common pathological phenomenon, which causes hepatic injury as well as remote organ injuries such as the lung. Several mediators, such as oxidative stress, Ca^{2+} overload and neutrophil infiltration, have been implied in the pathogenesis of liver and remote organ injuries following reperfusion. WNT1 inducible signaling pathway protein 1 (WISP1) is an extracellular matrix protein that has been associated with the onset of several malignant diseases. Previous work in our group has demonstrated WISP1 is upregulated and contributes to proinflammatory cascades in hepatic IRI. However, the role of WISP1 in the pathogenesis of lung injury after hepatic IRI still remains unknown.

Methods: Male C57BL/6 mice were used to examine the expression and role of WISP1 in the pathogenesis of lung injuries after hepatic IRI and explore its potential mechanisms in mediating lung injuries.

Results: We found WISP1 was upregulated in lung tissues following hepatic IRI. Treatment with anti-WISP1 antibody ameliorated lung injuries with alteration of cytokine profiles. Administration with rWISP1 aggravated lung injuries following hepatic IRI through excessive production of proinflammatory cytokines and inhibition of anti-inflammatory cytokines.

Conclusions: In this study, we concluded that WISP1 contributed to lung injuries following hepatic IRI through TLR4 pathway.

Keywords: Hepatic ischemia-reperfusion injury, WNT1 inducible signaling pathway protein 1, Inflammatory cascades, Toll like receptor

Introduction

Hepatic ischemia-reperfusion injury (IRI) is a pathological phenomenon event when hypoxic liver undergoes oxygenic blood reperfusion. Usually IRI can be divided into two categories, namely warm ischemia which often occurs in trauma, shock, and liver transplantation with temporary blood interruption and cold ischemia which appears during organ preservation before transplantation. Recent studies have implied several pathological mechanisms in the pathogenesis of IRI including production of reactive oxygen species (ROS), synthesis of inducible nitric oxide synthase (iNOS), and secretion of proinflammatory cytokines and chemokines which leads to immune cell (especially neutrophil) recruitment and inflammatory cascades [1–3]. Excessive production of proinflammatory cytokines in the serum, including TNF-α, IL-1β and IL-6 in the early phase contribute to the local and remote organ damage [4, 5]. Previous studies have confirmed lung injury in the IRI model [6]. However, the exact mechanism of IRI induced remote organ injury still remains unclear.

Pattern recognition receptors (PRRs) have been demonstrated to participate in the pathogenesis of IRI, with one of the most important members being Toll-like receptor 4 (TLR4) [7]. TLR4 can recognize various kinds of endogenous antigens and is activated in IRI in liver and remote organs [8]. The functions of TLR4 on immune cells are more vital than on hepatocytes

* Correspondence: quanligene@126.com
[†]Yao Tong, Zhuang Yu and Renlingzi Zhang contributed equally to this work.
Department of Anesthesiology, Shanghai East Hospital, School of Medicine, Tongji University, 150 Jimo Road, Shanghai 200120, China

although the regulating mechanisms may be different [9, 10]. Besides TLR4 signaling, other PRRs, such as TLR2 and TLR9, have been reported to be involved in the pathogenesis of IRI [11–13].

WNT1 inducible signaling pathway protein 1 (WISP1) is a secreted extracellular matrix (ECM) protein which is ubiquitously expressed in multiple organs, such as lung, liver, kidney, heart and small intestine [14]. WISP1 belongs to the CCN family which contains 6 members, namely CCN1 (cysteine-rich protein 61, Cyr61), CCN2 (connective tissue growth factor, CTGF), CCN3 (nephroblastoma overexpressed gene, NOV), CCN4 (WNT1 inducible signaling pathway protein-1, WISP1), CCN5 (WISP2) and CCN6 (WISP3) [15]. The functions of WISP1 has been linked to cell proliferation, survival and differentiation [15]. Recent studies have demonstrated that WISP1 relative expression is significantly upregulated in some diseases, including lung carcinoma, hepatocellular carcinoma [16] and colon adenocarcinomas [17]. Interestingly, Li et al. have linked WISP1 to the progression of inflammation [18], that is, stimulation of recombinant WISP1 aggravates proinflammatory responses in LPS stimulated macrophages. Previous work in our group has demonstrated WISP1 is upregulated and contributes to proinflammatory cascades in hepatic IRI [19]. However, the role of WISP1 in the pathogenesis of lung injury after IRI still remains unknown.

In this study, we aimed to investigate the WISP1 expression in the lung tissue after hepatic IRI and determine the regulating mechanisms and functions of WISP1 in the lung injury after hepatic IRI.

Methods

Mice

C57BL/6 mice were purchased from Shanghai Laboratory Animal Co Ltd. (SLAC, Shanghai, China). TLR4 knockout (TLR4 KO) mice were kindly provided by Dr. Timothy R. Billiar (University of Pittsburgh, USA). All mice were raised in specific pathogen-free condition. Male mice of 8–10 weeks (weight 18.4.8 ± 1.8 g) old were used for experiments. Animal experiments were authorized by the Ethics Committee of Tongji University.

Induction of hepatic I/R injury model]

The induction of segmental (70%) hepatic hepatic warm I/R injury model was performed as previously described with minor modifications [8, 20, 21]. Mice were treated with isotype control IgG or neutralizing WISP1/WISP2 antibody (MyBioSource, 6 μg/g) intraperitoneally 1 h before ischemia and again at the time of reperfusion. In another experiment, mice were administered with recombinant WISP1 protein (rWISP1, 1 μg/g) or sterile phosphate-buffered saline (PBS, w/o Ca^{2+}/Mg^{2+}) intraperitoneally immediately after reperfusion. Sham mice were sufficiently anesthetized, and then a midline abdominal incision was made. The portal triad was exposed without further treatment for liver ischemia. Mice were sacrificed at the predetermined time points (0 h, 3 h, 6 h, 12 h and 24 h) after reperfusion for collecting serum and lung tissues.

Lung edema measurement

Lung edema was evaluated as previously reported by an increase in the wet-to-dry (W/D) weight ratio of the lungs [21, 22]. The left lung was dissected and weighted before and after drying in a micro oven at 65 °C for 48 h. W/D ratio was then detected.

Alveolar-capillary permeability assay

Evans blue albumin (EBA) was used to measure Alveolar-capillary permeability as previous illustrated [23]. Briefly, the internal jugular vein of mice was injected with EBA (25 mg/kg) 1 h before sacrificed. And then, the right lung and blood samples were available for further steps.

Evaluation of Bronchoalveolar lavage fluid (BALF)

BALF was evaluated as previously publications in our group [21]. Mice were instilled with 1 mL PBS and approximately 80% fluid was retrieved. BALF was kept on ice immediately after recovered and was then centrifuged at 1000×g, 4 °C for 5 min. Supernatants were used for total protein concentration examination and cytokine levels, which can keep at − 80 °C for long-term preservation. Total cell counts were determined using a hemocytometer.

RNA extraction, reverse transcription PCR, Quantative real-time PCR

Total RNA was extracted from lung tissues using TRIzol reagent (Sigma-Aldrich) according to established protocols in our group [21, 24]. The total concentration of RNA was measured at 260 nm with a spectrophotometer (BeckmanCoulter, Brea, CA, USA). First strand complementary DNA (cDNA) synthesis was performed using PrimerScript RT Master Mix (Takara Bio Inc., Shiga, Japan) according to the manufacturer's protocols. Real-time PCR for glyceraldehyde-3-phosphate dehydrogenase (GAPDH), WISP1, IL-6, TNF-α, IL-10 was performed using SYBR premix Ex Taq™ (Takara) with a Step One Plus real-time PCR system (Applied biosystems, USA), under the manufacturer's instructions. GAPDH was used as house-keeping gene to normalize the gene expression. Gene relative expression was calculated using the $2^{-\Delta\Delta}$Ct method. All of the primers were synthesized by Sangon Biotech (Shanghai, China). Primers sequence was as follows: mWISP1 forward 5′- CGCCCGAGGTACGCAATAG, reverse 5′- GCAGTTGGGTTGGAAGGACT, mIL-6 forward 5′- CTGCAAGAGACTTCCATCCAG, reverse 5′- AGTG GTATAGACAGGTCTGTTGG, mTNF-α forward 5′- CAGGCGGTGCCTATGTCTC, reverse 5′- CGAT CACCCCGAAGTTCAGTAG, mIL-10 forward 5′- CTTACTGACTGGCATGAGGATCA, reverse 5′- GCAGCTCTAGGAGCATGTGG.

Enzyme-linked immunosorbent assay (ELISA)

BALF supernatants were analyzed for mIL-6, mTNF-α and mIL-10 cytokines using a sensitive commercial ELISA kit (R&D Systems) according to the manufacturer's instructions.

Western blot analysis

Western blot analysis was performed as previously described in our studies [21, 24]. Lung tissues were dissected and lysed using iced-cold lysis buffer (Beyotime, catalog no. P0013G). Protein concentration was determined via standard BCA assay. After gel electrophoresis, protein was then transferred to a nitrocellulose membrane and blocked using 5% nonfat milk for 1 h. Membranes were incubated with rabbit anti-mouse WISP1 antibody (1:400, R&D systems) and β-actin antibody (1:10000, Proteintech) at 4 °C overnight, and then incubated with secondary antibody for 1 h at 37 °C. Odyssey image analysis system (Licor Biosciences) was used to quantify.

Immunofluorescence

Immunofluorescent staining was performed using standard protocols [25, 26]. Briefly, 4–6-mm frozen sections from murine lung tissues were incubated with anti-WISP1 antibody (abcom, 1:200) antibody overnight at 4 °C. Sections were then incubated with secondary Alexa Fluor 488-labelled rabbit anti-mouse antibody (CST, 1:200) for 1 h at room temperature. Nucleus was stained with DAPI for 5 min at room temperature. The positive signals were analysed using a confocal fluorescence microscope (Zeiss LSM510 Confocal).

Determination of myeloperoxidase (MPO) level

The lung MPO level was determined using a commercial mouse MPO ELISA kit (Hycult Biotech) according to the manufacturer's instructions.

Statistical analysis

Data were displayed as mean ± SEM. Statistical analysis was performed using GraphPad Prism 5 program. Differences between groups were compared using the Student *t*-test or one-way analysis of variance (ANOVA). Statistically significant differences were considered as $P < 0.05$.

Results

WISP1 is highly increased in lung tissue following hepatic IRI

Previous work in our group has demonstrated WISP1 facilitates proinflammatory cascades following hepatic IRI in the liver dependent on TLR4 signaling [24]. Since remote organ injuries, such as lung injury [8], have been reported following hepatic IRI, we next sought to detect whether WISP1 was involved in the pathogenesis of lung injury in hepatic IRI. Interestingly, WISP1 gene transcription was found to be highly increased in the lung tissue following hepatic IRI after reperfusion for 6 h, 12 h, and 24 h (Fig. 1a). Western blot analysis further confirmed WISP1 protein level was also significantly upregulated (Fig. 1b). To further analyze WISP1 expression in morphology, we also performed immunofluorescence and Immunohistochemistry assays to verify WISP1 expression. Consistent with previous results, WISP1 is a secreted extracellular matrix protein mainly expressed in cytoplasm (Fig. 1c and d). WISP1 was highly expressed in cytoplasm of the cells in lung tissue (Fig. 1c and d). Together, these results indicated that WISP1 was highly increased in lung tissue following hepatic IRI.

Treatment with anti-WISP1 antibody ameliorates lung injury following hepatic IRI

To further confirm the role of WISP1 in the pathogenesis of lung injury after hepatic IRI, we treated mice in sham and hepatic IRI group with neutralizing anti-WISP1 or control IgG antibody intraperitoneally 1 h before ischemia and again at the onset of reperfusion. After reperfusion for 6 h, mice were sacrificed and lung injury was assessed. Histopathology evaluation indicated treatment with anti-WISP1 antibody ameliorated liver injury, as showed by histopathological and biochemical (ALT/AST) evidence (Fig. 2a and b) and lung injury characterized by less diffuse interstitial edema and inflammatory cell infiltration (Fig. 2c), decreased W/D weight ratio (Fig. 2d) as well as decreased lung EBA permeability (Fig. 2e). Consistent with histopathology analysis, total cell counts (Fig. 2f) and total protein levels (Fig. 2g) were also decreased, indicating less severe inflammation compared with control group. MPO is a peroxidase enzyme which is abundantly expressed on polymorphonuclear neutrophils. The function of MPO has been associated with production of hypochlorous acid (HOCl) which is a subtype of ROS [27]. Consistently, we found MPO levels were also decreased in the lung tissue after anti-WISP1 antibody treatment following hepatic IRI (Fig. 2h). These results indicated that anti-WISP1 neutralizing antibody markedly ameliorated lung injury following hepatic IRI, further confirming the pathological role of WISP1.

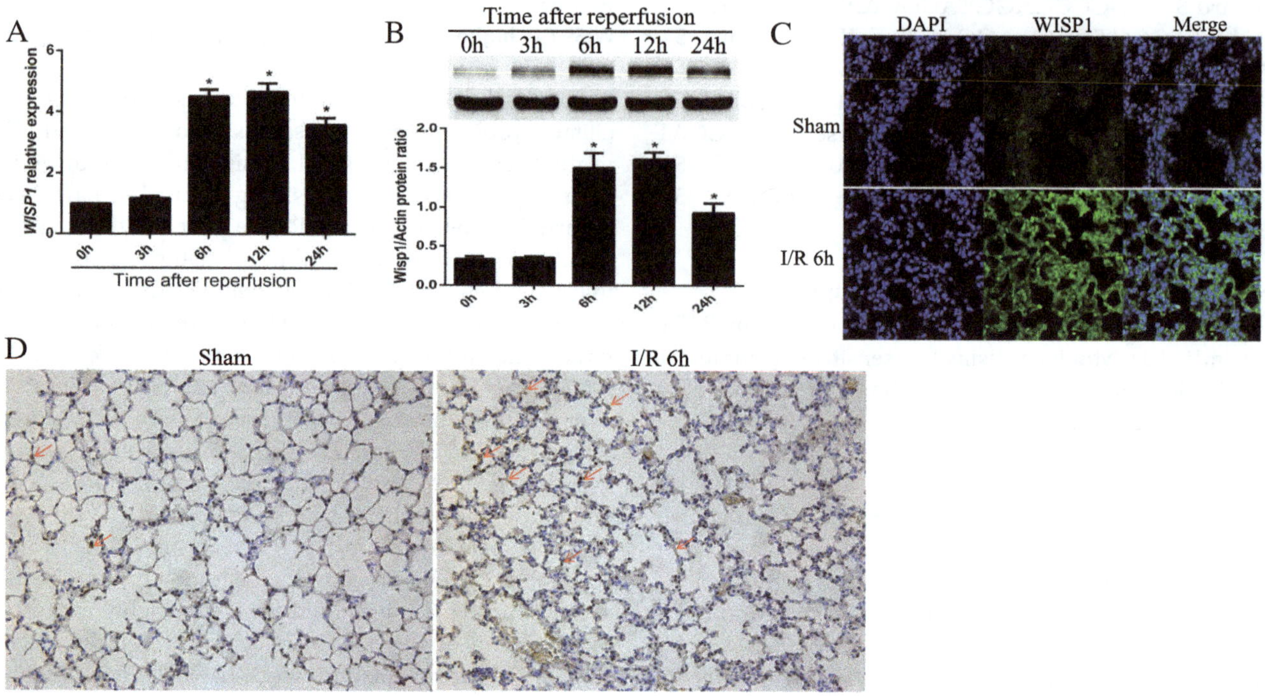

Fig. 1 WISP1 is Highly Increased in Lung Tissue Following Hepatic IRI. qRT-PCR (**a**) and western blot (**b**) analysis of WISP1 in lung samples from WT mice undergoing ischemia for 60 min and reperfusion (I/R) for 0 h, 6 h, 12 h, and 24 h ($n = 6$ respectively). **c** Immunofluorescence and (**d**) Immunohistochemistry assays of WISP1 in lung samples from WT mice in sham and IRI group undergoing ischemia for 60 min and reperfusion for 6 h. Gene expression was normalized to *β-actin* mRNA levels in each sample. $^{*}p < 0.05$ compared with 0 h of reperfusion, data are expressed as mean ± s.e.m. for all samples

Treatment with anti-WISP1 antibody alters cytokine profiles in lung tissue following hepatic IRI

Previous results indicated anti-WISP1 antibody ameliorated lung injury following hepatic IRI. We next sought in determine whether treatment with anti-WISP1 antibody augmented proinflammatory or anti-inflammatory cytokine profiles which contributed to the injury in the lung tissue. Mice were treated as previously described. qRT-PCR analysis demonstrated that proinflammatory cytokine IL-6 (Fig. 3a) and TNF-α (Fig. 3b) transcriptions were significantly downregulated in lung tissue following hepatic IRI. However, anti-inflammatory cytokine IL-10 (Fig. 3c) was markedly upregulated. To further determine such cytokine alterations in protein level, we next performed ELISA analysis for these cytokines. In accordance with qRT-PCR results, IL-6 (Fig. 3e) and TNF-α (Fig. 3f) protein level were highly elevated and IL-10 (Fig. 3g) level was decreased. Additionally, we used anti-WISP2 antibody as a control to detect whether it has the same effect. There were no significant changes in pro-inflammatory cytokines' transcription or release following neutralizing WISP2 antibody treatment during liver IRI (Fig. 3d and h). Together, these data suggested anti-WISP1 antibody led to decreased proinflammatory cytokine production and excessive anti-inflammatory cytokine secretion.

Administration with rWISP1 aggravates lung injury following hepatic IRI

To comprehensively study the pathological role of WISP1, mice in the sham and hepatic IRI group were administered with rWISP1 or control medium (sterile PBS) intraperitoneally once immediately after reperfusion. Lung injury was assessed as previously reported. Histopathology analysis suggested administration with rWISP1 aggravated lung injury characterized by more severe diffuse interstitial edema and more inflammatory cell infiltration (Fig. 4a), increased W/D weight ratio (Fig. 4b) as well as decreased lung EBA permeability (Fig. 4c). Total cell counts (Fig. 4d) and total protein levels (Fig. 4e) were also decreased, indicating severer inflammation compared with control group. Besides, MPO levels were also increased (Fig. 4f). These data indicated administration with rWISP1 aggravated lung injury following hepatic IRI, which contrasts with treatment with anti-WISP1 antibody.

rWISP1 facilitates Proinflammatory cytokine and inhibits anti-inflammatory cytokine production in lung tissue following hepatic IRI

Administration with rWISP1 significantly aggravated lung injury following hepatic IRI, we next wondered

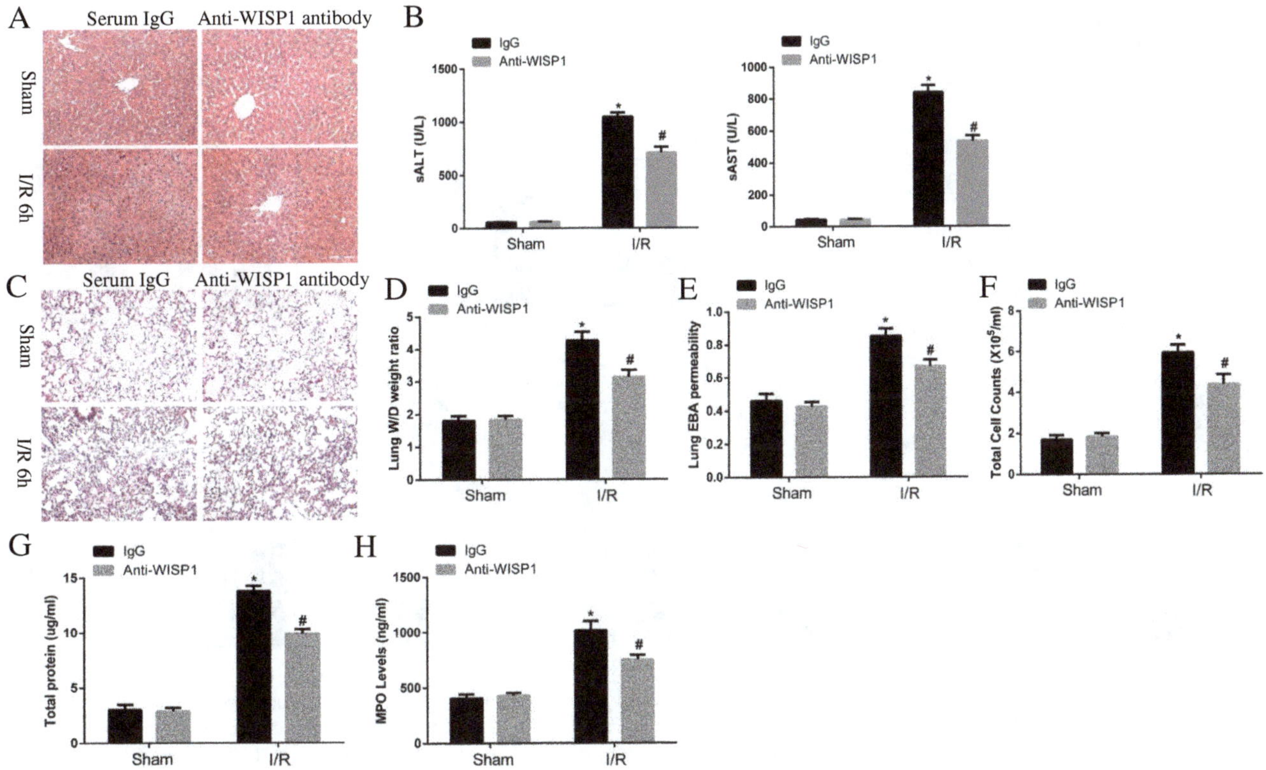

Fig. 2 Treatment with Anti-WISP1 Antibody Ameliorates Lung Injury Following Hepatic IRI. WT mice in sham and IRI group undergoing ischemia for 60 min and reperfusion for 6 h were treated intraperitoneally with either control IgG antibody or anti-WISP1 antibody (6 μg/g) 1 h before ischemia and at the onset of reperfusion ($n = 6$ respectively). H&E staining (**a** and **c**), ALT and AST levels (**b**), W/D weight ratio (**d**), EBA permeability analysis (**e**), total cell counts (**f**) and proteins (**g**) in BALF and MPO levels (**h**) of lung samples from WT mice in sham and IRI group were performed. $^{*}p < 0.05$ compared with sham group, $^{\#}p < 0.05$ compared with IgG group, data are expressed as mean ± s.e.m. for all samples

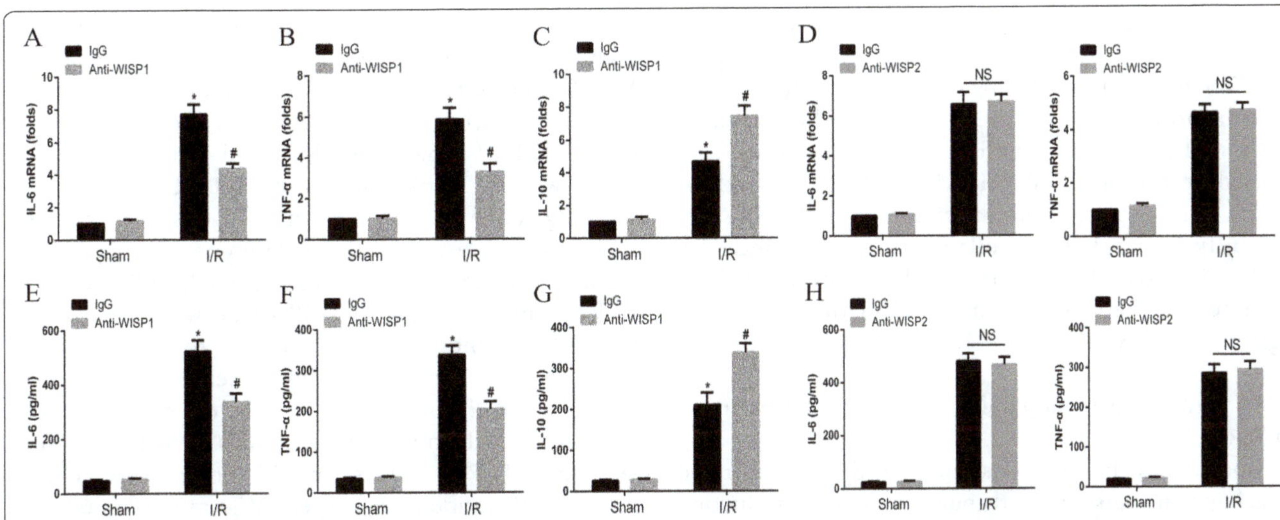

Fig. 3 WISP1 facilitates the expression of pro-inflammatory cytokines in IBD LPMCs. WT mice in sham and IRI group undergoing ischemia for 60 min and reperfusion for 6 h were treated intraperitoneally with either control IgG antibody or neutralizing WISP1/WISP2 antibody (6 μg/g) 1 h before ischemia and at the onset of reperfusion ($n = 6$ respectively). qRT-PCR for IL-6 (**a** and **d**), TNF-α (**b** and **d**), and IL-10 (**c**) from lung tissues in all groups was performed. ELISA for IL-6 (**e** and **h**), TNF-α (**f** and **h**), and IL-10 (**g**) from BALF supernatants in all groups was performed. $^{*}p < 0.05$ compared with sham group, $^{\#}p < 0.05$ compared with IgG group, data are expressed as mean ± s.e.m. for all samples

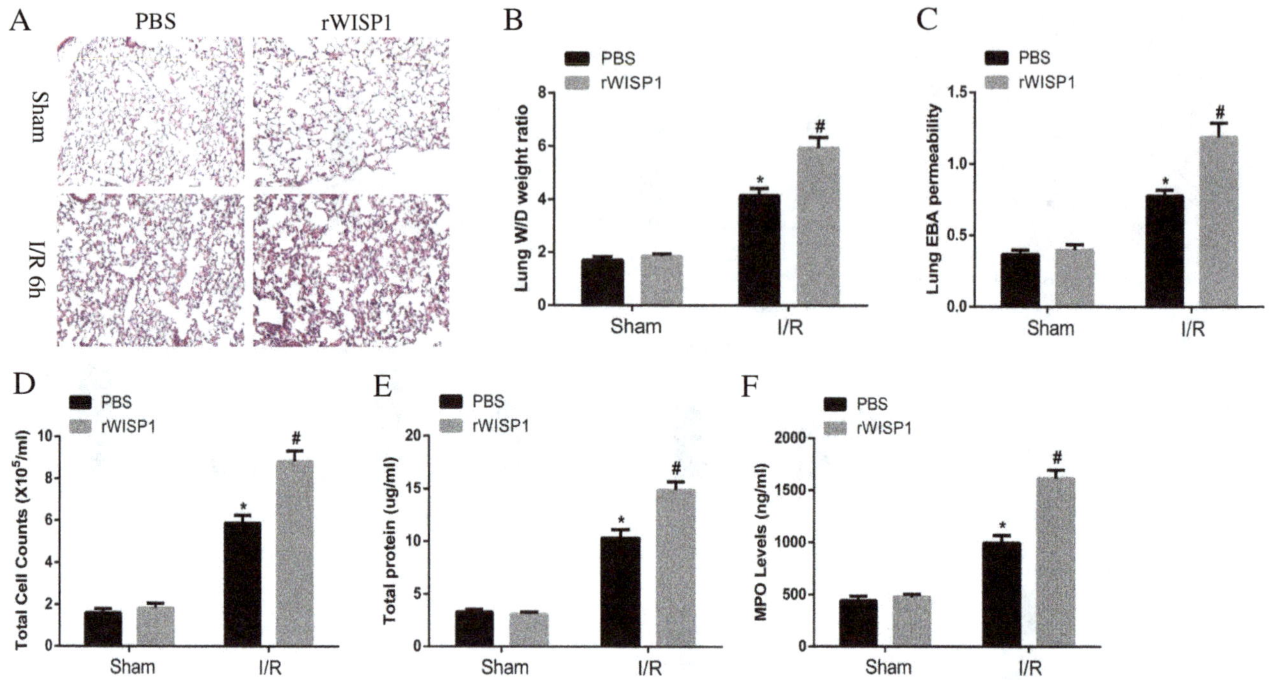

Fig. 4 Administration with rWISP1 Aggravates Lung Injury Following Hepatic IRI. WT mice in sham and IRI group undergoing ischemia for 60 min and reperfusion for 6 h were treated intraperitoneally with either sterile PBS or rWISP1 (1 μg/g) at the onset of reperfusion ($n = 6$ respectively). H&E staining (**a**), W/D weight ratio (**b**), EBA permeability analysis (**c**), total cell counts (**d**) and proteins (**e**) in BALF and MPO levels (**f**) of lung samples from WT mice in sham and IRI group were performed.$^{*}p < 0.05$ compared with sham group, $^{\#}p < 0.05$ compared with PBS group, data are expressed as mean ± s.e.m. for all samples

whether rWISP1 could alter inflammatory cytokine production in the lung tissue. Mice were treated as previously described. Lung tissues were harvested, and then qRT-PCR and ELISA analysis were performed. Consistently, qRT-PCR analysis suggested IL-6 (Fig. 5a) and TNF-α (Fig. 5b) transcript levels were significantly upregulated in lung tissue following hepatic IRI. IL-10 (Fig. 5c) was markedly downregulated. ELISA evaluation in protein level further confirmed the increased levels of IL-6 (Fig. 5d) and TNF-α (Fig. 5e) and decreased levels of IL-10 (Fig. 5f). Collectively, these results demonstrated administration with rWISP1 significantly facilitated proinflammatory cytokine and inhibited anti-inflammatory cytokine production in the lung after hepatic IRI, further validating the pathological role of WISP1.

WISP1 contributes to lung injury in hepatic IRI dependent on TLR4

Previous work has demonstrated WISP1 ameliorated lung injury in hepatic IRI through increased production of proinflammatory cytokines and inhibition of anti-inflammatory cytokines. We next sought to determine the specific mechanism of WISP1 in regulating inflammatory cascades in the lung. Previous studies have demonstrated that WISP1 interacted with TLR4 and contributed to ventilator-induced lung injury (VILI) dependent on TLR4 signaling [18]. However, the underlying mechanism of WISP1 in mediating lung injury following hepatic IRI still remains unknown. C57BL/6 WT ($TLR^{+/+}$ in the Fig. 6) and $TLR4^{-/-}$ mice were adopted in the experiment. Both mice were treated with control and IRI operation to determine the expression of WISP1. Interestingly, in IRI (I/R in the Fig. 6) group, WISP1 transcripts (Fig. 6a) and protein expression (Fig. 6a) in $TLR4^{-/-}$ mice was decreased significantly compared with WT mice, indicating WISP1 expression in the lung tissue following hepatic IRI was dependent on TLR4. Next, we would like to examine whether WISP1 mediates inflammatory cascades through TLR4. WT and $TLR4^{-/-}$ mice in sham and IRI group were treated with anti-WISP1 antibody and rWISP1 to evaluate lung injury. $TLR4^{-/-}$ mice displayed decreased W/D ratio (Fig. 6b) and EBA permeability (Fig. 6c) compared with WT mice while no significance was detected between WT and $TLR4^{-/-}$ mice in IRI group treated with anti-WISP1 antibody. However, W/D ratio (Fig. 6d) and EBA permeability (Fig. 6e) of $TLR4^{-/-}$ mice in IRI group administered with rWISP1 were significantly decreased compared with those in WT mice, indicating rWISP1 could not induce lung injury in $TLR4^{-/-}$ mice. Collectively, these date demonstrated WISP1 expression was

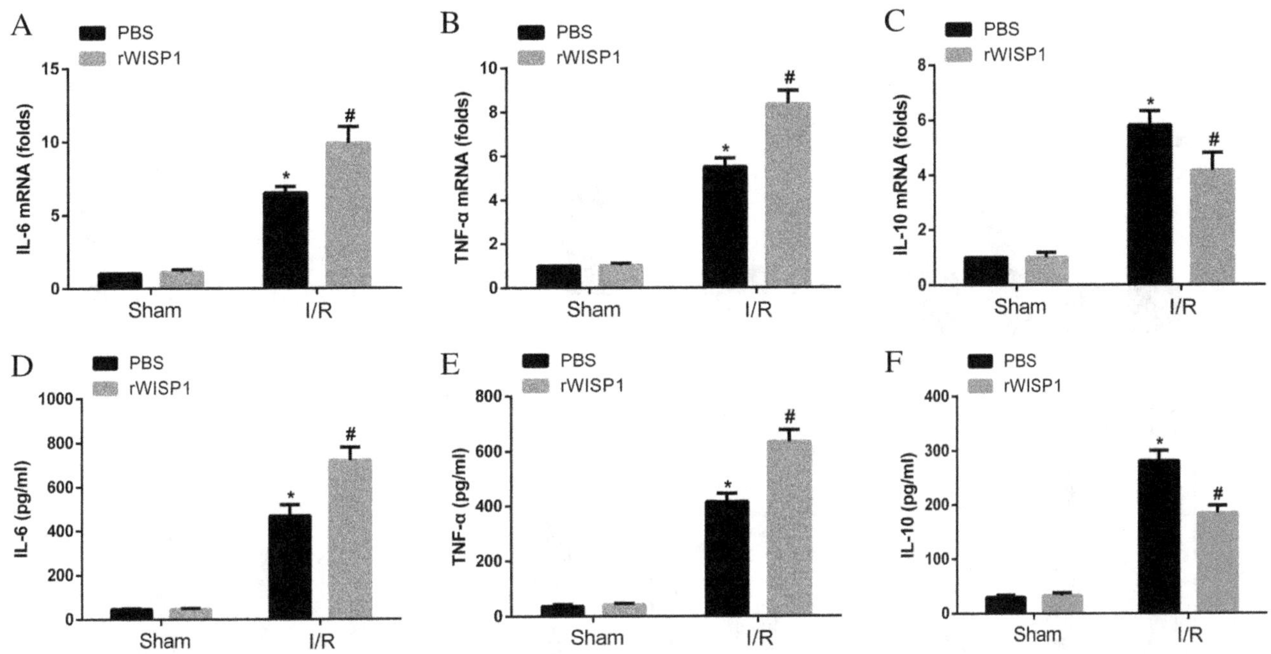

Fig. 5 rWISP1 Facilitates Proinflammatory Cytokine and Inhibits Anti-inflammatory Cytokine Production in Lung Tissue Following Hepatic IRI. WT mice in sham and IRI group undergoing ischemia for 60 min and reperfusion for 6 h were treated intraperitoneally with either sterile PBS or rWISP1 (1 μg/g) at the onset of reperfusion ($n = 6$ respectively). qRT-PCR for IL-6 (**a**), TNF-α (**b**), and IL-10 (**c**) from lung tissues in all groups was performed. ELISA for IL-6 (**d**), TNF-α (**e**), and IL-10 (**f**) from BALF supernatants in all groups was performed.$^{*}p < 0.05$ compared with sham group, $^{\#}p < 0.05$ compared with PBS group, data are expressed as mean ± s.e.m. for all samples

dependent on TLR4 and WISP1 contributed to lung injury in hepatic IRI through TLR4.

Discussion

Hepatic IRI is a common injury followed by liver transplantation, trauma, shock, etc. Besides liver injury, hepatic IRI also induce remote organ injuries, such as lung injury [8]. The underlying mechanisms of hepatic IRI still remain unclear, of which some mediators have been found playing indispensable roles in liver IRI induced lung injury, including high mobility group box-1 protein (HMGB1), adrenaline and N-acetyl-cysteine [28–30]. In the current study, we reported a new mediator, WISP1, plays a pivotal effect on hepatic IRI induced lung injury.

WNT1 inducible signaling pathway protein 1 (WISP1), one of the most important members in the CCN family, is a secreted extracellular matrix (ECM) which is ubiquitously expressed in various organs and tissues. The molecular function of CCN family has been associated with wound healing, organ fibrosis, cell survival and proliferation [31, 32]. WISP1 has been identified to be involved in the onset of several malignant diseases, such as breast cancer, hepatocellular carcinoma, colon adenocarcinomas, and lung carcinoma, osteoarthritis and lung fibrosis [16, 17, 33, 34]. In addition, we have demonstrated that WISP1 interacts with TLR4 by co-immunoprecipitation and mediates ventilator-induced lung injury (VILI) dependent on TLR4 signaling [18]. We also find WISP1 might contribute to hepatic ischemia reperfusion injury in mice and possibly depends on TLR4/TRIF signaling [24]. However, the role of WISP1 in the lung injury after IRI remains unknown.

This study aims to confirm the role of WISP1 in the lung injury following hepatic IRI and explore the possible regulating mechanisms. Interestingly, we found WISP1 transcript and protein expression were highly increased in the lung tissue following reperfusion for 6 h, 12 h and 24 h compared with sham mice. Immunofluorescence further confirmed WISP1 expression in the cytoplasm of cell in the lung. These results preliminarily indicated that WISP1 not only participated in the liver injury but also was involved in the pathogenesis of lung injury after hepatic IRI. To further validate the role of WISP1 in the lung injury, mice in the sham and IRI group were treated with anti-WISP1 antibody intraperitoneally to neutralize WISP1 in vivo. Fortunately, we found WISP1 neutralization significantly ameliorated lung injury after hepatic IRI compared to control IgG group characterized by less diffuse interstitial edema and inflammatory cell infiltration. Consistently, treatment with anti-WISP1 antibody markedly inhibited TNF-α and IL-6 production and enhanced IL-10 expression, further confirming the ameliorated lung injury. Conversely, administration with rWISP1

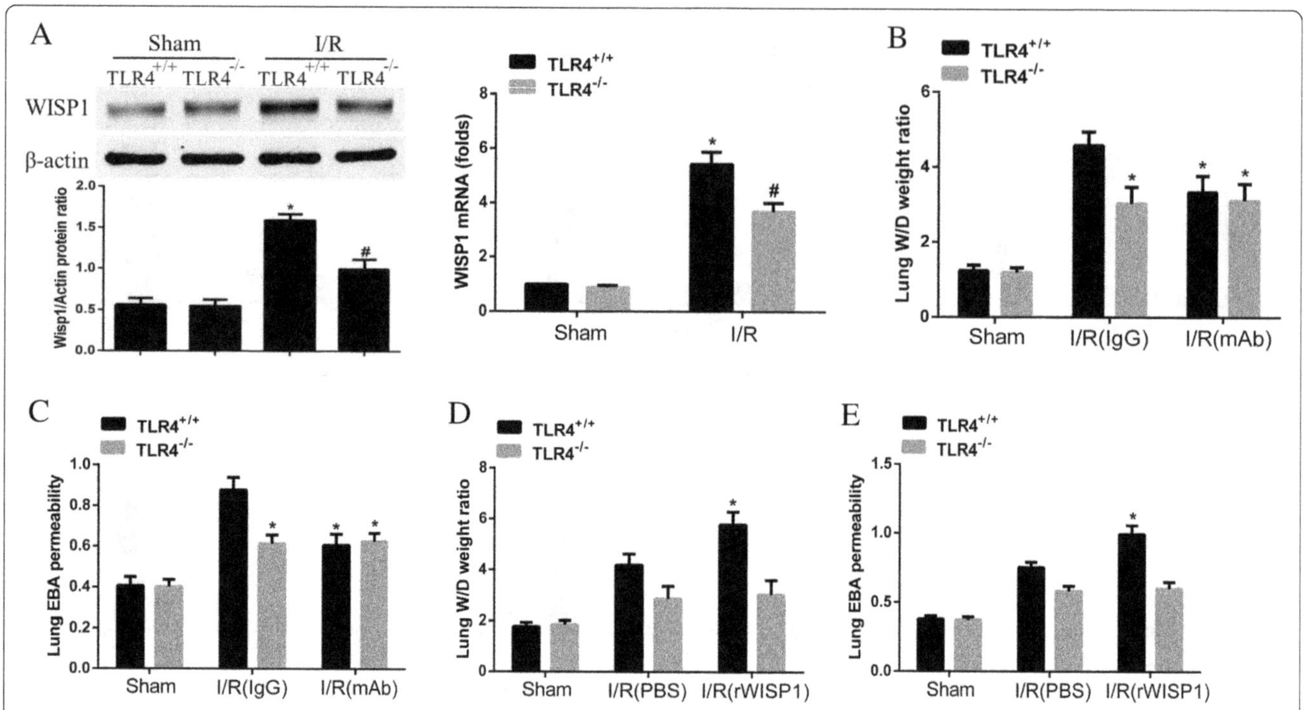

Fig. 6 WISP1 Contributes to Lung Injury in Hepatic IRI Dependent on TLR4. WT and $TLR4^{-/-}$ mice in sham and IRI group undergoing ischemia for 60 min and reperfusion for 6 h were treated intraperitoneally with either control IgG antibody or anti-WISP1 antibody (6 µg/g) 1 h before ischemia and at the onset of reperfusion ($n = 6$ respectively). In another experiment, WT and $TLR4^{-/-}$ mice were treated intraperitoneally with either sterile PBS or rWISP1 (1 µg/g) at the onset of reperfusion ($n = 6$ respectively). Western blot and qRT-PCR analysis (**a**) of WISP1 in the lung tissue from all groups were performed. W/D weight ratio (**b**), EBA permeability (**c**) for mice treated with control IgG antibody or anti-WISP1 antibody were analyzed. W/D weight ratio (**d**) and EBA permeability (**e**) for mice administered with sterile PBS or rWISP1 were analyzed. **a** $^{*}p < 0.05$ compared with sham group, $^{\#}p < 0.05$ compared with I/R($TLR4^{+/+}$) group, (**b**, **c**) $^{*}p < 0.05$ compared with I/R (IgG) group, (**d**, **e**) $^{*}p < 0.05$ compared with I/R (PBS) group, data are expressed as mean ± s.e.m. for all samples

aggravated lung injury together with excessive expression of TNF-α and IL-6 as well as inhibition of IL-10 production. Since the expression and function of WISP1 has been closely linked to TLR4 pathway, we next sought to explore the potential relationship between WISP1 and TLR4. Interestingly, we found $TLR4^{-/-}$ mice in IRI group displayed less transcript and protein expression of WISP1 compared with WT mice, preliminarily suggesting that WISP1 expression in lung injury after hepatic IRI was dependent on TLR4. Besides, rWISP1 could not induce lung injury in $TLR4^{-/-}$ mice of IRI group compared with WT mice, further indicating that WISP1-mediated lung injury and inflammatory cascades might also dependent on TLR4. These data suggested there might be a circulatory regulating mechanism between WISP1 and TLR4 in the lung injury following hepatic IRI. However, the specific mechanisms how TLR4 regulates WISP1 expression and how WISP1 mediates inflammatory cascades through TLR4 need to be further elucidated in future studies.

In conclusion, our study demonstrated that WISP1 expression is upregulated in lung tissue following hepatic IRI. Anti-WISP1 antibody ameliorated lung injury with alterations in cytokine profiles. rWISP1 aggravated lung injury through excessive proinflammatory cytokine production and inhibition of anti-inflammatory cytokines. WISP1 contributes to lung injury through TLR4 pathway after hepatic IRI. Medications targeting WISP1 might be a promising approach for patients with lung injury following hepatic IRI.

Abbreviations

BALF: Bronchoalveolar Lavage Fluid; ECM: Extracellular matrix; HMGB1: High mobility group box-1 protein; iNOS: Inducible nitric oxide synthase; IRI: Ischemia-reperfusion injury; MPO: Myeloperoxidase; PRRs: Pattern recognition receptors; ROS: reactive oxygen species; TLR4: Toll-like receptor 4; VILI: Ventilator-induced lung injury; WISP1: WNT1 inducible signaling pathway protein 1

Acknowledgements

We thank Prof. Timothy R. Billiar (M.D., Ph.D. Professor, Department of Surgery, University of Pittsburgh Medical Center, Pittsburgh, PA) for providing suggestions of this study and supplying us the TLR4 knockout mice.

Funding

We are very grateful for the support from the National Natural Science Foundation of China (No. 81571927 to Li Q).

Authors' contributions

QL, YT and ZC designed the study; YT and ZY wrote the manuscript; YT and RZ collected the data; XD, ZY and YT performed the experiments and analyzed the data; ZC helped to review the analysis of data; QL and ZC discussed the results and reviewed the manuscript before submission. All authors read and approved the final version of the manuscript.

Consent for publication

All authors read and approved the final version of the manuscript.

Competing interests

The authors declare that they have no competing interests.

References

1. Bilzer M, Gerbes AL. Preservation injury of the liver: mechanisms and novel therapeutic strategies. J Hepatol. 2000;32:508–15.
2. Caldwell-Kenkel JC, Currin RT, Tanaka Y, Thurman RG, Lemasters JJ. Reperfusion injury to endothelial cells following cold ischemic storage of rat livers. Hepatology. 1989;10:292–9.
3. Lentsch AB, Kato A, Yoshidome H, McMasters KM, Edwards MJ. Inflammatory mechanisms and therapeutic strategies for warm hepatic ischemia/reperfusion injury. Hepatology. 2000;32:169–73.
4. Colletti LM, Burtch GD, Remick DG, Kunkel SL, Strieter RM, et al. The production of tumor necrosis factor alpha and the development of a pulmonary capillary injury following hepatic ischemia/reperfusion. Transplantation. 1990;49:268–72.
5. Colletti LM, Remick DG, Burtch GD, Kunkel SL, Strieter RM, et al. Role of tumor necrosis factor-alpha in the pathophysiologic alterations after hepatic ischemia/reperfusion injury in the rat. J Clin Invest. 1990;85:1936–43.
6. Chan KC, Lin CJ, Lee PH, Chen CF, Lai YL, et al. Propofol attenuates the decrease of dynamic compliance and water content in the lung by decreasing oxidative radicals released from the reperfused liver. Anesth Analg. 2008;107:1284–9.
7. Chang WJ, Toledo-Pereyra LH. Toll-like receptor signaling in liver ischemia and reperfusion. J Invest Surg. 2012;25:271–7.
8. Kaczorowski DJ, Tsung A, Billiar TR. Innate immune mechanisms in ischemia/reperfusion. Front Biosci. 2009;1:91–8.
9. Tsung A, Hoffman RA, Izuishi K, Critchlow ND, Nakao A, et al. Hepatic ischemia/reperfusion injury involves functional TLR4 signaling in nonparenchymal cells. J Immunol. 2005;175:7661–8.
10. Hui W, Jinxiang Z, Heshui W, Zhuoya L, Qichang Z. Bone marrow and non-bone marrow TLR4 regulates hepatic ischemia/reperfusion injury. Biochem Biophys Res Commun. 2009;389:328–32.
11. Bamboat ZM, Balachandran VP, Ocuin LM, Obaid H, Plitas G, et al. Toll-like receptor 9 inhibition confers protection from liver ischemia-reperfusion injury. Hepatology. 2010;51:621–32.
12. Jin X, Wang L, Wu HS, Zhang L, Wang CY, et al. N-acetylcysteine inhibits activation of toll-like receptor 2 and 4 gene expression in the liver and lung after partial hepatic ischemia-reperfusion injury in mice. Hepatobiliary Pancreat Dis Int. 2007;6:284–9.
13. Zhang JX, Wu HS, Wang H, Zhang JH, Wang Y, et al. Protection against hepatic ischemia/reperfusion injury via downregulation of toll-like receptor 2 expression by inhibition of Kupffer cell function. World J Gastroenterol. 2005;11:4423–6.
14. Pennica D, Swanson TA, Welsh JW, Roy MA, Lawrence DA, et al. WISP genes are members of the connective tissue growth factor family that are up-regulated in Wnt-1-transformed cells and aberrantly expressed in human colon tumors. Proc Natl Acad Sci U S A. 1998;95:14717 22.
15. Berschneider B, Konigshoff M. WNT1 inducible signaling pathway protein 1 (WISP1): a novel mediator linking development and disease. Int J Biochem Cell Biol. 2011;43:306–9.
16. Margalit O, Eisenbach L, Amariglio N, Kaminski N, Harmelin A, et al. Overexpression of a set of genes, including WISP-1, common to pulmonary metastases of both mouse D122 Lewis lung carcinoma and B16-F10.9 melanoma cell lines. Brit J Cancer. 2003;89:314–9.
17. Calvisi DF, Conner EA, Ladu S, Lemmer ER, Factor VM, et al. Activation of the canonical Wnt/beta-catenin pathway confers growth advantages in c-Myc/E2F1 transgenic mouse model of liver cancer. J Hepatol. 2005;42:842–9.
18. Li HH, Li Q, Liu P, Liu Y, Li J, et al. WNT1-inducible signaling pathway protein 1 contributes to ventilator-induced lung injury. Am J Respir Cell Mol Biol. 2012;47:528–35.
19. Murahovschi V, Pivovarova O, Ilkavets I, Dmitrieva RM, Docke S, et al. WISP1 is a novel adipokine linked to inflammation in obesity. Diabetes. 2015;64:856–66.
20. Nace GW, Huang H, Klune JR, Eid RE, Rosborough BR, et al. Cellular-specific role of toll-like receptor 4 in hepatic ischemia-reperfusion injury in mice. Hepatology. 2013;58:374–87.
21. Ding X, Wang X, Zhao X, Jin S, Tong Y, et al. RGD peptides protects against acute lung injury in septic mice through Wisp1-integrin beta6 pathway inhibition. Shock. 2015;43:352–60.
22. Zhu GF, Sun B, Niu SF, Cai YY, Lin K, et al. Combined surfactant therapy and inhaled nitric oxide in rabbits with oleic acid-induced acute respiratory distress syndrome. Am J Respir Crit Care Med. 1998;158:437–43.
23. Li H, Su X, Yan X, Wasserloos K, Chao W, et al. Toll-like receptor 4-myeloid differentiation factor 88 signaling contributes to ventilator-induced lung injury in mice. Anesthesiology. 2010;113:619–29.
24. Tong Y, Ding XB, Chen ZX, Jin SQ, Zhao X, et al. WISP1 mediates hepatic warm ischemia reperfusion injury via TLR4 signaling in mice. Sci Rep. 2016;6:20141.
25. de Jong PR, Takahashi N, Harris AR, Lee J, Bertin S, et al. Ion channel TRPV1-dependent activation of PTP1B suppresses EGFR-associated intestinal tumorigenesis. J Clin Invest. 2014;124:3793–806.
26. Bertin S, Aoki-Nonaka Y, de Jong PR, Nohara LL, Xu H, et al. The ion channel TRPV1 regulates the activation and proinflammatory properties of CD4(+) T cells. Nat Immunol. 2014;15:1055–63.
27. Klebanoff SJ. Myeloperoxidase: friend and foe. J Leukoc Biol. 2005;77:598–625.
28. Yang Z, Deng Y, Su D, Tian J, Gao Y, et al. TLR4 as receptor for HMGB1-mediated acute lung injury after liver ischemia/reperfusion injury. Lab Investig. 2013;93(7):792–800.
29. Castro AP, Castro Junior MA, Lauz S, Facin E, Simões Mde J, et al. The role of N-acetyl-cysteine in the lung remote injury after hepatic ischemia and reperfusion in rabbits. Acta Cir Bras. 2012;27(1):49–55.
30. Ota S, Yazawa T, Tojo K, Baba Y, Uchiyama M, et al. Adrenaline aggravates lung injury caused by liver ischemia-reperfusion and high-tidal-volume ventilation in rats. J Intensive Care. 2016;4:8.
31. Chen CC, Lau LF. Functions and mechanisms of action of CCN matricellular proteins. Int J Biochem Cell B. 2009;41:771–83.
32. Jun JI, Lau LF. The matricellular protein CCN1 induces fibroblast senescence and restricts fibrosis in cutaneous wound healing. Nat Cell Biol. 2010;12:676–85.
33. Blom AB, Brockbank SM, van Lent PL, van Beuningen HM, Geurts J, et al. Involvement of the Wnt signaling pathway in experimental and human osteoarthritis prominent role of Wnt-induced signaling protein 1. Arthritis Rheum. 2009;60:501–12.
34. Konigshoff M, Kramer M, Balsara N, Wilhelm J, Amarie OV, et al. WNT1-inducible signaling protein-1 mediates pulmonary fibrosis in mice and is upregulated in humans with idiopathic pulmonary fibrosis. J Clin Invest. 2009;119:772–87.

Lung hyperinflation and functional exercise capacity in patients with COPD

Linn T. Aalstad[1], Jon A. Hardie[1], Birgitte Espehaug[2], Einar Thorsen[1,3], Per S. Bakke[1], Tomas M. L. Eagan[1,4] and Bente Frisk[5,6*]

Abstract

Background: Lung hyperinflation contributes to dyspnea, morbidity and mortality in chronic obstructive pulmonary disease (COPD). The inspiratory-to-total lung capacity (IC/TLC) ratio is a measure of lung hyperinflation and is associated with exercise intolerance. However, knowledge of its effect on longitudinal change in the 6-min walk distance (6MWD) in patients with COPD is scarce. We aimed to study whether the IC/TLC ratio predicts longitudinal change in 6MWD in patients with COPD.

Methods: This prospective cohort study included 389 patients aged 40–75 years with clinically stable COPD in Global Initiative for Chronic Obstructive Lung Disease stages II-IV. The 6MWD was measured at baseline, and after one and 3 years. We performed generalized estimating equation regression analyses to examine predictors for longitudinal change in 6MWD. Predictors at baseline were: IC/TLC ratio, age, gender, pack years, fat mass index (FMI), fat-free mass index (FFMI), number of exacerbations within 12 months prior to inclusion, Charlson index for comorbidities, forced vital capacity (FVC), forced expiratory volume in 1 s (FEV_1), and light and hard self-reported physical activity.

Results: Reduced IC/TLC ratio ($p < 0.001$) was a statistically significant predictor for decline in 6MWD. With a 0.1-unit decrease in baseline IC/TLC ratio, the annual decline in 6MWD was 12.7 m ($p < 0.001$). Study participants with an IC/TLC ratio in the upper quartiles maintained their 6MWD from baseline to year 3, while it was significantly reduced for the patients with an IC/TLC ratio in the lower quartiles. Absence of light and hard physical activity, increased age and FMI, decreased FEV_1 and FVC, more frequent exacerbations and higher Charlson comorbidity index were also predictors for lower 6MWD at any given time, but did not predict higher rate of decline over the timespan of the study.

Conclusion: Our findings demonstrated that patients with less lung hyperinflation at baseline maintained their functional exercise capacity during the follow-up period, and that it was significantly reduced for patients with increased lung hyperinflation.

Keywords: COPD, 6-min walk distance, IC/TLC ratio, Functional exercise capacity, Lung hyperinflation

* Correspondence: bente.frisk@hvl.no
[5]Department of Health and Functioning, Western Norway University of Applied Sciences, Inndalsveien 28, 5063 Bergen, Norway
[6]Department of Physiotherapy, Haukeland University Hospital, Bergen, Norway
Full list of author information is available at the end of the article

Background

Chronic obstructive pulmonary disease (COPD) is a major cause of morbidity and mortality, and is predicted to become the third leading cause of death worldwide in 2030 [1]. Expiratory flow limitation is generally regarded as the hallmark feature of COPD [2], but lung hyperinflation is also a manifestation of COPD with major clinical consequences [3].

Lung hyperinflation is clinically relevant in COPD, mostly because of its contribution to dyspnea [4] and morbidity associated with the disease [5]. Hyperinflation has also shown to be related to exercise limitation [4], which is a significant component of quality of life [6]. The inspiratory capacity (IC) and inspiratory-to-total lung capacity (IC/TLC) ratio are indirect measures of lung hyperinflation reflecting the end-expiratory lung volume [5, 7]. IC and IC/TLC ratio progressively declines as COPD advances [7, 8], mirroring the rise in lung hyperinflation [9].

The 6-min walk test (6MWT) is widely used in the assessment of functional exercise capacity in patients with COPD [10]. The 6-min walk distance (6MWD) gives valuable information that can be used in the clinical staging of COPD patients, as it correlates well with dyspnea, lung hyperinflation and airway obstruction [11]. In addition, longitudinal changes in 6MWD have demonstrated to be important predictors of mortality [12–14]. However, there is limited knowledge about the effect of IC/TLC ratio on longitudinal changes in 6MWD in patients with COPD.

To our knowledge, only one previous study has examined the relationship between lung hyperinflation and functional exercise capacity, using IC/TLC ratio and 6MWD in the assessment. Ramon et al. [15] demonstrated that IC/TLC ratio and subjective dyspnea predicted decline in exercise capacity. However, Ramon et al. [15] only included patients recruited during their first hospitalization due to a COPD exacerbation, and may not be representative for COPD patients in general. The observation time was 1.7 years [15].

The aim of the present study was to examine whether lung hyperinflation measured as IC/TLC ratio predicts longitudinal change in 6MWD in patients with COPD. We hypothesized that increased hyperinflation predicts longitudinal decline in functional exercise capacity in patients with COPD.

Methods

Study population

The current study was a prospective cohort study that included 389 of a total of 433 patients from the Bergen COPD Cohort Study (BCCS), aged 44–75 years, with an average follow-up time of 3 years (2006–2010). Details of sampling procedures and data collection for the BCCS have been described previously [16]. In brief, all patients had a clinically stable COPD in Global Initiative for Chronic Obstructive Lung Disease (GOLD) stages II-IV [17], a smoking history of ≥10 pack years, a post-bronchodilation forced expiratory volume in 1 s (FEV_1)/forced vital capacity (FVC) ratio < 0.7 and a post-bronchodilation FEV_1 < 80% of predicted value according to Norwegian reference values [18]. Exacerbations that required medical treatment and/or hospitalization during the last 4 weeks prior to inclusion led to postponement of inclusion. There were no restrictions to treatment during the study period, and the patients received medications and therapies prescribed by their physician. Active cancer or inflammatory disorders like rheumatoid arthritis, systemic lupus erythematosus or other connective tissue disorders and inflammatory bowel disease in the last 5 years were reasons for exclusion from the study. The patients were recruited through outpatient clinics from several hospitals in Western Norway and from three private specialist practices in Bergen, Norway [16].

Measurements

Six-min walk test

Functional exercise capacity was assessed by the 6MWT with 6MWD as the primary outcome measure. The 6MWT was performed at baseline and after one and 3 years after inclusion in the study. The test was supervised by a trained technician and performed according to the American Thoracic Society (ATS) guidelines [10]. However, the 6MWT was performed only once at each visit without a prior practice test. The 6MWD and use of oxygen during the test were registered. Measurements of heart rate and oxygen saturation, as well as evaluation of dyspnea and fatigue according to the Borg CR10 Scale [19], were done before and immediately after the test.

Self-reported physical activity

Level of habitual physical activity was registered by a questionnaire with two questions related to spare time physical activity, one for hard and one for light physical activity. Sweating and breathlessness were used as the delineation between hard and light physical activity. The possible response categories were none, less than 1 h per week, 1–2 h per week and 3 or more hours per week. These questions are validated previously [20, 21], and have been used in a large Norwegian general population study [22].

Body composition, spirometry, dyspnea, exacerbations and Charlson index for comorbidities

We measured height and body mass, and the study participants underwent bioelectrical impedance measurements of fat mass and fat-free mass after an overnight fast (Bodystat 1500, Isle of man, England). Fat mass index (FMI) and fat-free mass index (FFMI) were calculated as fat mass and fat-free mass, respectively, divided by the square of height.

The study participants underwent complete lung function tests at baseline, including spirometry and plethysmography, according to the ATS/ERS Standardization of Lung Function Testing [23, 24]. We performed spirometry before and after inhalation of 0.4 mg salbutamol on a Viasys Masterscope (Viasys, Hoechberg, Germany). The FVC and FEV_1 were taken as the highest values from at least three acceptable and repeatable maneuvers. Lung volumes were obtained by plethysmography and lung hyperinflation was assessed by the IC/TLC ratio. The spirometers were calibrated twice daily with a 3-L calibration syringe.

The modified Medical Research Council (mMRC) dyspnea scale [25] was used to measure symptoms of dyspnea. A physician examined all the patients at baseline and registered number of exacerbations the last 12 months prior to inclusion, comorbidities and smoking habits. The Charlson index for comorbidities was calculated.

Statistics

Descriptive statistics were used to characterize the study population (mean, standard deviation and percent). Normal distribution was assessed by histogram, Q-Q-plot and Shapiro Wilks test. We compared the continuous and categorical variables across gender by independent t-tests and chi-square tests, respectively.

We performed generalized estimating equations (GEE) regression analyses [26] to examine IC/TLC ratio as predictor for change in 6MWD. Time was included in the model as a categorical variable with three measurements: baseline, 1 and 3 years, and in addition as a continuous variable to examine yearly change in 6MWD. Age, gender, pack years, FMI, FFMI, more than two exacerbations within 12 months prior to inclusion (yes/no), Charlson index for comorbidity (level 1, 2, 3 and 4), FVC, FEV_1 and light or hard self-reported physical activity (yes/no, yes = ≥1 h/week) at baseline were included as potential confounders. To account for within-patient correlation we applied an unstructured working correlation structure. GEE regression analysis provides an approach for analyzing correlated measurements without excluding subjects with an incomplete dataset.

We performed bivariate GEE analysis for each predictor variable. In an additional analysis, time was investigated as a continuous variable. Multivariate GEE analyses were performed in three stages, first including all variables as main effects, and secondly, expanding with all possible interaction terms between predictor and time. Based on the latter, the third and final model included all variables and the statistically significant interaction terms. Analyses for multicollinearity between FMI and FFMI, and between IC/TLC ratio, FVC and FEV_1 did not demonstrate multicollinearity, and therefore all variables were included in the same model.

In addition, we performed multivariate GEE analyses with baseline IC/TLC ratio categorized into quartiles, and the variable was included in the analysis as the interaction term with time. The IC/TLC groups were named IC/TLC 1, 2, 3 and 4, respectively, with IC/TLC 1 representing the lower quartile.

A power analysis for a simple group comparison with three repeated measures [26] informed that 174 patients were needed to detect a difference in mean 6MWD of 30 m [27] as statistically significant at a 5% significance level and a power of 80%. The calculation was based on an assumption of a within-subject correlation coefficient of 0.25 and a SD for 6MWD of 100 m. A within-subject correlation coefficient of 0.5 increased the number of patients to 232.

IBM SPSS Statistics version 24 was used to conduct the analyses. Estimated regression coefficients obtained in the GEE analyses are presented with confidence intervals and p-values. Statistical significance level was set at 0.05.

Results

Study population

At baseline, 389 patients completed the 6MWT, and 319 (82%) and 264 (68%) completed the 6MWT at 1 year and 3-years, respectively. Of the remaining 125 participants, 104 were disabled and 21 were deceased. The patients who dropped out were older ($p < 0.001$), had lower FEV_1 ($p < 0.001$), FVC ($p < 0.001$) and IC/TLC ratio ($p < 0.001$) compared to the patients who completed the study, and the 6MWD were 87 m ($p < 0.001$) shorter at baseline. Baseline characteristics of the study population are presented in Table 1. The mean age of the patients was 64 ± 7 years, and 61% were male. Airflow limitation was moderate to very severe with a mean FEV_1 of 49 ± 14% of predicted value. Measurements of IC/TLC ratio at baseline were available for 371 patients. The patients had a mean IC/TLC ratio of 0.35 ± 0.09 and approximately 15% of the patients had an IC/TLC ratio below the critical threshold of 0.25. The cut points for the quartiles were 0.29 (25th percentile), 0.34 (median) and 0.40 (75th percentile).

Longitudinal change in 6MWD

Estimated unadjusted mean (SE) 6MWD at baseline and after 1 and 3 years were 429 (6), 437 (6) and 408 (8) m, respectively. There was a statistically significant annual decrease in 6MWD during the follow-up period of – 10.9 m (95% CI: -15.3 – -6.6, $p < 0.001$). However, mean 6MWD increased slightly from baseline to year 1 (B = 8.1, $p = 0.05$) (Table 2), and was significantly reduced from year 1 to year

Table 1 Baseline characteristics of the study population

Predictors	Total	Female	Male	*P*-value
Sex, n (%)	389 (100)	153 (39.3)	236 (60.7)	
Age (years)	63.6 ± 6.8	62.6 ± 6.3	64.2 ± 7.0	0.028
6MWD (m)	423 ± 112	406 ± 104	434 ± 115	0.015
SpO_2 before 6MWT (%)	94.2 ± 2.7	94.1 ± 2.9	94.3 ± 2.6	0.621
SpO_2 after 6MWT (%)	91.0 ± 5.7	90.9 ± 6.1	91.0 ± 5.4	0.804
Borg dyspnea score after 6MWT (median)	4.0	4.0	3.0	0.085
mMRC	2.2 ± 2.3	2.3 ± 2.4	2.1 ± 2.2	0.410
BMI (kg/m^2)	25.4 ± 5.2	24.5 ± 5.7	25.9 ± 4.8	0.016
FMI (kg/m^2)	8.4 ± 3.3	9.8 ± 3.7	7.4 ± 2.6	< 0.001
FFMI (kg/m^2)	17.0 ± 3.2	14.7 ± 2.4	18.5 ± 2.8	< 0.001
Smoking status n (%)				0.215
Current	167 (43)	72 (47)	95 (40)	
Former	222 (57)	81 (53)	141 (60)	
Pack years	40.9 ± 22.8	33.5 ± 16.6	45.6 ± 24.9	< 0.001
GOLD category, n %				0.283
II	179 (46)	76 (50)	103 (44)	
III	169 (43)	65 (42)	104 (44)	
IV	41 (11)	12 (8)	29 (12)	
Charlson comorbidity index, n (%)				0.011
1	225 (58)	99 (65)	126 (53)	
2	93 (24)	38 (25)	55 (23)	
3	46 (12)	12 (8)	34 (15)	
4	25 (6)	4 (2)	21 (9)	
Experienced > 2 exacerbations, n (%)	75 (20)	38 (25)	37 (16)	0.036
FEV_1 (L)	1.5 ± 0.5	1.3 ± 0.4	1.7 ± 0.5	< 0.001
FEV_1 (% pred.)	48.7 ± 14.0	49.6 ± 13.5	48.1 ± 14.4	0.315
FVC (L)	3.3 ± 0.9	2.7 ± 0.6	3.7 ± 0.8	< 0.001
FVC (% pred.)	85.5 ± 16.6	85.2 ± 17.1	85.6 ± 16.4	0.791
FEV_1/FVC (%)	45.7 ± 11.1	47.6 ± 11.0	44.5 ± 11.0	0.006
TLC (L)	7.1 ± 1.4	6.1 ± 0.9	7.8 ± 1.3	< 0.001
TLC (% pred.)	115.9 ± 18.0	121.4 ± 17.8	112.3 ± 17.1	< 0.001
IC (L)	2.4 ± 0.7	2.0 ± 0.5	2.7 ± 0.7	< 0.001
IC/TLC ratio	0.35 ± 0.09	0.36 ± 0.08	0.33 ± 0.09	0.002
TLCO	5.2 ± 1.9	4.4 ± 1.6	5.6 ± 2.0	< 0.001
TLCO (% pred.)	59.1 ± 18.8	57.2 ± 18.5	60.3 ± 19.0	0.143
Physical activity ≥1 h/week				
Light physical activity	263 (73.0)	104 (73.7)	159 (72.6)	0.691
Hard physical activity	141 (39.6)	54 (38.9)	88 (40.6)	0.139

Data are presented as mean ± SD, unless otherwise stated. Independent samples T-test for continuous variables and Chi square for categorical variables
6MWD 6-min walking distance, *BMI* body mass index, *FMI* fat mass index, *FFMI* fat free mass index, *GOLD* Global Initiative for Chronic Obstructive Lung Disease, *FEV_1* forced expiratory volume in 1 s, *FVC* forced vital capacity, *IC* inspiratory capacity, *TLC* total lung capacity, *IC/TLC ratio* inspiratory-to-total lung capacity ratio, *TLCO* transfer factor for carbon monoxide

3 (B = − 29, $p < 0.001$) indicating a non-linear relationship. This pattern was most evident in patients with an IC/TLC ratio in the lower quartiles (Fig. 1).

Predictors for longitudinal change in 6MWD

A 0.1 unit increase in baseline IC/TLC ratio was associated with an increase in 6MWD both in the

Table 2 Predictors for mean 6MWD estimated with GEE regression analysis

Predictors	Bivariate		Multivariate[a]		
	Beta	p	Beta	95% CI	p
Time		< 0.001			< 0.001[b]
1 year vs. baseline	8.1	0.052	6.0	- 1.9 – 13.4	0.134
3 years vs. baseline	- 21.0	< 0.001	- 24.1	- 35.1 – - 13.9	< 0.001
Sex, (male vs. female)	35.1	0.002	- 28.8	- 60.1 – 2.5	0.072
Age (years)	- 5.3	< 0.001	- 1.8	- 3.4 – - 0.3	0.019
FEV_1 (L)	107.3	< 0.001	47.5	21.7–73.2	< 0.001
FVC (L)	57.1	< 0.001	20.9	5.2–36.7	0.009
IC/TLC ratio (at 0.35)	489.4	< 0.001			< 0.001[c]
At baseline			116.3	−10.0 – 242.7	0.071
At 1 year			175.2	25.1–325.4	0.022
At 3 years			454.2	263.3–645.2	< 0.001
FMI (kg/m^2)	- 8.2	< 0.001	- 8.3	- 12.2 – - 4.4	< 0.001
FFMI (kg/m^2)	5.2	0.008	1.3	- 3.6 – 6.3	0.592
Pack years	- 0.2	0.577	- 0.2	- 0.7 – 0.3	0.421
Experienced > 2 exacerbations last year	- 66.4	< 0.001	- 32.1	- 53.5 – - 10.7	0.003
Charlson comorbidity index; score		0.001			0.006[b]
2 vs. 1	- 30.6	0.025	- 12.1	- 33.5 – 9.2	0.266
3 vs. 1	- 56.6	0.003	- 37.4	- 68.7 – - 6.1	0.019
4 vs. 1	- 58.9	0.016	- 54.8	- 91.6 – - 18.0	0.004
Light physical activity ≥1 h/week	69.9	< 0.001	34.2	7.5–60.8	0.012
Hard physical activity ≥1 h/week	66.4	< 0.001	37.0	18.6–55.4	< 0.001

Beta estimated regression coefficient, *P* *p*-value, *CI* confidence interval, *6MWD* 6-min walk distance, *GEE* generalized estimated equation, *FEV_1* forced expiratory volume in one second, *FVC* forced vital capacity, *IC/TLC ratio* inspiratory-to-total lung capacity ratio, *FMI* fat mass index, *FFMI* fat free mass index
[a] The model included all predictors and interaction terms for time x IC/TLC ratio centered at mean value (0.35). [b] Test for overall effect. [c] Test for time as effect modifier (test of interaction)

bivariate (B = 489 m, $p < 0.001$) and multivariate (B = 229 m, $p = 0.001$) analysis (Table 2). In the final model, we allowed for a time-dependent effect of the IC/TLC ratio, and found that it gained importance as predictor of 6MWD with longer follow-up (Table 2). Among all included factors, only IC/TLC ratio demonstrated a statistically significant time-dependent effect on 6MWD ($p < 0.001$). However, several other baseline factors had a statistically significant impact on 6MWD irrespective of follow-up. We observed that not performing light and hard physical activity, decreasing values of FEV_1 or FVC, increasing age or FMI, Charlson comorbidity index of 3 or higher, and having more than two exacerbations the last 12 months prior to study inclusion, predicted a statistically significant decrease in 6MWD (Table 2).

Discussion

The main findings of this study were: 1) Increased lung hyperinflation measured as IC/TLC ratio predicted longitudinal decline in 6MWD, with time as an effect modifier. Absence of light and hard physical activity, increased age and FMI, decreased FEV_1 and FVC, more frequent exacerbations and higher Charlson comorbidity index were also predictors for lower 6MWD at any given time, but did not predict higher rate of decline over the timespan of the study. 2) Study participants with an IC/TLC ratio in the upper quartiles maintained their 6MWD from baseline to year 3, while it was significantly reduced for study participants with an IC/TLC ratio in the lower quartiles.

Longitudinal change in 6MWD

The analysis of data with repeated outcome measurements over time is complicated. Baseline predictor variables can be associated to the outcome at any given time point without actually predicting the time-related change in the outcome. It is the interaction of time and the baseline variable (effect modification) which shows whether there is a prediction of change in the outcome over time. In our study, only IC/TLC ratio interacted significantly with time, and as such, was the only variable to actually predict a change in the 6MWD.

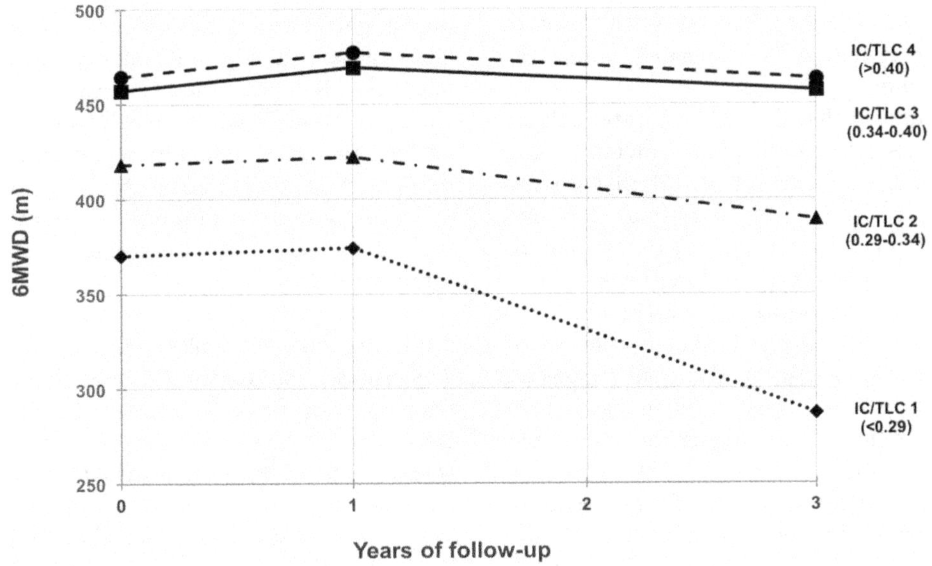

Fig. 1 Estimated mean 6-min walk distance (6MWD) by quartiles of inspiratory-to-total lung capacity (IC/TLC) ratio at baseline and during 3 years of follow-up. IC/TLC ratio at baseline was divided into approximate quartiles. IC/TLC ratio and the interaction term with time was included in an unadjusted generalized estimating equations regression analyses

To our knowledge, only four previous studies have investigated risk factors for decline in functional exercise capacity assessed by the 6MWT in patients with COPD [12, 15, 28, 29]. Of these, only one study has examined the relationship between lung hyperinflation and functional exercise capacity. Ramon et al. [15] conducted a prospective cohort study with 342 patients with a clinically stable COPD, and a mean follow-up period of 1.7 years. The study demonstrated that IC/TLC ratio and dyspnea score predicted decline in functional exercise capacity measured by 6MWD.

We confirmed the findings from Ramon et al. by demonstrating that IC/TLC ratio predicted longitudinal change in functional exercise capacity. However, patients in the study by Ramon et al. [15] were recruited during their first hospitalization due to a COPD exacerbation, and performed two 6MWTs, the first at least 3 months after discharge from hospital and the second 18–24 months after the first test. The period of follow-up was relatively short. Our study included a wide spectrum of patients with clinically stable COPD in GOLD stages II-IV that performed the 6MWT three times during a follow-up period of 3 years. We also demonstrated, irrespective of follow-up, associations between a decrease in 6MWD and a decrease in FEV_1 and FVC, increased age, FMI, comorbidity and number of exacerbations and absence of light and hard physical activity.

Previous studies have demonstrated that airflow limitation (lower FEV_1) and older age were risk factors for longitudinal decline in functional exercise capacity [12, 28, 29]. In addition, Spruit et al. [29] found that lower body mass index (BMI) was a predictor for longitudinal change in functional exercise capacity. Our group has previously demonstrated in the same cohort as in this study, that lower levels of habitual hard physical activity is associated with an increased deterioration in functional exercise capacity [28]. In consistency with previous research [12, 28, 29], we demonstrated in this study that lower FEV_1 and older age were associated with a lower 6MWD. A lower FEV_1 is related to reduced maximal expiratory flow rates and impaired ventilatory capacity, being a limiting factor for functional exercise capacity.

Lung hyperinflation predisposes for a mechanical constraint on expansion of the tidal volume as the need for ventilation increases during exercise, resulting in exercise intolerance [9, 30]. Performing light and hard habitual physical activity demonstrated a positive association with 6MWD. However, these results were not significant when analyzing for time as an effect modifier. Physical activity improves exercise capacity and the function of the skeletal and muscle system, but it does not improve the bronchial obstruction in patients with COPD [31].

We did not examine whether BMI was a predictor for change in 6MWD, but included FMI in the analysis, which was a statistically significant predictor at 1 and 3 years. A novel finding from our study is that a higher frequency of COPD exacerbations and a higher Charlson comorbidity index were predictors for a lower 6MWD. As previously demonstrated by Park et al. [8], progression of lung hyperinflation is associated with more frequent exacerbations.

Studies have demonstrated that IC/TLC ratio declines over time in patients with COPD [7, 32], including a recent study conducted by Park et al. [8] that demonstrated a decline in IC/TLC ratio over time at a mean rate of 0.70% per year. As such, one expects that the patients experience a progression of lung hyperinflation during the study period, associated with a decline in IC/TLC ratio [8]. Patients in the lower quartiles of IC/TLC ratio experienced a higher decrease in 6MWD during the follow-up period compared to participants with an IC/TLC ratio in the higher quartiles, who maintained their 6MWD.

Different variables show up as significant predictors in different studies. Whether it is FEV_1 or IC/TLC ratio, or markers of clinical severity or body composition, they all reflect status of the lung mechanics and clinical condition, which are the two most important factors describing the severity of the disease.

Functional exercise capacity

Functional exercise capacity is determined by central and peripheral factors, and the mechanism is complex [33]. In patients with COPD, exercise capacity is mainly limited by peripheral muscle fatigue, impaired ventilatory mechanics and gas exchange [33, 34]. With an increased lung hyperinflation, the patients experiences increased work of breathing. The respiratory muscles are placed at mechanical disadvantage due to adaptation of the diaphragm to chronic overload of the respiratory muscles [28, 35, 36]. This results in impaired inspiratory muscle strength [37] and endurance [38], leading to dyspnea [39, 40] and reduced exercise capacity [41]. Breathing becomes more energy demanding and physical activity becomes increasingly uncomfortable, resulting in a decreased level of habitual physical activity, and secondly, a deterioration in functional exercise capacity.

Our results demonstrates that performing habitual physical activity at baseline was associated with 6MWD in a positive manner.

Lung hyperinflation

IC can be measured by spirometry, and lung hyperinflation is therefore an easy way to evaluate the patient's disease severity and risk for functional exercise capacity deterioration. Recent studies have demonstrated that IC can be within the normal range in patients with mild airway obstruction in GOLD stage I, although residual volume (RV) and functional residual capacity (FRC) can be increased [8, 42], pointing towards early hyperinflation. To be able to detect early hyperinflation, we chose to analyze IC/TLC ratio, instead of IC alone. We could also have used the RV/TLC ratio as an explanatory variable, which is another widely used index for lung hyperinflation. In order to compare our findings with those of Ramon et al. [15], we chose to use IC/TLC ratio. We performed additional analyses with RV/TLC instead of IC/TLC ratio, yielding approximately the same results.

Study strengths and limitations

The current study was a large cohort consisting of patients with clinically stable COPD in GOLD stages II-IV. The large sample size, wide spectrum of disease severity and quite even distribution among gender are clear strengths of our study. This prospective study is also one of few to consider the relationship between longitudinal change in 6MWD and IC/TLC ratio.

The 6MWT with 6MWD as main outcome is a widely used measure of functional exercise capacity in COPD, but the cardiopulmonary exercise test (CPET) performed on cycle ergometer or treadmill, is considered as the gold standard for evaluating causes of exercise intolerance in patients with COPD [43]. Peak oxygen uptake (VO_{2peak}) is the main outcome of CPET. The association between 6MWD and VO_{2peak} has shown to be moderate to strong [44, 45] and the 6MWD a reliable measure of walking capacity [46, 47].

In healthy persons and patients with mild COPD, the 6MWT often shows a ceiling effect where it is the maximal walking speed rather than the ventilatory capacity that limits the 6MWD [28]. For some of our patients, the 6MWD was not different from the normal population. A longitudinal decline in 6MWD has been demonstrated in previous studies [12, 29], but this finding was only evident in patients with severe airflow obstruction. Even though there was a decline in 6MWD for patients in GOLD stages III and IV, the mean annual decline was less than 30 m that is considered the minimal clinically significant change [27].

The patients were evaluated three times during the follow-up period of 3 years, performing one 6MWT at each visit. Since the test-battery in the BCCS was comprehensive and demanding for the patients, only one 6MWT was performed at each visit rather than two, which is recommended by the ATS guidelines. By doing two tests, any learning effect is reduced. A decline in 6MWD could therefore have been concealed by the learning effect, and could explain our finding of no change in 6MWD after 1 year. However, it is more unlikely that this effect influenced the results after 3 years.

This study was a subsample of the BCCS, in which patients with inflammatory diseases were excluded. However, patients with chronic diseases like heart failure were included in the study. A possible limitation of our study is the possible effect that such comorbid disease could influence longitudinal change in 6MWD. Regardless, our findings are likely generalizable because comorbid diseases are common among patients with COPD and our study population is assumedly representative for common COPD patients. This is also accounted for by including Charlson comorbidity index in the analyses.

Patients were free to receive medication and therapy, such as pulmonary rehabilitation, during the study. This may have influenced the longitudinal change in 6MWD. Frisk et al. [28] reported that patients participating in a pulmonary rehabilitation program during the study period reported a higher level of habitual physical activity at 3 years follow-up. However, hard physical activity and FEV_1 remained as significant predictors for change in 6MWD when separate analyses were done for patients who did participate in pulmonary rehabilitation and those who did not [28].

Our study had a dropout rate of 32% from baseline to year 3. Most patients were lost to follow-up because of increased disease severity or death. Our dropout rate is comparable to the dropout rate of 31% in the study by Spruit et al. [29], which also had a study period of 3 years. The study by Casanova et al. [12] had a dropout rate of 34% during a study period of 5 years. In studies with COPD patients, an increasing dropout rate is hard to avoid due to progression of the disease during longitudinal studies.

Conclusion

Baseline IC/TLC ratio was a statistically significant predictor for longitudinal change in 6MWD over a period of 3 years. Patients with less lung hyperinflation at baseline maintained their functional exercise capacity in the follow-up period, while it declined significantly in those with increased hyperinflation.

Clinical implications

Decline in functional exercise capacity can to a certain degree be prevented by therapeutic interventions such as pulmonary rehabilitation [48]. It is useful to be able to identify patients that are at particular risk for such deterioration, in order to modify the course of disease.

Abbreviations

6MWD: 6-min walk distance; 6MWT: 6-min walk test; ATS: American Thoracic Society; BCCS: Bergen COPD Cohort Study; BMI: Body mass index; COPD: Chronic obstructive pulmonary disease; CPET: Cardiopulmonary exercise test; FEV_1: Forced expiratory volume in 1 s; FFMI: Fat-free mass index; FMI: Fat mass index; FRC: Functional residual capacity; FVC: Forced vital capacity; GEE: Generalized estimating equations; GOLD: Global Initiative for Chronic obstructive lung disease; IC: Inspiratory capacity; IC/TLC: Inspiratory-to-total lung capacity; mMRC: Modified Medical Research Council; RV: Residual volume; VO_{2peak}: Peak oxygen uptake

Acknowledgements

Not applicable.

Funding

This research did not receive any specific grant from funding agencies in the public, commercial, or not-for-profit sectors.

Authors' contributions

Concept and design (LTA, BF, ET, JAH, TMLE, PSB). Data collection (LTA, BF, JAH, TMLE, PSB, ET). Data analyses and interpretation (LTA, BF, BE, JAH, ET). Drafting the manuscript (LTA, BF, ET, BE, JAH). All the authors have revised and approved the final manuscript.

Consent for publication

Not applicable.

Competing interests

PSB has received speakers' fees from AstraZeneca, Boehringer Ingelheim, Pfizer unrelated to the current work, and received advisory board fees from Mundipharma, AstraZeneca, Boehringer Ingelheim, GlaxoSmithKline unrelated to the current work the last 36 months. TMLE reports speakers' fees from AstraZeneca and Boehringer Ingelheim unrelated to the current work, within the last 36 months. All other authors declare no competing interests.

Author details

[1]Department of Clinical Science, University of Bergen, Bergen, Norway. [2]Centre for Evidence-Based Practice, Western Norway University of Applied Sciences, Bergen, Norway. [3]Department of Occupational Medicine, Haukeland University Hospital, Bergen, Norway. [4]Department of Thoracic Medicine, Haukeland University Hospital, Bergen, Norway. [5]Department of Health and Functioning, Western Norway University of Applied Sciences, Inndalsveien 28, 5063 Bergen, Norway. [6]Department of Physiotherapy, Haukeland University Hospital, Bergen, Norway.

References

1. World Health Organization. Chronic obstructive pulmonary disease (COPD). 2017. Available from: http://www.who.int/respiratory/copd/en/.
2. O'Donnell DE. Hyperinflation, dyspnea, and exercise intolerance in chronic obstructive pulmonary disease. Proc Am Thorac Soc. 2006;3(2):180–4.
3. Laveneziana PWK, O'Donnell DE. Static and Dynamic Hyperinflation in Chronic Obstructive Pulmonary Disease. In: Mechanics of Breathing. 2nd ed; 2014. p. 73–97.
4. O'Donnell DE, Laveneziana P. Dyspnea and activity limitation in COPD: mechanical factors. COPD. 2007;4(3):225–36.
5. Tantucci C, Donati P, Nicosia F, Bertella E, Redolfi S, De Vecchi M, et al. Inspiratory capacity predicts mortality in patients with chronic obstructive pulmonary disease. Respir Med. 2008;102(4):613–9.

6. Jones PW. Activity limitation and quality of life in COPD. COPD. 2007;4(3):273–8.
7. Celli BR, Decramer M, Lystig T, Kesten S, Tashkin DP. Longitudinal inspiratory capacity changes in chronic obstructive pulmonary disease. Respir Res. 2012;13:66.
8. Park J, Lee CH, Lee YJ, Park JS, Cho YJ, Lee JH, et al. Longitudinal changes in lung hyperinflation in COPD. Int J Chron Obstruct Pulmon Dis. 2017;12:501–8.
9. O'Donnell DE, Guenette JA, Maltais F, Webb KA. Decline of resting inspiratory capacity in COPD: the impact on breathing pattern, dyspnea, and ventilatory capacity during exercise. Chest. 2012;141(3):753–62.
10. Laboratories ATSCoPSfCPF. ATS statement: guidelines for the six-minute walk test. Am J Respir Crit Care Med. 2002;166(1):111–7.
11. Casanova C, Cote C, de Torres JP, Aguirre-Jaime A, Marin JM, Pinto-Plata V, et al. Inspiratory-to-total lung capacity ratio predicts mortality in patients with chronic obstructive pulmonary disease. Am J Respir Crit Care Med. 2005;171(6):591–7.
12. Casanova C, Cote CG, Marin JM, de Torres JP, Aguirre-Jaime A, Mendez R, et al. The 6-min walking distance: long-term follow up in patients with COPD. Eur Respir J. 2007;29(3):535–40.
13. Oga T, Nishimura K, Tsukino M, Sato S, Hajiro T, Mishima M. Exercise capacity deterioration in patients with COPD: longitudinal evaluation over 5 years. Chest. 2005;128(1):62–9.
14. Pinto-Plata VM, Cote C, Cabral H, Taylor J, Celli BR. The 6-min walk distance: change over time and value as a predictor of survival in severe COPD. Eur Respir J. 2004;23(1):28–33.
15. Ramon MA, Ferrer J, Gimeno-Santos E, Donaire-Gonzalez D, Rodriguez E, Balcells E, et al. Inspiratory capacity-to-total lung capacity ratio and dyspnoea predict exercise capacity decline in COPD. Respirology. 2016;21(3):476–82.
16. Eagan TM, Ueland T, Wagner PD, Hardie JA, Mollnes TE, Damas JK, et al. Systemic inflammatory markers in COPD: results from the Bergen COPD cohort study. Eur Respir J. 2010;35(3):540–8.
17. Vestbo J, Hurd SS, Agusti AG, Jones PW, Vogelmeier C, Anzueto A, et al. Global strategy for the diagnosis, management, and prevention of chronic obstructive pulmonary disease: GOLD executive summary. Am J Respir Crit Care Med. 2013;187(4):347–65.
18. Johannessen A, Lehmann S, Omenaas ER, Eide GE, Bakke PS, Gulsvik A. Post-bronchodilator spirometry reference values in adults and implications for disease management. Am J Respir Crit Care Med. 2006;173(12):1316–25.
19. Borg GA. Psychophysical bases of perceived exertion. Med Sci Sports Exerc. 1982;14(5):377–81.
20. Kurtze N, Rangul V, Hustvedt BE, Flanders WD. Reliability and validity of self-reported physical activity in the Nord-Trondelag health study (HUNT 2). Eur J Epidemiol. 2007;22(6):379–87.
21. Kurtze N, Rangul V, Hustvedt BE, Flanders WD. Reliability and validity of self-reported physical activity in the Nord-Trondelag health study: HUNT 1. Scand J Public Health. 2008;36(1):52–61.
22. Holmen J, Midthjell K, Krüger Ø, Langhammer A, Holmen TL, Bratberg GH, et al. The Nord-Trøndelag health study 1995-97 (HUNT 2): objectives, contents, methods and participation. Norsk Epidemiologi. 2003;13(1):19–32.
23. Miller MR, Hankinson J, Brusasco V, Burgos F, Casaburi R, Coates A, et al. Standardisation of spirometry. Eur Respir J. 2005;26(2):319–38.
24. Wanger J, Clausen JL, Coates A, Pedersen OF, Brusasco V, Burgos F, et al. Standardisation of the measurement of lung volumes. Eur Respir J. 2005; 26(3):511–22.
25. Bestall JC, Paul EA, Garrod R, Garnham R, Jones PW, Wedzicha JA. Usefulness of the Medical Research Council (MRC) dyspnoea scale as a measure of disability in patients with chronic obstructive pulmonary disease. Thorax. 1999;54(7):581–6.
26. Twisk JW. Applied Longitudinal Data Analysis for Epidemiology: A Practical Guide. 2nd ed. Cambridge: Cambridge University Press; 2013.
27. Singh SJ, Puhan MA, Andrianopoulos V, Hernandes NA, Mitchell KE, Hill CJ, et al. An official systematic review of the European Respiratory Society/American Thoracic Society: measurement properties of field walking tests in chronic respiratory disease. Eur Respir J. 2014;44(6): 1447–78.
28. Frisk B, Espehaug B, Hardie JA, Strand LI, Moe-Nilssen R, Eagan TM, et al. Physical activity and longitudinal change in 6-min walk distance in COPD patients. Respir Med. 2014;108(1):86–94.
29. Spruit MA, Polkey MI, Celli B, Edwards LD, Watkins ML, Pinto-Plata V, et al. Predicting outcomes from 6-minute walk distance in chronic obstructive pulmonary disease. J Am Med Dir Assoc. 2012;13(3):291–7.
30. Guenette JA, Webb KA, O'Donnell DE. Does dynamic hyperinflation contribute to dyspnoea during exercise in patients with COPD? Eur Respir J. 2012;40(2):322–9.
31. Casaburi R, ZuWallack R. Pulmonary rehabilitation for management of chronic obstructive pulmonary disease. N Engl J Med. 2009;360(13):1329–35.
32. Cortopassi F, Celli B, Divo M, Pinto-Plata V. Longitudinal changes in handgrip strength, hyperinflation, and 6-minute walk distance in patients with COPD and a control group. Chest. 2015;148(4):986–94.
33. Pepin V, Saey D, Laviolette L, Maltais F. Exercise capacity in chronic obstructive pulmonary disease: mechanisms of limitation. COPD. 2007;4(3):195–204.
34. Killian KJ, Leblanc P, Martin DH, Summers E, Jones NL, Campbell EJ. Exercise capacity and ventilatory, circulatory, and symptom limitation in patients with chronic airflow limitation. Am Rev Respir Dis. 1992;146(4):935–40.
35. Levine S, Gregory C, Nguyen T, Shrager J, Kaiser L, Rubinstein N, et al. Bioenergetic adaptation of individual human diaphragmatic myofibers to severe COPD. J Appl Physiol (1985). 2002;92(3):1205–13.
36. Levine S, Kaiser L, Leferovich J, Tikunov B. Cellular adaptations in the diaphragm in chronic obstructive pulmonary disease. N Engl J Med. 1997; 337(25):1799–806.
37. Rochester DF, Braun NM. Determinants of maximal inspiratory pressure in chronic obstructive pulmonary disease. Am Rev Respir Dis. 1985;132(1):42–7.
38. Perez T, Becquart LA, Stach B, Wallaert B, Tonnel AB. Inspiratory muscle strength and endurance in steroid-dependent asthma. Am J Respir Crit Care Med. 1996;153(2):610–5.
39. Killian KJ. Sense of effort and dyspnoea. Monaldi Arch Chest Dis. 1998;53(6):654–60.
40. Hamilton AL, Killian KJ, Summers E, Jones NL. Muscle strength, symptom intensity, and exercise capacity in patients with cardiorespiratory disorders. Am J Respir Crit Care Med. 1995;152(6 Pt 1):2021–31.
41. Maltais F, Simard AA, Simard C, Jobin J, Desgagnes P, LeBlanc P. Oxidative capacity of the skeletal muscle and lactic acid kinetics during exercise in normal subjects and in patients with COPD. Am J Respir Crit Care Med. 1996;153(1):288–93.
42. Deesomchok A, Webb KA, Forkert L, Lam YM, Ofir D, Jensen D, et al. Lung hyperinflation and its reversibility in patients with airway obstruction of varying severity. COPD. 2010;7(6):428–37.
43. Force ERST, Palange P, Ward SA, Carlsen KH, Casaburi R, Gallagher CG, et al. Recommendations on the use of exercise testing in clinical practice. Eur Respir J. 2007;29(1):185–209.
44. Oga T, Nishimura K, Tsukino M, Hajiro T, Ikeda A, Mishima M. Relationship between different indices of exercise capacity and clinical measures in patients with chronic obstructive pulmonary disease. Heart Lung. 2002;31(5):374–81.
45. Hill K, Jenkins SC, Cecins N, Philippe DL, Hillman DR, Eastwood PR. Estimating maximum work rate during incremental cycle ergometry testing from six-minute walk distance in patients with chronic obstructive pulmonary disease. Arch Phys Med Rehabil. 2008;89(9):1782–7.
46. Hernandes NA, Wouters EF, Meijer K, Annegarn J, Pitta F, Spruit MA. Reproducibility of 6-minute walking test in patients with COPD. Eur Respir J. 2011;38(2):261–7.
47. Eiser N, Willsher D, Dore CJ. Reliability, repeatability and sensitivity to change of externally and self-paced walking tests in COPD patients. Respir Med. 2003;97(4):407–14.
48. Spruit MA, Singh SJ, Garvey C, ZuWallack R, Nici L, Rochester C, et al. An official American Thoracic Society/European Respiratory Society statement: key concepts and advances in pulmonary rehabilitation. Am J Respir Crit Care Med. 2013;188(8):e13–64.

21

Randomized controlled trial to evaluate the utility of suction and inner-stylet of EBUS-TBNA for mediastinal and hilar lymphadenopathy

Xiaoxiao Lin[1], Min Ye[1], Yuping Li[1], Jing Ren[1], Qiyan Lou[1], Yangyang Li[2], Xiaohui Jin[3], Ko-Pen Wang[4] and Chengshui Chen[1*]

Abstract

Background: The optimal procedure for maximizing the diagnostic yield and minimizing the procedural complexity of endobronchial ultrasound-guided transbronchial needle aspiration (EBUS-TBNA) is controversial. We conducted a prospective randomized controlled trial to determine the optimal procedure of EBUS-TBNA for mediastinal and hilar lymphadenopathy, with a particular focus on the roles of the inner-stylet and suction.

Methods: Consecutive patients with enlarged mediastinal and hilar lymph nodes (LNs), detected by computed tomography (CT) or positron emission tomography-CT (PET-CT), who underwent EBUS-TBNA were included. Each LN was sampled with three needle passes using suction–stylet, suction–no stylet, and stylet–no suction procedures. The samples were smeared onto glass slides for cytological evaluation. A single, blinded cytopathologist evaluated each set of slides. The primary outcomes were cytological specimen adequacy rate and diagnostic yield of malignant LNs. The secondary outcomes were tissue-core acquisition rate, procedural time, and the amount of bleeding.

Results: This study evaluated 97 patients with a total of 255 LNs. The final LN diagnosis was benign in 144, malignant in 104, and inadequate in 7 cases. There were no significant differences among the suction–stylet, suction–no stylet, and stylet–no suction groups in specimen adequacy rate (87.1, 88.2, 85.9%, respectively) or diagnostic yield of malignancy (32.2, 31.8, 31.0%, respectively). However, the use of suction was associated with an increase in tissue-core acquisition rate ($P < 0.001$). The no-stylet procedure decreased the average procedural time by 14 s ($P < 0.001$). There was no significant difference in the amount of bleeding among the procedures.

Conclusions: The use of suction or non-use of an inner-stylet does not make a significant difference in cytological specimen adequacy or diagnostic yield when performing EBUS-TBNA. While omitting the stylet can simplify the procedure, applying suction can increase the tissue-core acquisition rate. These findings may assist endoscopic physicians in determining the optimal EBUS-TBNA procedure and warrant clinical verification in a future multicentre study.

Keywords: Endobronchial ultrasound-guided transbronchial needle aspiration, Clinical trial, Lymphadenopathy, Malignant

* Correspondence: wzchencs@163.com
[1]Department of Pulmonary and Critical Care Medicine, The First Affiliated Hospital of Wenzhou Medical University, Ouhai District, Wenzhou, China
Full list of author information is available at the end of the article

Background

Endobronchial ultrasound-guided transbronchial needle aspiration (EBUS-TBNA) is a technique that is highly effective for diagnosing enlarged mediastinal and hilar lymph nodes (LNs) detected on computed tomography (CT) or positron emission tomography-CT (PET-CT), in patients with benign or malignant conditions. Some clinical studies have demonstrated that EBUS-TBNA is a cost-effective [1] and safe diagnostic technique for acquiring specimens, with a diagnostic yield similar to or even higher than that of surgical mediastinoscopy [2–4]. However, the optimal procedure of EBUS-TBNA for maximizing the diagnostic yield and minimizing the procedural complexity is controversial. In the past decade, various modifications of the EBUS-TBNA procedure [5–9] have been described for optimizing diagnostic yield, procedural efficiency, and specimen adequacy. Nevertheless, there has been limited discussion on how to simplify the procedure without decreasing its diagnostic yield.

The conventional EBUS-TBNA technique requires that a metal stylet within the inner lumen of a fine needle be inserted and removed during every needle pass, which increases the procedural time and complicates the procedure. Therefore, we considered the possibility of omitting the inner-stylet during EBUS-TBNA. In addition, because there is considerable controversy regarding whether it is necessary to apply suction during EBUS-TBNA, we here conducted a prospective randomized controlled trial to determine the optimal EBUS-TBNA procedure for detection of mediastinal and hilar malignant lymphadenopathy, with a particular focus on the effect of using an inner-stylet and suction.

Methods

Trial subjects

Consecutive patients with enlarged mediastinal and hilar LNs who underwent EBUS-TBNA between October 2016 and May 2017 were enrolled. An LN with a short-axis diameter > 5 mm on a chest CT image was considered as an enlarged LN. Lymph-node stations were classified in accordance with the international lymph-node map by the International Association for the Study of Lung Cancer [10]. All patients provided written informed consent. The EBUS-TBNA procedure was performed by the same experienced endoscopic physician for all patients. It was performed if an enlarged LN was identified by using a convex-probe echoendoscope (EB-530, FUJIFILM, Tokyo, Japan). The trial protocol was approved by the Clinical Research Ethics Committee of our hospital (YJLCYJ2016–216), and the trial was registered at www.chictr.org.cn (ChiCTR-IOR-17010616).

Trial procedure

TBNA was performed with a 22-gauge needle (NA-201SX-4022, Olympus, Tokyo, Japan) under EBUS and real-time color Doppler guidance with a convex-probe echoendoscope. After puncturing an LN, the fine needle was moved to and fro within the LN 10–20 times and then withdrawn. Each LN was sampled with three needle passes using suction–stylet, suction–no stylet, and stylet–no suction procedures (each process was performed once). To adjust for the effects of some potential confounding factors, including passes made using different procedures, the order of the procedure for each target site was randomized by a senior biostatistician from the School of Public Health, Wenzhou Medical University, using SAS 9.4 for Windows (Cary, North Carolina State, America).

During the conventional EBUS-TBNA procedure (the suction–stylet group), the inner lumen of the fine needle was first occluded with a metal stylet, which was removed after the needle entered the target LN. Once the stylet was withdrawn, a 20-mL syringe was applied to the needle for providing suction. For the no-stylet procedure, the stylet was omitted throughout the procedure, and the syringe was applied to the needle before the latter was inserted into the working channel of the echoendoscope. In the no-suction procedure, after the needle was inserted into the target LN, the stylet was withdrawn by 10 cm without using suction. During each pass, the physician assessed the amount of bleeding from the puncture site on the bronchial wall.

Each needle-pass specimen was extruded onto a separate glass slide using a 10-mL air-filled syringe, and a direct smear was made by an experienced EBUS nurse. Rapid on-site cytological evaluation was not performed. The residual contents of the needle from a single LN were flushed into the same container and consolidated by formalin to obtain a single cell block or tissue core for histological examination (in accordance with the handing and preparation procedures for histological specimens of our pathology department). After flushing the needle, the outside of the needle and the stylet were vigorously wiped with sterile gauze to reduce cross contamination between passes. A related on-site trial assistant recorded whether or not a visible tissue core was acquired with each needle pass and calculated the procedural time for each pass from the time of insertion of the fine needle through the working channel of the echoendoscope to the retrieval of the needle during each pass, excluding the time for reinsertion of the stylet into the fine needle. If insufficient specimen for a cell block or tissue core was obtained after the third pass, additional passes were permitted, with the choice of procedures and number of passes left to the discretion of the endoscopic physician.

The smears on glass slide were alcohol-fixed (95% ethanol) and stained with hematoxylin and eosin. A cytopathologist, who was blinded to the procedural order for EBUS-TBNA, characterized each individual needle pass for cytological specimen adequacy and made a specific diagnosis as follows: malignancy, benign (including normal lymphoid tissue and granulomatous inflammation), and inadequate. Specimens with > 40 lymphocytes per high power field [11] in the more cellular areas of the smeared slide was interpreted as adequate, as were those that exhibited malignant cells. Samples with insufficient diagnostic cellular materials or lymphocytes were deemed inadequate.

Assessment of procedural outcomes

The final diagnosis of each LN was determined using all available cytological and histological findings from three EBUS-TBNA procedures. The primary outcomes of the trial were the cytological specimen adequacy rate and the diagnostic yield for malignant lymphadenopathy. A sample size of 225 LNs would provide sufficient power for a 10% non-inferiority margin upon performing non-inferiority analysis. The secondary outcomes were tissue-core acquisition rate, procedural time and amount of bleeding during each procedure. The amount of bleeding was categorized on the basis of the following scores: 0 (major hemorrhage, resulting in termination of subsequent procedure); 1 (light hemorrhage that could be stopped using cold saline or norepinephrine); 2 (no or little hemorrhage occurred, even without treatment).

Statistical analysis

Statistical analysis was performed with the IBM SPSS Statistics Version 22.0 software (Chicago, IL, USA). The analysis evaluated only the first three passes for each LN. Descriptive statistics were used to summarize the characteristics of all patients and all LNs in the trial. Data on continuous variables were presented as mean ± standard deviation. McNemar tests were performed to determine the difference in specimen adequacy rate, diagnostic yield and tissue-core acquisition rate between suction–stylet and suction–no stylet or suction–stylet and stylet–no suction procedures. The paired t-test was employed to compare procedural time. In addition, the amount of bleeding was analyzed using Wilcoxon's test. A subgroup analysis was performed to determine the association of different EBUS-TBNA procedures with specimen adequacy rate and diagnostic yield, for LNs > 10 mm or ≤ 10 mm in diameter. A two-sided P value of < 0.05 was considered to indicate statistical significance.

Results

The trial evaluated 97 patients with a total of 255 mediastinal and hilar LNs. Randomization ensured that each third of the suction–stylet, suction–no stylet, and stylet–no suction passes were first, second, and third passed (Fig. 1). The baseline characteristics of the patients and LNs are summarized in Table 1. The mean age of patients was 61.2 years (range, 20–79 years); 71 (73.2%) of the patients were male. Of 57 inpatients for whom we could record clinical symptoms after the EBUS-TBNA procedure, 9 (15.8%) had transient fever; these 9 patients recovered within 24 h without treatment or with temporary antifebrile medication. There were no instances of procedure-related major hemorrhage in the present trial.

Two or three LNs were sampled for most patients. For the 255 LNs, the mean short-axis diameter on chest CT images was 14.7 mm, and the most common enlarged LN stations were 4R and 7. The final pathologic diagnoses for the 255 LNs were as follows: 104 malignancies, 144 benign diagnoses, and 7 inadequate samples.

The cytological specimen adequacy rates were 87.1, 88.2, and 85.9% in the suction–stylet, suction–no stylet, and stylet–no suction groups, respectively; the corresponding values for diagnostic yield of malignancy were 32.2, 31.8, and 31.0%, respectively, which showed no statistically significant difference among the three groups. The results of statistical analysis of specimen adequacy rate and diagnostic yield are detailed in Table 2. Subgroup analysis did not show a statistically significant association between the EBUS-TBNA procedures and specimen adequacy rate or diagnostic yield for LNs > 10 mm or LNs ≤ 10 mm (Table 3).

Comparison of secondary outcomes among the three procedures (Table 4) revealed that the use of suction was associated with an increase in the tissue-core acquisition rate (suction–stylet vs. stylet–no suction group; 47.1% [120/255] vs. 32.5% [83/255]; $P <$ 0.001). Non-use of the stylet did not decrease or increase the tissue-core acquisition rate (suction–stylet vs. suction–no stylet group: 47.1% vs. 49.4%; $P = 0.576$). In terms of procedural time, the no-stylet procedure was on average 14 s shorter than the suction–stylet procedure (87.1 s vs. 101.1 s; $P <$ 0.001). However, in terms of amount of bleeding, the use or non-use of suction yielded similar scores; similar results were observed for procedures with and without the stylet.

Discussion

This prospective randomized controlled trial demonstrated that the traditional procedure of applying suction during EBUS-TBNA did not make a statistically significant difference in cytological specimen adequacy or diagnostic yield of malignant lymphadenopathy, although it increased the rate of tissue-core acquisition for histological examination. Compared to procedures performed with a stylet, not using a stylet did not decrease the specimen adequacy or diagnostic yield. Upon comparing EBUS-TBNA procedures with or without suction and with or without stylet for LNs ≤ 10 mm and > 10 mm in short-axis diameter, we found no difference in the adequacy or diagnostic yield of cytological specimens. Although more data may be needed

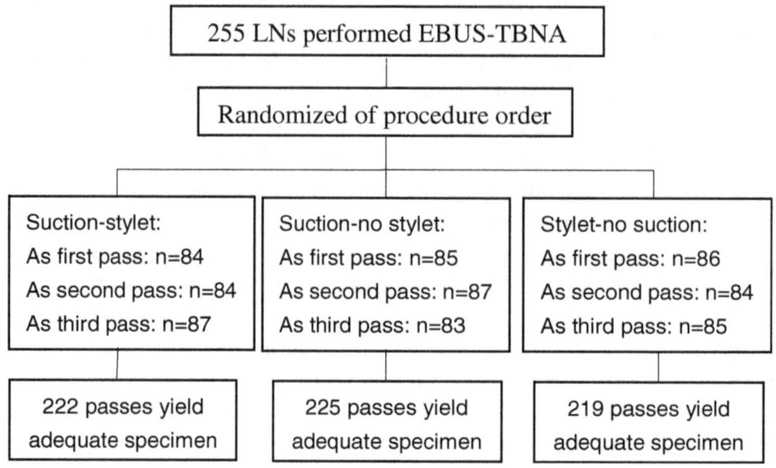

Fig. 1 The number of each pass order and adequate specimen for different EBUS-TBNA procedures. EBUS-TBNA: Endobronchial ultrasound-guided transbronchial needle aspiration; LN: Lymph node

Table 1 Characteristics of patients and lymph nodes included in the final analysis

Characteristics	Data
Patients, No.	97
Age, years	61.2 ± 13.2
Gender, No.	
Male	71
Female	26
Origin of patient, No.	
Outpatient	40
Inpatient	57
Lymph nodes, No.	255
Mean nodule size, mm	14.7 ± 7.6
≤ 10 mm, No.	86
> 10 mm, No.	169
Location of lymph nodes, No.	
2 L	1
4 L	29
4R	72
7	77
10 L	6
10R	3
11 L	28
11R	26
12R	1
mediastinal mass	12

to confirm these specific conclusions, our findings may assist endoscopic physicians in determining the optimal EBUS-TBNA procedure.

Mediastinal and hilar lymphadenopathy may be caused by various inflammatory, infectious, or malignant factors, and it is important to ascertain the diagnosis or to determine the disease stage in case of malignancy before deciding on treatment. Mediastinoscopy has long been the reference standard of mediastinal and hilar LN sampling; however, it has several disadvantages, including its relatively high complexity and invasiveness [12]. Over the last decade, EBUS-TBNA has provided a more readily available and safer alternative than mediastinoscopy for acquiring specimens [2, 3]. It has emerged as the best first-diagnostic tool for collecting tissue for diagnosis and staging of lung cancer [13] and has also come to be approved for use in other lymphadenopathies, such as tuberculosis, sarcoidosis and lymphoma [14–16].

However, EBUS-TBNA has several limitations. Although its median sensitivity for detecting malignant lymphadenopathy (89%) [13] is better than that of imaging examinations alone, EBUS-TBNA leads to misdiagnosis of malignant LNs

Table 2 Comparison of primary outcomes of EBUS-TBNA procedures

EBUS-TBNA procedure	The primary outcome	P^a value
	Specimen adequacy rate	
suction–stylet vs. suction–no stylet	87.1% vs. 88.2%	0.629
suction–stylet vs. stylet–no suction	87.1% vs. 85.6%	0.728
	Diagnostic yield	
suction–stylet vs. suction–no stylet	32.2% vs. 31.8%	> 0.999
suction–stylet vs. stylet–no suction	32.2% vs. 31.0%	0.711

[a]: Determined by McNemar test; *EBUS-TBNA* Endobronchial ultrasound-guided transbronchial needle aspiration

Table 3 Result of subgroup analysis among EBUS-TBNA procedures for LNs > 10 mm and ≤ 10 mm in diameter

Compared procedures	Subgroup	P[a] value	
	LN size, mm	adequacy rate	diagnostic yield
suction–stylet vs. no-stylet	≤ 10	> 0.999	> 0.999
	> 10	0.754	> 0.999
suction–stylet vs. no-suction	≤ 10	> 0.999	0.289
	> 10	0.523	> 0.999

[a]Determined by McNemar test; *EBUS-TBNA* Endobronchial ultrasound-guided transbronchial needle aspirationm, *LN* Lymph node

in an average of 11% of patients. Additionally, physicians need to obtain sufficient tissue specimens from EBUS-TBNA for molecular testing for diagnosis of malignancy or microbe cultivation for diagnosis of infectious diseases. Additionally, the EBUS-TBNA technique is time-consuming, especially when multiple LNs are identified and multiple needle passes are made. In our trial, we found that the procedure mainly required an additional 1–3 min for every needle pass and up to 10–15 min additionally per LN. Lastly, given the recommendations for combining EBUS-TBNA and endoscopic ultrasound-guided fine needle aspiration (EUS-FNA) for diagnosis of mediastinal and hilar lymphadenopathy [17], the operating physician should be skilled in both procedures. Consequently, it is important to simplify the EBUS-TBNA procedure and acquire adequate specimens without decreasing its diagnostic yield.

The use of an inner-stylet during EBUS-TBNA is somewhat controversial. It has commonly been used because it can theoretically prevent bronchial mucosa and cartilage filling the inner lumen and protect the fine needle by increasing its stiffness upon entry into the target LN. However, the inner-stylet has to be inserted and removed through the fine needle during every needle pass, which increases the procedural time and complicates the EBUS-TBNA procedure. Moreover, conventional TBNA is performed without an inner-stylet in the fine needle. Evaluation of the use of the inner-stylet in EBUS-TBNA has been limited to a single recent study. Scholten and colleagues [18] found no significant differences in diagnostic yield, specimen adequacy, or cytological quality between with-stylet and no-stylet procedures; these conclusions agreed with our findings. However, these previous authors failed to quantify the procedural time saved by omitting the stylet. In our trial, we found that non-use of the stylet statistically significantly decreased the procedural time; relative to the suction-stylet procedure, the no-stylet procedure was on an average 14 s shorter, excluding the time spent on inserting the inner-stylet into the fine needle. In addition, during the entire trial, there was no instance of needle breakage when the inner-stylet was not used. Moreover, from the patient's perspective, omitting the inner-stylet might help reduce the cost of EBUS needles. Although the clinical value of the time saved with the no-stylet procedure merits further study, it is evident that omitting the stylet could simplify the EBUS-TBNA procedure, without reducing the cytological specimen adequacy or diagnostic yield.

Application of suction during FNA has been a standard practice for many decades in various medical specialties, including pathology and gastroenterology. However, there is considerable controversy about the need to apply suction during EBUS-TBNA. Some clinicians believe that suction might increase tissue trauma at the biopsy site and result in more bleeding into the specimen, thus decreasing the diagnostic yield of EBUS-TBNA. Others have argued that suction helps to acquire more specimen material. Wallace et al. [19] reported that, compared to FNA without suction, the traditional method of applying suction during EUS-FNA did not show any difference in diagnostic yield but provided worse specimen quality because of excessive blood in the specimen. Recently, Casal et al. [20] conducted a randomized trial for comparing the with-suction and no-suction procedures of EBUS-TBNA and found no difference in diagnostic yield, adequacy or quality of cytological specimens. However, they did not analyze the histological specimen adequacy of each procedure. A retrospective nonrandomized study showed that high suction pressures during EBUS-TBNA might be useful for safe collection of sufficient tissue specimens [21]. Our trial data support the conclusion that suction does not influence cytological specimen adequacy, diagnostic yield or the amount of bleeding.

Rapid advances in oncologic therapy have necessitated further ancillary studies, including immunohistochemical

Table 4 Statistical results of the three procedures in secondary outcomes

Secondary outcome	Group A[b]	Group B[c]	Group C[d]	P value[a]	
				A vs. B	A vs. C
Procedural time (second)	101.1 ± 31.3	87.1 ± 34.7	89.3 ± 33.6	< 0.001	< 0.001
Tissue-core acquisition (%)	47.1	49.4	32.5	0.576	< 0.001
The amount of bleeding (score)	1.97 ± 0.17	1.96 ± 0.20	1.97 ± 0.17	0.366	> 0.999

[a]Procedural time, tissue-core acquisition rate, and the amount of bleeding were analyzed by the paired t-test, McNemar test, and the Wilcoxon's test, respectively
[b]A, suction–stylet procedure
[c]B, suction–no stylet procedure
[d]C, stylet–no suction procedure

and molecular analyses for subtyping and genotyping of lung cancer, during the diagnostic workup of small tissue specimens. A guideline from the College of American Pathologists, International Association for the Study of Lung Cancer, and Association for Molecular Pathology, states that tissue samples should be prioritized for molecular analysis and that cytological samples are also suitable for studies, with cell blocks being preferred over smeared material [22]. In our trial, the suction procedure assisted in obtaining a greater volume of tissue specimens, which could be processed for cell block or tissue histology analyses. However, another guideline for the acquisition and preparation of EBUS-TBNA specimens for the diagnosis of lung cancer suggests that cell blocks and core tissue are both good materials for mutational analysis [23]. Numerous studies have reported on preparation of cell blocks for ancillary studies [24–26]. Therefore, further investigations may be needed to explore whether the amount of tissue-core obtained during EBUS-TBNA with or without suction would influence the diagnosis and subtyping of lung cancer.

The most frequent complication associated with EBUS-TBNA is hemorrhage; other rare complications of the procedure are infection, pneumothorax, and device breakage [27]. In 2014, a systematic review on adverse events in 16,181 patients who underwent endosonography for mediastinal and hilar LNs or central lung masses reported 23 (0.14%) serious adverse events (0.3 and 0.05% with EUS-FNA and EBUS-TBNA, respectively), with no mortality [28]. In the present trial, there were no instances of severe infectious disease, need for ICU admission, or death after EBUS-TBNA. The incidence of fever was 15.8% (9/57) among inpatients in our trial, and all febrile patients recovered in 24 h without treatment or with temporary antifebrile medication. In addition, there was no significant difference in the amount of bleeding with each pass between EBUS-TBNA procedures with and without suction or with and without stylet, and there was no instance of major hemorrhage. These results suggest that EBUS-TBNA is a safe method in general and that the probability of complications is similar among the different EBUS-TBNA procedures.

An advantage of the present prospective trial, which involved randomization of the procedure order and blinding of the cytopathologist, is its self-contrast design, which could control for the effects of size, location, density, and pathological type of different LNs, as well as other unknown factors. Furthermore, in our trial, an on-site assistant recorded the procedural time for each pass; this has not been evaluated in other previous studies.

A limitation of our trial, however, is its single-centre and single-operator design. A multicentre trial would be ideal to confirm the statistical significance of the results obtained with different EBUS-TBNA procedures. Additionally, we compared tissue-core acquisition rate among different procedures but, regrettably, failed to analyze the specimen quality for cell block or tissue histological examination, which might have decreased the chance of identifying differences among the procedures.

Conclusions

In summary, the use of suction or non-use of the inner-stylet does not make a significant difference in cytological specimen adequacy or diagnostic yield when performing EBUS-TBNA. Omitting the stylet can simplify the procedure, and applying suction can help increase the tissue-core acquisition rate. These findings may assist endoscopic physicians in determining the optimal EBUS-TBNA procedure and warrant clinical verification in a future multicentre study.

Abbreviations

CT: computed tomography; EBUS-TBNA: endobronchial ultrasound-guided transbronchial needle aspiration; EUS-FNA: endoscopic ultrasound-guided fine needle aspiration; LN: lymph node; PET-CT: positron emission tomography-computed tomography

Acknowledgements

We would like to thank Prof. Guangyun Mao from the School of Public Health, Wenzhou Medical University, for his assistance with statistical analysis, and acknowledge all medical workers from the department of Endoscopy and the department of Pathology, The First Affiliated Hospital of Wenzhou Medical University, for their coordination to carry out the clinical trial.

Funding

The collection of date was supported by grants from the International Pulmonary Key Laboratory of Zhejiang Province to CSC, the Interventional Pulmonology Key Laboratory of Wenzhou City to CSC, the Interventional Pulmonology Innovation Subject of Zhejiang Province to CSC, the National Nature Science Foundation of China (81270313 to CSC, 81770074 to CSC, 81570075 to CSC), the Natural Science Foundation of Zhejiang Province (LZ15H010001 to CSC), the Science Technology Department Foundation of Zhejiang Province (WKJ-ZJ-1526 to CSC) and the National Key R&D Program of China (2016YFC1304000 to CSC).

Authors' contributions

XXL analyzed data and was a major contributor in writing the manuscript; CSC designed the trial and analyzed data; MY performed the trial. YPL and KPW designed the trial. JR, QYL, YYL and XHJ collected data; all authors read and approved the final manuscript.

Consent for publication

Not applicable.

Competing interests

The authors declare that they have no competing interests.

Author details

[1]Department of Pulmonary and Critical Care Medicine, The First Affiliated Hospital of Wenzhou Medical University, Ouhai District, Wenzhou, China. [2]Department of Pathology, The First Affiliated Hospital of Wenzhou Medical University, Ouhai District, Wenzhou, China. [3]Department of Endoscopy, The First Affiliated Hospital of Wenzhou Medical University, Ouhai District, Wenzhou, China. [4]Division of Pulmonary and Critical Care Medicine, Johns Hopkins University School of Medicine, Baltimore, USA.

References

1. Rintoul RC, Glover MJ, Jackson C, et al. Cost effectiveness of endosonography versus surgical staging in potentially resectable lung cancer: a health economics analysis of the ASTER trial from a European perspective. Thorax. 2014;69:679–81.
2. Annema JT, van Meerbeeck JP, Rintoul RC, et al. Mediastinoscopy vs endosonography for mediastinal nodal staging of lung cancer: a randomized trial. JAMA. 2010;304:2245–52.
3. Sehgal IS, Dhooria S, Aggarwal AN, et al. Endosonography versus Mediastinoscopy in mediastinal staging of lung Cancer: systematic review and meta-analysis. Ann Thorac Surg. 2016;102:1747–55.
4. Ernst A, Anantham D, Eberhardt R, et al. Diagnosis of mediastinal adenopathy-real-time endobronchial ultrasound guided needle aspiration versus mediastinoscopy. J Thorac Oncol. 2008;3:577–82.
5. Muthu V, Gupta N, Dhooria S, et al. A prospective, randomized, double-blind trial comparing the diagnostic yield of 21- and 22-gauge aspiration needles for performing endobronchial ultrasound-guided Transbronchial needle aspiration in sarcoidosis. Chest. 2016;149:1111–3.
6. Konge L, Clementsen PF, Ringsted C, et al. Simulator training for endobronchial ultrasound: a randomised controlled trial. Eur Respir J. 2015; 46:1140–9.
7. Lee HS, Lee GK, Lee HS, et al. Real-time endobronchial ultrasound-guided transbronchial needle aspiration in mediastinal staging of non-small cell lung cancer: how many aspirations per target lymph node station? Chest. 2008;134:368–74.
8. Casal RF, Lazarus DR, Kuhl K, et al. Randomized trial of endobronchial ultrasound-guided transbronchial needle aspiration under general anesthesia versus moderate sedation. Am J Respir Crit Care Med. 2015;191: 796–803.
9. Guo H, Liu S, Guo J, et al. Rapid on-site evaluation during endobronchial ultrasound-guided transbronchial needle aspiration for the diagnosis of hilar and mediastinal lymphadenopathy in patients with lung cancer. Cancer Lett. 2016;371:182–6.
10. Rusch VW, Asamura H, Watanabe H, et al. The IASLC lung cancer staging project: a proposal for a new international lymph node map in the forthcoming seventh edition of the TNM classification for lung cancer. J Thorac Oncol. 2009;4:568–77.
11. Alsharif M, Andrade RS, Groth SS, et al. Endobronchial ultrasound-guided transbronchial fine-needle aspiration: the University of Minnesota experience, with emphasis on usefulness, adequacy assessment, and diagnostic difficulties. Am J Clin Pathol. 2008;130:434–43.
12. Detterbeck FC, Jantz MA, Wallace M, et al. Invasive mediastinal staging of lung cancer: ACCP evidence-based clinical practice guidelines (2nd edition). Chest. 2007;132:202S–20S.
13. Silvestri GA, Gonzalez AV, Jantz MA, et al. Methods for staging non-small cell lung cancer: diagnosis and management of lung cancer, 3rd ed: American College of Chest Physicians evidence-based clinical practice guidelines. Chest. 2013;143:e211S–50S.
14. Navani N, Molyneaux PL, Breen RA, et al. Utility of endobronchial ultrasound-guided transbronchial needle aspiration in patients with tuberculous intrathoracic lymphadenopathy: a multicentre study. Thorax. 2011;66:889–93.
15. Davis GS. The role of endobronchial ultrasound-guided transbronchial needle aspiration (EBUS TBNA) in the diagnosis of sarcoidosis. Cancer Cytopathol. 2014;122:239–40.
16. Kheir F, Itani A, Assasa O, et al. The utility of endobronchial ultrasound-transbronchial needle aspiration in lymphoma. Endosc Ultrasound. 2016;5:43–8.
17. Vilmann P, Clementsen PF, Colella S, et al. Combined endobronchial and esophageal endosonography for the diagnosis and staging of lung cancer: European Society of Gastrointestinal Endoscopy (ESGE) guideline, in cooperation with the European Respiratory Society (ERS) and the European Society of Thoracic Surgeons (ESTS). Endoscopy. 2015;47:545–59.
18. Scholten EL, Semaan R, Illei P, et al. Stylet use does not improve diagnostic outcomes in endobronchial Ultrasonographic Transbronchial needle aspiration: a randomized clinical trial. Chest. 2017;151:636–42.
19. Wallace MB, Kennedy T, Durkalski V, et al. Randomized controlled trial of EUS-guided fine needle aspiration techniques for the detection of malignant lymphadenopathy. Gastrointest Endosc. 2001;54:441–7.
20. Casal RF, Staerkel GA, Ost D, et al. Randomized clinical trial of endobronchial ultrasound needle biopsy with and without aspiration. Chest. 2012;142:568–73.
21. Shiroyama T, Okamoto N, Suzuki H, et al. Usefulness of high suction pressure for sufficient tissue collection during endobronchial ultrasound guided transbronchial needle aspiration. PLoS One. 2013;8:e82787.
22. Lindeman NI, Cagle PT, Beasley MB, et al. Molecular testing guideline for selection of lung cancer patients for EGFR and ALK tyrosine kinase inhibitors: guideline from the College of American Pathologists, International Association for the Study of Lung Cancer, and Association for Molecular Pathology. J Thorac Oncol. 2013;8:823–59.
23. van der Heijden EH, Casal RF. Trisolini Rocco et al. Guideline for the acquisition and preparation of conventional and endobronchial ultrasound-guided transbronchial needle aspiration specimens for the diagnosis and molecular testing of patients with known or suspected lung cancer. Respiration. 2014;88(6):500–17.
24. Neal N, Brown James M, Matthew N, et al. Suitability of endobronchial ultrasound-guided transbronchial needle aspiration specimens for subtyping and genotyping of non-small cell lung cancer: a multicenter study of 774 patients. Am J Respir Crit Care Med. 2012;185(12):1316–22.
25. Abhishek B, Leon Marino E, Peter D, et al. Clinical performance of endobronchial ultrasound-guided transbronchial needle aspiration for assessing programmed death ligand-1 expression in nonsmall cell lung cancer. Diagn Cytopathol. 2018;46(5):378–83.
26. Emily H, David M, Ian P, et al. Cell block samples from endobronchial ultrasound transbronchial needle aspiration provide sufficient material for ancillary testing in lung cancer-a quaternary referral centre experience. J Thorac Dis. 2016;8(9):2544–50.
27. Asano F, Aoe M, Ohsaki Y, et al. Complications associated with endobronchial ultrasound-guided transbronchial needle aspiration: a nationwide survey by the Japan Society for Respiratory Endoscopy. Respir Res. 2013;14:50.
28. von Bartheld MB, van Breda A, Annema JT. Complication rate of endosonography (endobronchial and endoscopic ultrasound): a systematic review. Respiration. 2014;87:343–51.

22

Pulmonary carcinosarcoma showing an obvious response to pazopanib

Azusa Tanimoto[1*], Shinji Takeuchi[1], Hiroshi Kotani[1], Kaname Yamashita[1], Tadaaki Yamada[2], Koushiro Ohtsubo[1], Hiromichi Ebi[1], Hiroko Ikeda[3] and Seiji Yano[1]

Abstract

Background: Pulmonary carcinosarcoma (PCS) is a rare primary lung malignancy and has a poor prognosis among lung tumor histological subtypes. However, an appropriate treatment strategy has not been developed for unresectable PCS.

Case presentation: A 65-year-old man who was diagnosed with PCS was treated by surgical removal of the primary lung lesion, followed by six cycles of adjuvant chemotherapy with cisplatin plus irinotecan. Following the chemotherapy, he experienced a relapse with brain metastasis, which induced the rapid onset of left leg paralysis. Radical surgical resection and stereotactic radiosurgery to the resection cavity were performed. However, meningeal dissemination and new lung metastases occurred after a year and half. To control these multiple metastatic lesions, the patient was treated with the multiple kinase inhibitor pazopanib. No change was observed in the meningeal dissemination, while the metastatic lung lesions were prominently reduced in size following treatment with pazopanib. Consequently, the patient showed a partial response to pazopanib treatment, although the dose of pazopanib was reduced by half as a result of thrombocytopenia.

Conclusion: This is the first report of metastatic PCS showing an evident therapeutic response to tumor-targeted therapy. We suggest that pazopanib may be a therapeutic option for patients with metastatic PCS.

Keywords: Pulmonary carcinosarcoma, Pazopanib, Thrombocytopenia, VEGFR

Background

Pulmonary carcinosarcoma (PCS), which accounts for only 0.3% of all lung tumors, is a rare histological subtype of non-small lung cancer (NSCLC) [1]. PCS is defined by the presence of epithelial elements (squamous or adenocarcinoma) combined with sarcomatous elements such as rhabdomyosarcoma, osteosarcoma, or chondrosarcoma [2]. A few studies have demonstrated the presence of common chromosomal abnormalities in the epithelial and sarcomatous components of PCS [3, 4], suggesting a monoclonal origin of PCS tumors. Standard therapy for PCS has not yet been established owing to the low incidence of this type of tumor. Pazopanib, a multi-targeted tyrosine kinase inhibitor against the proto-oncogene c-Kit (c-KIT), platelet-derived growth factor receptor (PDGFR), fibroblast growth factor receptor (FGFR), and vascular endothelial growth factor receptor (VEGFR), has been reported to show beneficial outcomes in patients with metastatic non-adipocytic soft-tissue sarcoma and renal cell carcinoma, and superior safety and quality-of-life profiles compared with sunitinib, which is a similar targeted drug [5, 6]. Here, we report the first case of metastatic PCS that showed a remarkable response to pazopanib despite the necessity of dose reduction owing to thrombocytopenia.

Case report

A 65-year-old man who never smoked and had consulted a local hospital 3 years earlier presented to our hospital, where he was diagnosed with PCS and treated with right pneumonectomy, followed by six cycles of adjuvant chemotherapy with cisplatin plus irinotecan, because the pTNM stage was pT3N1M0 stage IIIA according to the 7 th lung cancer TNM classification. One year later, he experienced the rapid onset of left lower extremity paralysis, and brain gadolinium contrast-enhanced magnetic resonance imaging (MRI) performed in our hospital revealed a

* Correspondence: atanimoto@staff.kanazawa-u.ac.jp
[1]Division of Medical Oncology, Cancer Research Institute, Kanazawa University, 13-1, Takara-machi, Kanazawa, Ishikawa 920-0934, Japan
Full list of author information is available at the end of the article

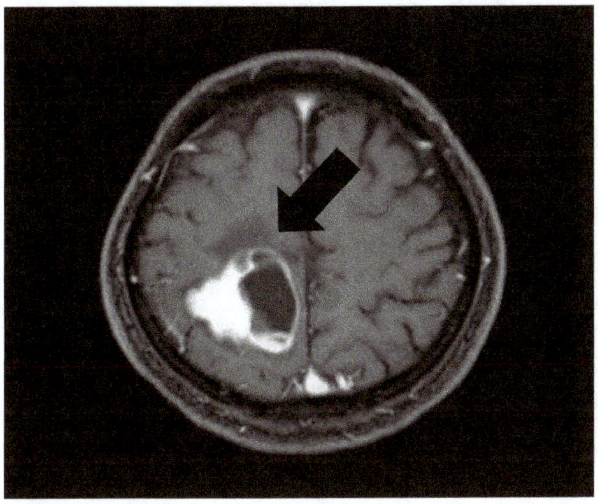

Fig. 1 Brain magnetic resonance imaging (MRI) reveals a cerebral ring-enhancing lesion with hemorrhage (arrow)

new brain mass with active bleeding in the right parietal lobe (Fig. 1). The patient was treated with surgical resection, followed by stereotactic radiosurgery to the resection cavity. Immunohistochemical analysis of resected tissue samples revealed sarcomatous tumors composed of spindle cells and cartilage and epithelial tumors expressing cytokeratin AE1/AE3 (Fig. 2a, b). These histological findings were quite similar to those observed with tissue from pneumonectomy specimens (Fig. 2c, d). Therefore, we made a definitive histological diagnosis of metastatic PCS on the brain tumor specimens. A year and a half after this operation, brain gadolinium contrast-enhanced MRI revealed meningeal dissemination (Fig. 3a), and chest radiography identified two nodules in the left lower lung field (Fig. 3b) which were diagnosed with lung recurrence although the lesions were not verified histologically for fear of fatal iatrogenic pneumothorax because of right pneumonectomy. The patient began treatment for PCS with pazopanib (Votrient®, GlaxoSmithKline, Uxbridge, Middlesex, UK) 800 mg orally once a day on the basis of the histological diagnosis because pazopanib has been approved for the treatment of soft tissue sarcoma in Japan. Two weeks after treatment initiation, the patient was withdrawn from the drug because his platelet count was reduced to 60,000/μL. Since the platelet count recovered to above the lower limit of normal 2 weeks later, he was permitted to resume pazopanib at 400 mg orally once a day. Although a brain MRI scan showed no change in the meningeal dissemination, a chest and abdominal computed tomography scan demonstrated a reduction in size of 60% in the lung metastatic lesions of PCS according to Response Evaluation Criteria In Solid Tumors (RECIST) version 1.1 after 2 months of treatment (Fig. 4a-d). His quality of life during the pazopanib treatment had kept adequate because there was little adverse event by pazopanib except thrombocytopenia. 6 months later, the patient showed consciousness disorder due to the progression of the meningeal dissemination and stopped taking pazopanib despite the lung metastatic lesions kept shrinking.

Discussion and conclusions

Complete surgical resection is the first choice for standard treatment for PCS, if possible. On the other hand,

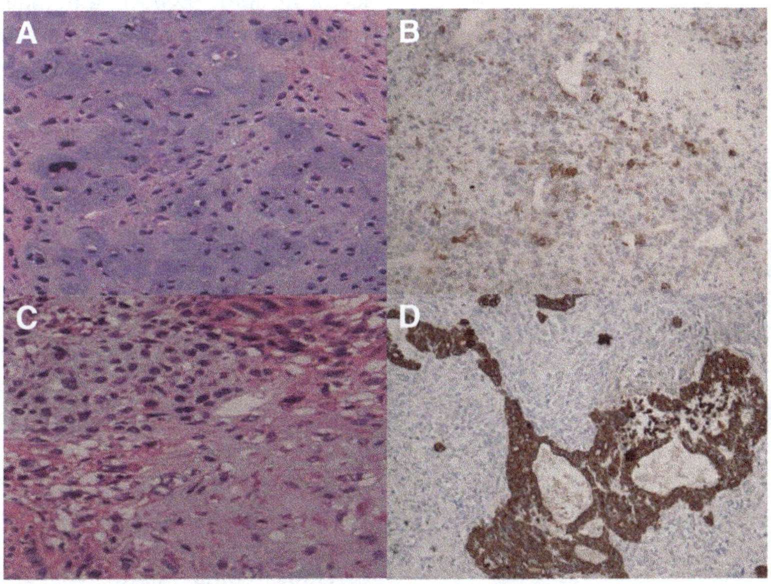

Fig. 2 Histological findings: Photomicrograph of resected specimen from brain metastases demonstrates cartilage compositions (**a**) (hematoxylin and eosin [HE] staining, × 100) and epithelial tumors (**b**) (cytokeratin AE1/AE3 staining, × 100). **c**, **d** Photomicrograph of HE and cytokeratin AE1/AE3 stained specimen demonstrates findings conformable with resected specimen from primary lung lesion (magnification, × 100)

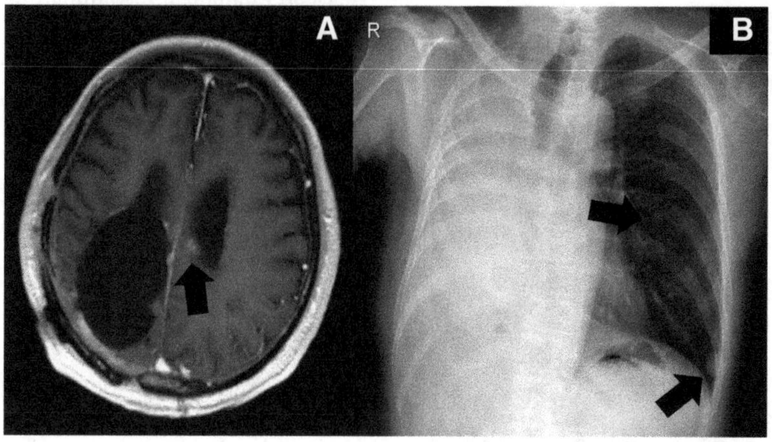

Fig. 3 **a** Brain magnetic resonance imaging (MRI) shows meningeal dissemination in left lateral ventricle (arrow). **b** Chest x-ray scan shows two nodule shadows in left lower lung field (arrow)

effective systemic chemotherapy in patients with inoperable PCS has not yet been developed [7] although the prognosis of PCS is poorer than that of other types of NSCLC [8]. In the present report, the multiple kinase inhibitor pazopanib showed an obvious effect in a case of metastatic PCS.

Several papers have reported that the prognosis of patients with PCS was poor, with a median survival of approximately 1 year [9, 10]. Although a few reports showed that doxorubicin-based regimens had some effect on metastatic PCS [1, 11], standard chemotherapy for metastatic PCS has not yet been developed [12]. Therefore, pazopanib has the potential to become one of the new treatment options for inoperable PCS.

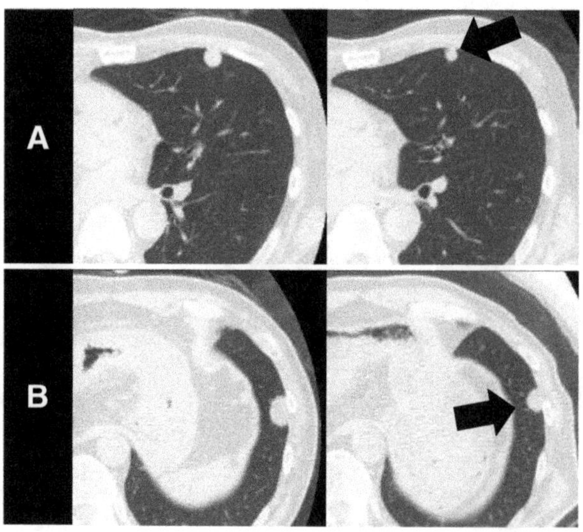

Fig. 4 Computed tomography (CT) image illustrates two nodules in left upper lobe (**a**) and lower lobe (**b**) prior to treatment. The size of the nodules (arrow) was reduced following treatment (right panel)

In-frame deletions at exon 19 in the *EGFR* gene in both the carcinomatous component and the sarcomatous component have been detected in resected PCS specimens [13], indicating the potential to identify oncogenic driver mutations for targeting in PCS tumors. We performed mutational analysis of *KIT Proto-Oncogene Receptor Tyrosine Kinase* (*KIT*) and *Platelet-Derived Growth Factor Receptor-A* (*PDGFRA*) genes in the present case, because pazopanib has inhibitory activity on PDGFR-α/β and c-Kit [14]. We found no active mutations of these genes, suggesting that the tumor regression in the present case might be attributable to inhibition by pazopanib of VEGFR instead of that of KIT and PDGFR. Previous research demonstrated that VEGF, but not c-KIT, epidermal growth factor receptor (EGFR), or human epidermal growth factor receptor 2 (HER-2), was strongly expressed in both the carcinomatous component and the sarcomatous component in 30 cases of uterine carcinosarcoma [15]. Clinical analysis revealed that increased VEGF and VEGFR-3 expression indicated poor survival in uterine and ovarian carcinosarcomas from analysis of 25 patient samples [16]. Therefore, it would be valuable if the expression of VEGF and VEGFR in PCS tumors could be surveyed, which could indicate the possibility of a novel treatment strategy via the VEGF/VEGFR axis in PCS. Further clinical study is needed to elucidate the crucial signals for PCS.

In the present case, the pulmonary metastatic lesions from PCS showed a marked reduction in size in response to pazopanib treatment. This is the first case of PCS demonstrating a good clinical response to molecular targeted therapy. Although a phase II clinical study found that the response rate to pazopanib in uterine carcinosarcoma was 0% (0/19) [17], another study reported the first cases of positive clinical response to pazopanib in patients with uterine carcinosarcoma and ovarian carcinosarcoma [18].

These findings would indicate the heterogeneity of dominant survival signals in carcinosarcoma regardless of the primary lesions. Therefore, the attempt should be made to identify a predictive biomarker, such as VEGF/VEGFR, for response to certain specific drugs in types of carcinosarcoma including PCS.

We have reported the case of a patient with PCS who showed a good response to pazopanib, albeit with dose reduction by half owing to adverse effects. Pazopanib may have potential in the treatment of PCS. Although PCS is extremely rare, continued study of the clinical benefits of pazopanib may aid in the development of a new therapeutic strategy for patients with metastatic PCS.

Abbreviations
c-KIT: Proto-oncogene c-Kit; PCS: Pulmonary carcinosarcoma; PDGFR: Platelet-derived growth factor receptor; VEGFR: Vascular endothelial growth factor receptor

Acknowledgements
The authors wish to thank Mitsutoshi Nakada, Katsuyoshi Miyashita for operating the patient.

Funding
Not applicable.

Authors' contributions
AT and SY were involved with concept and design of this manuscript. AT, ST and SY were involved with making treatment decisions. AT and TY were involved with drafting this manuscript. HK, KY, KO, HE and HI proofread the manuscript. All authors have read and approved the final version of the edited manuscript.

Consent for publication
Written informed consent was obtained from the patient for publication of this case report and any accompanying images. A copy of the written consent is available for review by the Editor of this journal.

Competing interests
The authors declare that they have no competing interests.

Author details
[1]Division of Medical Oncology, Cancer Research Institute, Kanazawa University, 13-1, Takara-machi, Kanazawa, Ishikawa 920-0934, Japan. [2]Department of Pulmonary Medicine, Graduate School of Medical Science, Kyoto Prefectural University of Medicine, Kyoto, Japan. [3]Division of Pathology, Kanazawa University Hospital, Kanazawa, Japan.

References
1. Davis MP, Eagan RT, Weiland LH, Pairolero PC. Carcinosarcoma of the lung: Mayo Clinic experience and response to chemotherapy. Mayo Clin Proc. 1984;59:598–603.
2. Koss MN, Hochholzer L, Frommelt RA. Carcinosarcomas of the lung: a clinicopathologic study of 66 patients. Am J Surg Pathol. 1999;23:1514–26.
3. Dacic S, Finkelstein SD, Sasatomi E, Swalsky PA, Yousem SA. Molecular pathogenesis of pulmonary carcinosarcoma as determined by microdissection-based allelotyping. Am J Surg Pathol. 2002;26:510–6.
4. Pardo J, Aisa G, de Alava E, Sola JJ, Panizo A, Rodriguez-Spiteri N, et al. Primary mixed squamous carcinoma and osteosarcoma (carcinosarcomas) of the lung have a CGH mapping similar to primitive squamous carcinomas and osteosarcomas. Diagnostic Mol Pathol B. 2008;17:151–8.
5. van der Graaf WT, Blay JY, Chawla SP, Kim DW, Bui-Nguyen B, Casali PG, et al. Pazopanib for metastatic soft-tissue sarcoma (PALETTE): a randomised, double-blind, placebo-controlled phase 3 trial. Lancet (London, England). 2012;379:1879–86.
6. Motzer RJ, Hutson TE, Cella D, Reeves J, Hawkins R, Guo J, et al. Pazopanib versus sunitinib in metastatic renal-cell carcinoma. N Engl J Med. 2013;369:722–31.
7. Pelosi G, Sonzogni A, De Pas T, Galetta D, Veronesi G, Spaggiari L, et al. Review article: pulmonary sarcomatoid carcinomas: a practical overview. Int J Surg Pathol. 2010;18:103–20.
8. Martin LW, Correa AM, Ordonez NG, Roth JA, Swisher SG, Vaporciyan AA, et al. Sarcomatoid carcinoma of the lung: a predictor of poor prognosis. Ann Thorac Surg. 2007;84:973–80.
9. Wick MR, Ritter JH, Humphrey PA. Sarcomatoid carcinomas of the lung: a clinicopathologic review. Am J Clin Pathol. 1997;108(1):40–53.
10. Weissferdt A, Moran CA. Malignant biphasic tumors of the lungs. Adv Anat Pathol. 2011;18:179–89.
11. Langer F, Wintzer HO, Werner M, Weber C, Brummendorf TH, Bokemeyer C. A case of pulmonary carcinosarcoma (squamous cell carcinoma and osteosarcoma) treated with cisplatin and doxorubicin. Anticancer Res. 2006;26:3893–7.
12. Huang SY, Shen SJ, Li XY. Pulmonary sarcomatoid carcinoma: a clinicopathologic study and prognostic analysis of 51 cases. World J Surg Oncol. 2013;11:252.
13. Toyokawa G, Takenoyama M, Taguchi K, Arakaki K, Inamasu E, Toyozawa R, et al. The first case of lung carcinosarcoma harboring in-frame deletions at exon19 in the EGFR gene. Lung Cancer (Amsterdam, Netherlands). 2013;81:491–4.
14. Sonpavde G, Hutson TE. Pazopanib: a novel multitargeted tyrosine kinase inhibitor. Curr Oncol Rep. 2007;9:115–9.
15. Cimbaluk D, Rotmensch J, Scudiere J, Gown A, Bitterman P. Uterine carcinosarcoma: immunohistochemical studies on tissue microarrays with focus on potential therapeutic targets. Gynecol Oncol. 2007;105:138–44.
16. Nayha V, Stenback F. Angiogenesis and expression of angiogenic agents in uterine and ovarian carcinosarcomas. APMIS. 2008;116:107–17.
17. Campos SM, Brady WE, Moxley KM, O'Cearbhaill RE, Lee PS, DiSilvestro PA, et al. A phase II evaluation of pazopanib in the treatment of recurrent or persistent carcinosarcoma of the uterus: a gynecologic oncology group study. Gynecol Oncol. 2014;133:537–41.
18. Nishikawa T, Hasegawa K, Yabuno A, Yoshida H, Yasuda M, Kozawa E, et al. Pazopanib as a second line treatment for uterine and ovarian carcinosarcoma: a single institutional study. J Gynecol Oncol. 2017;28:e25.

23

Clinical expression of cystic fibrosis in a large cohort of Italian siblings

Vito Terlizzi[1*], Marco Lucarelli[2], Donatello Salvatore[3], Adriano Angioni[4], Arianna Bisogno[5], Cesare Braggion[1], Roberto Buzzetti[6], Vincenzo Carnovale[7], Rosaria Casciaro[8], Giuseppe Castaldo[9,10], Natalia Cirilli[11], Mirella Collura[12], Carla Colombo[5], Antonella Miriam Di Lullo[13], Ausilia Elce[14], Vincenzina Lucidi[15], Elisa Madarena[16], Rita Padoan[17], Serena Quattrucci[18], Valeria Raia[19], Manuela Seia[20], Lisa Termini[21] and Federica Zarrilli[22]

Abstract

Background: A clinical heterogeneity was reported in patients with Cystic Fibrosis (CF) with the same *CFTR* genotype and between siblings with CF.

Methods: We investigated all clinical aspects in a cohort of 101 pairs of siblings with CF (including 6 triplets) followed since diagnosis.

Results: Severe lung disease had a 22.2% concordance in sib-pairs, occurred early and the FEV_1% at 12 years was predictive of the severity of lung disease in the adulthood. Similarly, CF liver disease occurred early (median: 15 years) and showed a concordance of 27.8% in sib-pairs suggesting a scarce contribution of genetic factors; in fact, only 2/15 patients with liver disease in discordant sib-pairs had a deficiency of alpha-1-antitrypsin (a known modifier gene of CF liver phenotype). CF related diabetes was found in 22 pairs (in 6 in both the siblings). It occurred later (median: 32.5 years) and is strongly associated with liver disease. Colonization by *P. aeruginosa* and nasal polyposis that required surgery had a concordance > 50% in sib-pairs and were poorly correlated to other clinical parameters. The pancreatic status was highly concordant in pairs of siblings (i.e., 95.1%) but a different pancreatic status was observed in patients with the same *CFTR* mutations. This suggests a close relationship of the pancreatic status with the "whole" *CFTR* genotype, including mutations in regulatory regions that may modulate the levels of *CFTR* expression. Finally, a severe course of CF was evident in a number of patients with pancreatic sufficiency.

Conclusions: Physicians involved in care of patients with CF and in genetic counseling must be aware of the clinical heterogeneity of CF even in sib-pairs that, at the state of the art, is difficult to explain.

Keywords: CFTR, Genotype, Phenotype, Modifier genes, FEV_1, Pseudomonas aeruginosa

Background

Cystic fibrosis (CF) is the most common, severe, autosomal recessive inherited disease among Caucasians [1]. It is usually characterized by elevated sweat chloride levels (SCL), pancreatic insufficiency (PI), progressive lung disease with chronic bacterial infections of lower airways and male infertility due to obstructive azoospermia. More than 2000 variants have been identified in the *cystic fibrosis transmembrane conductance regulator* (*CFTR*) gene so far (www.genet.sickkids.on.ca), but only few have been functionally characterized [2]. Some of them may be grouped in six classes according to the known effect on CFTR synthesis and/or function [2, 3]. However, although life-expectance and severity of the disease depend on the class of mutations [4, 5], there is a wide clinical heterogeneity in CF patients carrying the same *CFTR* genotype and even between siblings and twins with CF [6]. Several sources contribute to such variability as mutations in non-coding regions of the *CFTR* gene [7–9], intronic variants [9–11] and complex alleles [12, 13] making the genotype-phenotype relationship more complex.

* Correspondence: terlizzivito@libero.it
[1]Dipartimento di Pediatria, Centro Regionale Toscano per la Fibrosi Cistica, Azienda Ospedaliero-Universitaria Meyer, Viale Gaetano Pieraccini 24, 50139 Florence, Italy
Full list of author information is available at the end of the article

In the last decade several studies explored the role of modifier genes of CF phenotype [14] for meconium ileus (MI) [15–17], CF-related diabetes (CFRD) [18], CF liver disease (CFLD) [19], lung disease [20, 21] and the colonization by *P. aeruginosa* [22]. However, environmental factors, such as the quality of health care, compliance to therapy [23], lifestyle, and socio-economic status [24] play a pivotal role in the outcome of CF.

The strong heterogeneity of CF impacts on the genetic counseling and on the reproductive planning of families that have CF affected children. In the present study, we evaluated a series of pairs of siblings with CF monitored since diagnosis to study the degree of clinical heterogeneity of the CF phenotype, assessing and correlating clinical aspects and complications of the disease.

Methods

Patients

The study population consisted of patients followed since diagnosis at 12 CF specialized care centers in Italy who met diagnostic criteria for CF [25] and had at least one sibling suffering from CF. According to the current Italian legislation, we obtained from all patients (or from their legal guardian) the informed consent to use anonymously clinical data for research purposes.

Methods

Sweat chloride levels were tested according to guidelines [26]. We screened for a panel of mutations and for the most common *CFTR* rearrangements [27]; thus, we carried out gene sequencing (detection rate 95%) [28, 29] in patients in which one or both mutations resulted undetected after first level analysis [30]. We analyzed 7 intragenic *CFTR* short tandem repeats [31] to verify that both members of four sibling-pairs carrying only one known mutation had the same *CFTR* genotype. Molecular analysis revealed more than 50 different *CFTR* mutations in our patients and only for a half of them functional studies had defined the molecular effect and the class; furthermore, some of these latter mutations may combine more defects and can be attributed to more classes [2]. Thus, we did not perform correlations between the *CFTR* genotype and clinical parameters. However, Additional file 1: Table S1 provides the *CFTR* genotype of each patient included in the study.

Meconium ileus was defined using the criteria described [15]. The forced expiratory volume (FEV_1), expressed as the percentage of predicted value for age, according to standardized reference equations for spirometry [32] was recorded. To avoid age-related differences between siblings of each pair, we recorded as current FEV_1 the last value of the younger sibling and that of the older sibling at the same age. In the case of patients who had died or had undergone lung transplantation we recorded the last FEV_1 and the value of the living or non-transplanted member of the sibling-pair at the same age. Given the inter-individual variability of FEV_1 and the evolution of lung damage with age [33] the patients were classified as severe or mild according with the criteria by Schluchter et al., that take into account both the FEV_1 value and age [34, 35]. The airway colonization by *P. aeruginosa* was identified by sputum or oropharyngeal swab culture. Chronic infection was defined according to the modified Leeds criteria [36].

Fecal pancreatic elastase was evaluated annually and at least 3 months before enrollment. Pancreatic sufficiency was defined on the basis of fecal pancreatic elastase-1 higher than 200 mcg/g measured in the absence of acute pancreatitis or gastrointestinal diseases. Pancreatitis was defined as acute or chronic according to the report from International study group of pediatric pancreatitis [37] excluding all known causes of pancreatitis. Liver disease was evaluated by means of clinical, biochemical or ultrasonography abnormalities recorded in two consecutive examinations within a 3-month period, in the absence of other causes of congenital or acquired chronic liver disease [38]. Patients were considered as affected by CFLD when they had liver cirrhosis, considered as the extreme phenotype to define liver disease in our study, with imaging techniques showing nodular hepatic parenchyma and signs of portal hypertension [17]. A glucose tolerance test was performed annually in all patients with CF and the diagnosis of CFRD was made according to the standard American Diabetes Association criteria [39]. Finally, the history of nasal polyposis requiring surgery was evaluated.

Statistics

The concordance for disease (symptoms or complications) within sibling-pairs was calculated as the ratio between the number of pairs concordant for the symptom/complication and the number of pairs in which at least one member had the symptom/complication [15].

Results and discussion

Study population

We studied 208 patients with CF (median age: 30 years, range 12–61 years; 106 males); of these, 40 (19.2%) were diagnosed by newborn screening (NBS) and 168 (80.8%) by symptoms or by family history. All the 208 patients were over 12 years of age and 172/208 patients (82.7%) were over 18 years. The study included 95 pairs of siblings (22 pairs of females, 27 pairs of males and 46 pairs of one female and one male) and 6 sets of 3 siblings (2 including two males and one female, 2 including two females and one male and 2 including three females).

In 80/101 pairs (79.2%) all the siblings were above 18 years of age.

Pancreatic status

As shown in Table 1, in our pairs of siblings we found a concordance for PI of 95.1% (i.e., only in three sibling-pairs the pancreatic status resulted discordant) confirming the known correlation between the pancreatic status and the *CFTR* genotype. However, pairs of siblings with the same *CFTR* mutations may have PS or PI, and it is known that mutations like the R334W, the R347P, the 2789 + 5G > A [40], or the D1152H [41] may be associated with PS or PI. This means that the high degree of concordance for the pancreatic status found in siblings depends on the "whole" *CFTR* genotype (that is quite completely shared by siblings) including either mutations in the coding regions and variants in non-coding regions like the promoter or the intronic regions [7, 8] that together define the levels of residual activity of the CFTR protein at pancreatic level and thus may modulate the pancreatic status of each patient.

Table 1 compares the clinical characteristics and the complications in sib-pairs with different pancreatic status. In sib-pairs with PI, MI, severe lung disease, CFLD and CFRD occurred more frequently (even if the small number of cases preclude a statistical comparison) according to the current literature [42, 43].

Table 1 Concordance within sib-pairs for PI and correlation between the pancreatic status and meconium ileus (MI), severity of lung disease, CF liver disease (CFLD), CF related diabetes (CFRD) and recurrent panreatitis (RP) in 101 pairs of siblings with CF. N: absence of the symptom/complication

Concordance within sib-pairs for PI (%)95.1

		PI/PI	PI/PS	PS/PS
Number of sib-pairs		58	3	40
Meconium ileus:	MI/MI	4	0	0
	MI/N	5	0	2
	N/N	49	3	38
Lung disease:	Severe/severe	6	0	0
	Severe/mild	15	1	5
	Mild/mild	37	2	35
CF liver disease:	CFLD/CFLD	3	2	0
	CFLD/N	11	0	2
	N/N	44	1	38
CF related diabetes:	CFRD/CFRD	5	0	1
	CFRD/N	11	3	2
	N/N	42	0	37
Pancreatitis:	RP/RP	1	0	1
	RP/N	1	0	6
	N/N	56	3	33

Recurrent pancreatitis was significantly more frequent in sib-pairs with PS in agreement with the concept that recurrent pancreatitis in patients with CF is due to ductal plugging that typically occurs in patients with PS [43, 44]. On the other hand, modifier genes other than *CFTR* may enhance the risk to develop recurrent/chronic pancreatitis [45, 46] explaining some cases of patients with PI that developed recurrent pancreatitis (Additional file 1: Table S1).

Interestingly, among the patients with PS we found MI in 2 cases, severe lung disease in 6 and complications such CFLD in 5 or CFRD in 7 cases (Additional file 1: Table S1). We are confident that our patients with PS would not develop PI later either because most patients with PS have at least one mild mutation and because their age is higher than that of patients with PI (mean 34.6 years, median 33 years for patients with PS versus a mean age of 28.0 years and a median of 25 years of patients with PI). Thus, a severe clinical phenotype may occur in a percentage of patients with PS. Considering that most patients with CF and PS are nowadays diagnosed by NBS, the presence of these complicated cases suggests that patients with PS would be monitored with the same care of patients with PI.

Meconium ileus and DIOS

We found a 36.4% of concordance for MI in sib-pairs, i.e., 4 pairs were concordant for MI and 7 pairs were discordant suggesting that in addition to the *CFTR* genotype other non-genetic and genetic factors contribute to the development of MI. Among the genetic ones, in CFTR-deficient mice, that is an excellent model for human MI, three potential modifier loci for MI were found on chromosomes 1, 9 and 10, respectively [47]. Subsequent studies in humans identified at least 2 modifier loci for MI [15] and thus, the SLC4A4 gene was candidate as modifier genes for MI in patients with CF [48]. Furthermore, a role of KCNN4 as a modifier gene of MI was suggested [16, 17].

We found five patients with CF that had DIOS; such complication was revealed in both the members of two sib-pairs and in a member of a further pair (Additional file 1: Table S1). Interestingly, none of the five patients experienced MI, reinforcing the view that DIOS, once considered the adult equivalent of MI, has an independent etiology [15].

Lung disease

We found 34/208 patients (16.4%) with severe lung disease. The concordance for severe lung disease was 22.2%, i.e., in 21 pairs the lung status was discordant (i.e., severe versus mild) between siblings (Fig. 1) while in 6 pairs both the siblings had a severe lung disease suggesting that environmental factors and genes inherited

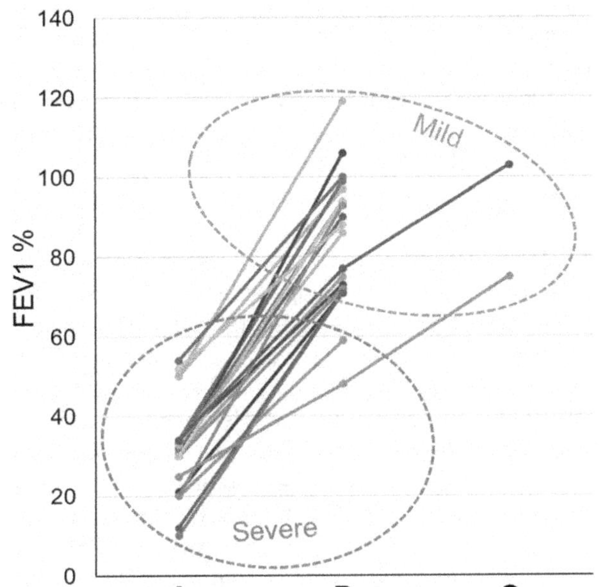

Fig. 1 FEV_1% of predicted for age in 21 pairs of siblings with cystic fibrosis discordant for the severity of lung disease. The classification as mild or severe was performed according to the criteria by Schluchter et al. [30] that take into account both the FEV_1 value and age

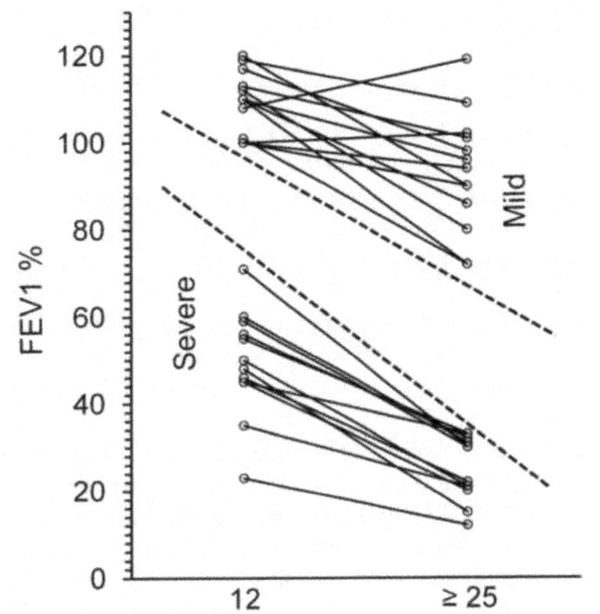

Fig. 2 FEV_1% of predicted for age in 25 patients with cystic fibrosis. For each patient we report the value measured at the age of 12 years and the current value at the age of 25 years or later. The classification of mild (13 cases) or severe (12 cases) was performed according to criteria by Schluchter et al. [30] that take into account both the FEV_1 value and age

independently by *CFTR* contribute to the pathogenesis of severe lung disease. This agree with the results of Vanscoy et al. on 231 pairs of siblings [49], and of Collaco et al. [21], that concluded that genetic and environmental factors contribute equally to lung function in patients with CF. Finally, an excellent study on 6365 patients with CF revealed five loci that modulate the severity of lung disease in patients with CF [20]. The severe lung disease correlated with PI (e.g., all the 6 pairs of siblings with severe lung disease had PI, see Additional file 1: Table S1) and with *P. aeruginosa* colonization (see below).

It is interesting to observe the longitudinal data of 25 patients from our study for which the values of FEV_1 at the age of 12 years and at the age of 25 years or later were available (Fig. 2). Even if the number of cases is small, the classification of severe ($n = 12$) or mild ($n = 13$) lung disease performed at 12 years invariably coincides with that obtained in the adulthood in the same patient, suggesting that the FEV_1% in young patients with CF is predictive of the lung function in the adult age.

On the other hand, it is known that structural lung damage is an early event in patients with CF [50]. This was revealed by high-resolution chest tomography [51] and by the presence of severe pulmonary inflammation and structural lung disease in still asymptomatic patients diagnosed by NBS [52].

Colonization by Pseudomonas aeruginosa

We found colonization by *P. aeruginosa* in 92/208 (44.2%) patients with CF. Among our 101 pairs of siblings, we found colonization by *P. aeruginosa* in all the members of 34 sibling-pairs, among which the three siblings of two triplets and only one member of 20 sibling-pairs (and in two of three members of a triplet), with a high concordance for colonization (i.e., 61.8%). This result agrees with previous studies on 50 [52] and 11 [19] pairs of siblings. Interestingly, among our siblings discordant for colonization, in 11/21 cases both the siblings lived in the same house, and the sibling colonized by *P. aeruginosa* was colonized since at least 3 years. These data indicate a limited role of the environment in the colonization and confirms a contribution of *CFTR* genotype and genes inherited independently by *CFTR* that may predispose to colonization by *P. aeruginosa,* as reviewed by Cutting [3]. Nevertheless, we cannot rule out an early intervention (e.g. antibiotics) to prevent nosocomial infection in non-colonized siblings.

In patients with colonization there is a significantly higher occurrence of severe lung disease (data not shown). However, colonization is likely a consequence of the severe pulmonary damage more than a causal contribution. Indeed, the mean age of colonization in our patients was 18.5 years (median 22.6), while the occurrence of the structural lung damage is an early event in patients with CF (as discussed in the previous paragraph).

CF liver disease

We found CFLD in 24/208 (11.5%) patients with CF. It is difficult to compare this figure with previous data because different parameters may be used to define CFLD (i.e., altered aminotransferase levels, focal biliary cirrhosis, US alterations, portal hypertension). As described in materials and methods, we used very stringent parameters to define CFLD and our results agree with the evidence that about 10% of patients with CF develop a severe liver damage and about 5% require liver transplantation. Our data confirm that CFLD is an early event since it was diagnosed at a mean age of 14.7 years (median 15 years old, range 7–27 years) in agreement with the view that CFLD peaks in adolescence [42].

CFLD was found in both the members of 5 sibling-pairs and in one member of 13 sibling-pairs (among which two triplets) and in two members of a further triplet. No previous data are available on the comparison of CFLD liver disease in siblings and in twins with CF, but the concordance for CFLD of 27.8% obtained in our sibling-pairs indicate a scarce contribution of genes in the pathogenesis of CFLD reinforcing the role of environmental, mostly still unknown, risk factors [38]. In fact, the largest two-stage control study (about 2000 patients with CF) on modifier genes of CFLD revealed mutations in the SERPIN1 gene encoding for alpha-1-antitrypsin only in about 2% of patients with CFLD [19]. In agreement, among the 15 sibling-pairs discordant for CFLD, only in 2 cases the sibling suffering from CFLD had levels of serum alpha-1-antitrypsin under the lower reference limit, compatible with the deficiency of the protein, while the siblings free from CFLD had normal levels of the protein.

Cystic fibrosis related diabetes (CFRD)

We found CFRD in all the members of 6/101 sibling-pairs (among which one triplet) and in one member of 16/101 sibling-pairs. The concordance for CFRD was 27.3% and this figure compares with that of 18.0% reported in a population of 588 sibling-pairs [53]. These data, added to the concordance for CFRD of 73.0% obtained in 68 pairs of monozygotic twins with CF [53] that share 100% of DNA, support the view that genetic modifiers play a marginal role in the development of diabetes in patients with CF. This is also confirmed by the observation that the occurrence of CFRD is not an early complication in patients with CF [39]. In fact, the diagnosis of CFRD in our patients was performed at the mean age of 32.2 years and in more than a half of patients > 30 years. Furthermore, we excluded also the gender as a risk factor for CFRD: we found such complication in 13/106 males and in 15/102 females (p not significant). Most studies on larger populations reported the female gender as a risk factor for CFRD [42], but a more recent study on 588 sibling-pairs did not find a statistically significant role of gender as risk factor for CFRD [53].

As shown in Table 1, PI was significantly more frequent in sib-pairs with CFRD, confirming PI as a risk factor for CFRD since it causes a progressive pancreatic fibrosis that gradually damages the insulae [54]. However, observing that 7/28 patients with CFRD had PS (Additional file 1: Table S1), we suggest that also CF patients with PS must be included in the annual screening for CFRD based on the glucose tolerance test [42].

In addition, CFLD contributes to the risk for CFRD [55] since we found a higher occurrence of CFLD among sib-pairs with CFRD than in those free from this complication. Finally, our data are in agreement with the view that severe lung disease is a risk factor for CFRD in turn [56, 57]. In fact, in 19 sib-pairs in which one or both patients had CFRD, in 12 cases one or both the siblings had a severe lung disease, a condition observed only in 15/79 pairs in which both the siblings were free from CFRD. This correlation is more evident in 16 sibling-pairs discordant for CFRD, in which the sibling with CFRD, at the same age, had the worst FEV_1% ($p = 0.004$, Wilcoxon signed rank test) in 14/16 cases (Fig. 3).

Nasal polyposis

We found nasal polyposis requiring surgery in both the siblings of 13 pairs and only in one sibling from 12 sibling-pairs (concordance for disease: 52.0%). There are no previous data on sibling pairs to which compare our results. The poor correlation of nasal polyposis to other clinical manifestations such as the pancreatic status and the severity of lung disease (data not shown) imply that modifier genes play a role in determining nasal polyposis. In fact, a recent study firstly described the potential role of interferon-related developmental regulator 1 (a known modifier gene for CF pulmonary disease severity) as a modifier gene of nasal polyposis in patients with CF [58].

Conclusions

Our study confirms the clinical heterogeneity of CF also in a percentage of pairs of siblings with CF. Physicians involved in genetic counseling must be aware of a so wide and mostly unpredictable variability. Stochastic, environmental and genetic factors also independent by *CFTR* contribute to such variability, even if with a different weight on each variable (i.e., nasal polyposis and *P. aeruginosa* colonization may be more influenced by genetic factors while CFRD and CFLD or the severe lung disease may be influenced either by genetic and by

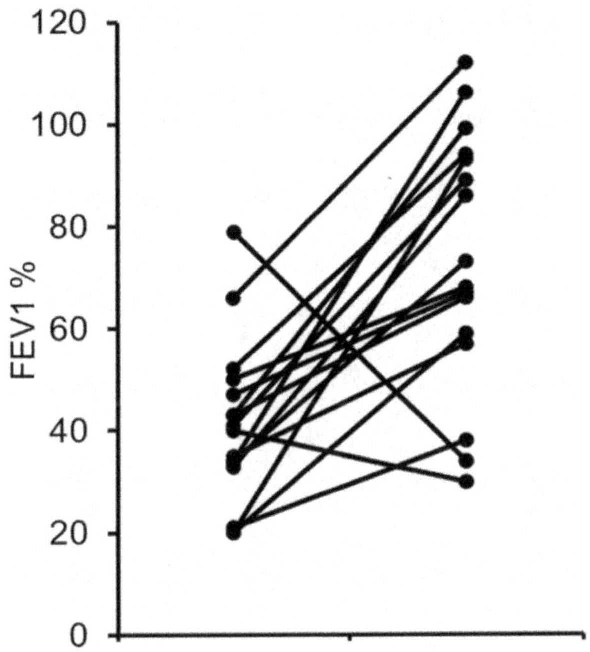

Fig. 3 Current FEV_1% of predicted for age in 15 pairs of siblings discordant for cystic fibrosis related diabetes (CFRD). **a** sibling with CFRD; **b** sibling free from CFRD. We reported as current FEV_1 the last value of the younger sibling and that of the older sibling at the same age

environmental factors). However other variables like medical care (that significantly improved in the last years), strongly influenced the clinical expression of each patient of our cohort that includes CF patients in the wide range between 12 to 61 years. Some working hypotheses emerged from our study: i) the classification of the lung damage as severe or mild based on the FEV_1% assessed at the age of 12 years coincides with that obtained in the adulthood; ii) CFRD is influenced by the severity of liver disease; iii) a severe course of the disease (including the occurrence of complications) may occur in a percentage of patients with CF and PS suggesting that also such cases, usually revealed by NBS and once classified as mild CF, should be monitored as the patients with PI.

Abbreviations

CF: Cystic fibrosis; CFLD: CF liver disease.; CFRD: CF-related diabetes; CFTR: Cystic fibrosis transmembrane conductance regulator; MI: Meconium ileus; PI: Pancreatic insufficiency; PS: Pancreatic sufficiency; SCL: Sweat chloride levels

Acknowledgements

We acknowledge the Società Italiana per lo studio della Fibrosi Cistica (SIFC) that stimulated this multicentric study, and the Ministero della Salute (Rome, Italy) L.548/93 for the regional research funding quote of years 2007-15. We thank Jean Ann Gilder (Scientific Communication srl., Naples, Italy) for editing the text.

Funding

This research did not receive any specific grant from funding agencies in the public, commercial or not-for-profit sectors.

Authors' contributions

V.T. and G.C conceived and designed the study, analyzed and interpreted the data and wrote the manuscript; M.L. and D.S. contributed to data interpretation and manuscript preparation, collected the data and revised the manuscript; RB analyzed statistically data; C.C., AM. DL.,V.L, V.C., C.B., N.C., R.P., R.C., L.T., E.M., M.C., S.Q., M.S., A.B., A.E., A.M.D.L., F.Z., A.A., V.R. collected and analyzed the data and revised the manuscript. All authors read and approved the final manuscript.

Consent for publication

Not applicable.

Competing interests

The authors declare that they have no competing interests.

Author details

[1]Dipartimento di Pediatria, Centro Regionale Toscano per la Fibrosi Cistica, Azienda Ospedaliero-Universitaria Meyer, Viale Gaetano Pieraccini 24, 50139 Florence, Italy. [2]Dipartimento di Biotecnologie Cellulari ed Ematologia, Istituto Pasteur Fondazione Cenci Bolognetti, Sapienza Università e Policlinico Umberto I, Rome, Italy. [3]Centro Regionale Fibrosi Cistica, Centro Pediatrico Bambino Gesù Basilicata, AOR San Carlo, Potenza, Italy. [4]Laboratorio di Genetica Medica, Ospedale Pediatrico Bambino Gesù, Rome, Italy. [5]Centro Regionale Fibrosi Cistica, Fondazione IRCCS Ca' Granda, Ospedale Maggiore Policlinico, Università degli Studi di Milano, Milan, Italy. [6]Freelance Epidemiologist, Bergamo, Italy. [7]Centro Regionale Fibrosi Cistica Adulti, Dipartimento di Scienze Mediche Traslazionali, Università di Napoli Federico II, Naples, Italy. [8]Centro Regionale Fibrosi Cistica, U.O.C. Pneumologia, IRCCS G. Gaslini, Genua, Italy. [9]Dipartimento di Medicina Molecolare e Biotecnologie Mediche, Università di Napoli Federico II, Naples, Italy. [10]CEINGE-Biotecnologie avanzate, Naples, Italy. [11]Centro Regionale Fibrosi Cistica, Dipartimento Materno-Infantile, Ospedali Riuniti Ancona, Ancona, Italy. [12]CRR Fibrosi Cistica, Ospedale dei Bambini, ARNAS Civico, Palermo, Italy. [13]Dipartimento di Neuroscienze, Scienze Riproduttive ed Odontostomatologica, Università di Napoli Federico II, Naples, Italy. [14]Università Telematica Pegaso, Naples, Italy. [15]Unità Regionale di Fibrosi Cistica, IRCCS Ospedale Pediatrico Bambino Gesù, Rome, Italy. [16]Centro Regionale Fibrosi Cistica, Ospedale Giovanni Paolo II, Lamezia, Italy. [17]Centro Regionale di supporto Fibrosi Cistica, Dipartimento di Pediatria, Università di Brescia, AO Spedali Civili, Brescia, Italy. [18]Centro Fibrosi Cistica Regione Lazio, Dipartimento di Pediatria e Neuropsichiatria Infantile, Sapienza Università-Policlinico Umberto I, Rome, Italy. [19]Centro Regionale Fibrosi Cistica, Sezione Pediatrica, Dipartimento di Scienze Mediche Traslazionali, Università di Napoli Federico II, Naples, Italy. [20]Laboratorio di Genetica Medica, Fondazione IRCCS Policlinico Ca' Granda Ospedale, Milan, Italy. [21]Ospedale dei Bambini G. Di Cristina, Centro Regionale Fibrosi Cistica, Palermo, Italy. [22]Dipartimento di Bioscienze e Territorio, Università del Molise, Isernia, Italy.

References

1. Jackson AD, Goss CH. Epidemiology of CF: how registries can be used to advance our understanding of the CF population. J Cyst Fibros. 2017;17: 30970. https://doi.org/10.1016/j.jcf.2017.11.013.
2. Veit G, Avramescu RG, Chiang AN, Houck SA, Cai Z, Peters KW, et al. From CFTR biology toward combinatorial pharmacotherapy: expanded classification of cystic fibrosis mutations. Mol Biol Cell. 2016;27:424–33.
3. Cutting GR. Cystic fibrosis genetics: from molecular understanding to clinical application. Nat Rev Genet. 2015;16:45–56.

4. Koch C, Cuppens H, Rainisio M, Madessani U, Harms H, Hodson M, et al. Investigators of the ERCF: comparison of major disease manifestations between patients with different classes of mutations. Pediatr Pulmonol. 2001;31:1–12.
5. McKone EF, Goss CH, Aitken ML. CFTR genotype as a predictor of prognosis in cystic fibrosis. Chest. 2006;130:1441–7.
6. Mekus F, Ballmann M, Bronsveld I, Bijman J, Veeze H, Tümmler B. Categories of delta F508 homozygous cystic fibrosis twin and sibling pairs with distinct phenotypic characteristics. Twin Res. 2000;3:277–93.
7. Giordano S, Amato F, Elce A, Monti M, Iannone C, Pucci P, et al. Molecular and functional analysis of the large 5' promoter region of CFTR gene revealed pathogenic mutations in CF and CFTR-related disorders. J Mol Diagn. 2013;15:331–40.
8. Amato F, Seia M, Giordano S, Elce A, Zarrilli F, Castaldo G, et al. Gene mutation in MicroRNA target sites of CFTR gene: a novel pathogenetic mechanism in cystic fibrosis? PlosONE. 2013;8:e60448.
9. Lucarelli M, Porcaro L, Biffignandi A, Costantino L, Giannone V, Alberti L, et al. A new targeted CFTR mutation panel based on next generation sequencing technology. J Mol Diagn. 2017;19:788–800.
10. Rossi T, Grandoni F, Mazzilli F, Quattrucci S, Antonelli M, Strom R, et al. High frequency of $(TG)_mT_n$ variant tracts in the cystic fibrosis transmembrane conductance regulator gene in men with high semen viscosity. Fertil Steril. 2004;82:1316–22.
11. Lucarelli M, Bruno SM, Pierandrei S, Ferraguti G, Stamato A, Narzi F, et al. A genotypic-oriented view of CFTR genetics highlights specific mutational patterns underlying clinical macro-categories of cystic fibrosis. Mol Med. 2015;21:257–75.
12. Lucarelli M, Narzi L, Pierandrei S, Bruno SM, Stamato A, d'Avanzo M, et al. A new complex allele of the CFTR gene partially explains the variable phenotype of the L997F mutation. Genet Med. 2010;12:548–55.
13. Terlizzi V, Castaldo G, Salvatore D, Lucarelli M, Raia V, Angioni A, et al. Genotype-phenotype correlation and functional studies in patients with cystic fibrosis bearing CFTR complex alleles. J Med Genet. 2017;54:224–35.
14. Salvatore F, Scudiero O, Castaldo G. Genotype-phenotype correlation in cystic fibrosis: the role of modifier genes. Am J Med Genet. 2002;111:88–95.
15. Blackman SM, Deering-Brose R, McWilliams R, Naughton K, Coleman B, Lai T, et al. Relative contribution of genetic and non-genetic modifiers to intestinal obstruction in cystic fibrosis. Gastroenterology. 2006;131:1030–9.
16. Zielenski J, Markiewicz D, Yuan X, Patel M, Sun L, Aznarez I, et al. Meconium ileus in cystic fibrosis neonates is associated with polymorphic markers in the calcium-activated potassium channel (KCNN4) gene. JPGN. 2004; 39:S405–6.
17. Philp AR, Riquelme TT, Millar-Büchner P, González R, Sepúlveda FV, Pablo Cid L, et al. Kcnn4 is a modifier gene of intestinal cystic fibrosis preventing lethality in the Cftr-F508del mouse. Sci Rep. 2018;8:9320.
18. Blackman SM, Hsu S, Vanscoy LL, Collaco JM, Ritter SE, Naughton K, et al. Genetic modifiers play a substantial role in diabetes complicating cystic fibrosis. J Clin Endocrinol Metab. 2009;94:1302–9.
19. Bartlett JR, Friedman KJ, Ling SC, Pace RG, Bell SC, Bourke B, et al. Genetic modifiers of liver disease in cystic fibrosis. JAMA. 2009;302:1076–83.
20. Corvol H, Blackman SM, Boëlle PY, Gallins PJ, Pace RG, Stonebraker JR, et al. Genome-wide association meta-analysis identifies five modifier loci of lung disease severity in cystic fibrosis. Nat Commun. 2015;6:8382.
21. Collaco JM, Blackman SM, McGready J, Naughton KM, Cutting GR. Quantification of the relative contribution of environmental and genetic factors to variation in cystic fibrosis lung function. J Pediatr. 2010;157:802–7.
22. Green DM, Collaco JM, KE MD, Naughton KM, Blackman SM, Cutting GR. Heritability of respiratory infection with Pseudomonas aeruginosa in cystic fibrosis. J Pediatr. 2012;161:290–5.
23. Eakin MN, Riekert KA. The impact of medication adherence on lung health outcomes in cystic fibrosis. Curr Opin Pulm Med. 2013;19:687–91.
24. Schechter MS. Nongenetic influences on cystic fibrosis outcomes. Curr Opin Pulm Med. 2011;17:448–54.
25. Farrell PM, White TB, Ren CL, Hempstead SE, Accurso F, Derichs N, et al. Diagnosis of cystic fibrosis: consensus guidelines from the Cystic Fibrosis Foundation. J Pediatr. 2017;181S:S4–S15.e1.
26. LeGrys VA, Yankaskas JR, Quittell LM, Marshall BC, Mogayzel PJ Jr. Cystic Fibrosis Foundation. Diagnostic sweat testing: the Cystic Fibrosis Foundation guidelines. J Pediatr. 2007;151:85–9.
27. Tomaiuolo R, Sangiuolo F, Bombieri C, Bonizzato A, Cardillo G, Raia V, et al. Epidemiology and a novel procedure for large scale analysis of CFTR rearrangements in classic and atypical CF patients: a multicentric Italian study. J Cyst Fibros. 2008;7:347–51.
28. Lucarelli M, Narzi L, Piergentili R, Ferraguti G, Grandoni F, Quattrucci S, et al. A 96-well formatted method for exon and exon/intron boundary full sequencing of the CFTR gene. Anal Biochem. 2006;353:226–35.
29. Ferraguti G, Pierandrei S, Bruno SM, Ceci F, Strom R, Lucarelli M. A template for mutational data analysis of the CFTR gene. Clin Chem Lab Med. 2011;49:1447–51.
30. Dequeker E, Stuhrmann M, Morris MA, Casals T, Castellani C, Claustres M, et al. Best practice guidelines for molecular genetic diagnosis of cystic fibrosis and CFTR-related disorders: updated European recommendations. Eur J Hum Genet. 2009;17:51–65.
31. Elce A, Boccia A, Cardillo G, Giordano S, Tomaiuolo R, Paolella G, et al. Three novel CFTR polymorphic repeats improve segregation analysis for cystic fibrosis. Clin Chem. 2009;55:1372–9.
32. Quanjer PH, Stanojevic S, Cole TJ, Baur X, Hall GL, Culver BH, et al. ERS global lung function initiative. Multi-ethnic reference values for spirometry for the 3–95 year age range: the global lung function 2012 equations. Eur Respir J. 2012;40:1324–43.
33. Schluchter MD, Konstan MW, Drumm ML, Yankaskas JR, Knowles MR. Classifying severity of cystic fibrosis lung disease using longitudinal pulmonary function data. Am J Respir Crit Care Med. 2006;174:780–6.
34. Wang X, Dockery DW, WypiJ D, Fay ME, Ferris BG. Pulmonary function between 6 and 18 years of age. Pediatr Pulmunol. 1993;15:75–88.
35. Konstan MW, Wagener JS, Van Devanter DR. Characterizing aggressiveness and predicting future progression of CF lung disease. J Cyst Fibros. 2009; 8(Suppl 1):S15–9.
36. Lee TW, Brownlee KG, Conway SP, Denton M, Littlewood JM. Evaluation of a new definition for chronic Pseudomonas aeruginosa infection in cystic fibrosis patients. J Cyst Fibros. 2003;2:29–34.
37. Morinville VD, Husain SZ, Bai H, Barth B, Alhosh R, Durie PR, et al. Definitions of pediatric pancreatitis and survey of present clinical practices. J Pediatr Gastroenterol Nutr. 2012;55:261–5.
38. Debray D, Kelly D, Houwen R, Strandvik B, Colombo C. Best practice guidance for the diagnosis and management of cystic fibrosis-associated liver disease. J Cyst Fibros. 2011;10:S29–36.
39. Kelly A, Moran A. Update on cystic fibrosis-related diabetes. J Cyst Fibros. 2013;12:318–31.
40. Castellani C, Cuppens H, Macek M, Cassiman JJ, Kerem E, Durie P, et al. Consensus on the use and interpretation of cystic fibrosis mutation analysis in clinical practice. J Cyst Fibros. 2008;7:179–96.
41. Terlizzi V, Carnovale V, Castaldo G, Castellani C, Cirilli N, Colombo C, et al. Clinical expression of patients with the D1152H CFTR mutation. J Cyst Fibrosis. 2015;14:447–52.
42. Castellani C, Assael BM. Cystic fibrosis: a clinical view. Cell Mol Life Sci. 2017; 74:129–40.
43. Walkowiak J, Lisowska A, Blaszczynski M. The changing face of the exocrine pancreas in cystic fibrosis: pancreatic sufficiency, pancreatitis and genotype. Eur J Gastroenterol Hepatol. 2008;20:157–60.
44. Terlizzi V, Tosco A, Tomaiuolo R, Sepe A, Amato N, Casale A, et al. Prediction of acute pancreatitis risk based on PIP score in children with cystic fibrosis. J Cyst Fibros. 2014;13:579–84.
45. Tomaiuolo AC, Sofia VM, Surace C, Majo F, Genovese S, Petrocchi S, et al. Relationship between CFTR and CTRC variants and the clinical phenotype in late-onset cystic fibrosis disease with chronic pancreatitis. J Mol Diagn. 2015; 17:171–8.
46. Sofia VM, Da Sacco L, Surace C, Tomaiuolo AC, Genovese S, Grotta S, et al. Extensive molecular analysis suggested the strong genetic heterogeneity of idiopathic chronic pancreatitis. Mol Med. 2016;26:22.
47. Norkina O, De Lisle RC. Potential genetic modifiers of the cystic fibrosis intestinal inflammatory phenotype on mouse chromosomes 1, 9, and 10. BMC Genet. 2005;6:29.
48. Dorfman R, Li W, Sun L, Wang Y, Sandford A, Paré PD, et al. Modifier gene study of meconium ileus in cystic fibrosis: statistical considerations and gene mapping results. Hum Genet. 2009;126:763–78.
49. Vanscoy LL, Balckman SM, Collaco JM, et al. Heriability of lung disease severity in cystic fibrosis. Am J Respir Crit Care Med. 2007;175:1036–43.

50. Kerem E, Viviani L, Zolin A, MacNeill S, Hatziagorou E, Ellemunter H, et al. Factors associated with FEV1 decline in cystic fibrosis: analysis of the ECFS patient registry. Eur Respir J. 2014;43:125–13.
51. Mott LS, Graniel KG, Park J, de Klerk NH, Sly PD, Murray CP, et al. Assessment of early bronchiectasis in young children with cystic fibrosis is dependent on lung volume. Chest. 2013;144:1193–8.
52. Sly PD, Brennan S, Gangell C, de Klerk N, Murray C, Mott L, et al. Lung disease at diagnosis in infants with cystic fibrosis detected by newborn screening. Am J Respir Crit Care Med. 2009;180:146–52.
53. Blackman SM, Commander CW, Watson C, et al. Genetic modifiers of cystic fibrosis-related diabetes. Diabetes. 2013;62:3627–35.
54. Picard E, Aviram M, Yahav Y, Rivlin J, Blau H, Bentur L, et al. Familial concordance of phenotype and microbial variation among siblings with CF. Ped Pulmunol. 2004;38:292–7.
55. Minicucci L, Lorini R, Giannattasio A, Colombo C, Iapichino L, Reali MF, et al. Liver disease as risk factor for cystic fibrosis-related diabetes development. Acta Pediatr. 2007;96:736–9.
56. Terliesner N, Vogel M, Steighardt A, Gausche R, Henn C, Hentschel J, et al. Cystic-fibrosis related-diabetes (CFRD) is preceded by and associated with growth failure and deteriorating lung function. J Pediatr Endocrinol Metab. 2017;30:815–21.
57. Hunt WR, Helfman BR, McCarty NA, Hansen JM. Advanced glycation end products are elevated in cystic fibrosis-related diabetes and correlate with worse lung function. J Cyst Fibros. 2016;15:681–8.
58. Baldan A, Lo Presti AR, Belpinati F, Castellani C, Bettin MD, Xumerle L, et al. IFRD1 gene polymorphisms are associated with nasal polyposis in cystic fibrosis patients. Rhinology. 2015;53:359–64.

24

Endothelial cells from pulmonary endarterectomy specimens possess a high angiogenic potential and express high levels of hepatocyte growth factor

Akira Naito[1,2†], Seiichiro Sakao[1*†], Irene M. Lang[3], Norbert F. Voelkel[4], Takayuki Jujo[1,5], Keiichi Ishida[6], Toshihiko Sugiura[1], Goro Matsumiya[6], Ichiro Yoshino[7], Nobuhiro Tanabe[1] and Koichiro Tatsumi[1]

Abstract

Background: Impaired angiogenesis is assumed to be an important factor in the development of chronic thromboembolic pulmonary hypertension (CTEPH). However, the role of endothelial cells (ECs) in CTEPH remains unclear. The aim of this study was to investigate the angiogenic potential of ECs from pulmonary endarterectomy (PEA) specimens.

Methods: We isolated ECs from PEA specimens (CTEPH-ECs) and control EC lines from the intact pulmonary arteries of patients with peripheral lung cancers, using a MACS system. These cells were analyzed in vitro including PCR-array analysis, and the PEA specimens were analyzed with immunohistochemistry. Additionally, the serum HGF levels were determined in CTEPH patients.

Results: A three-dimensional culture assay revealed that CTEPH-ECs were highly angiogenic. An angiogenesis-focused gene PCR array revealed a high expression of hepatocyte growth factor (HGF) in CTEPH-ECs. The high expression of HGF was also confirmed in the supernatant extracted from PEA specimens. The immunohistochemical analysis showed expression of HGF on the surface of the thrombus vessels. The serum HGF levels in CTEPH patients were higher than those in pulmonary thromboembolism survivors.

Conclusion: Our study suggests that there are ECs with pro-angiogenetic character and high expression of HGF in PEA specimens. It remains unknown how these results are attributable to the etiology. However, further investigation focused on the HGF pathway may provide novel diagnostic and therapeutic tools for patients with CTEPH.

Keywords: Chronic thromboembolic pulmonary hypertension, Pulmonary endarterectomy, Endothelial cell, Hepatocyte growth factor, Angiogenesis

Background

Chronic thromboembolic pulmonary hypertension (CTEPH) is a form of pulmonary hypertension that is related to unresolved organizing clots and it is generally acknowledged that pulmonary endarterectomy (PEA) is the gold standard for CTEPH treatment. Various etiological factors, including infection, inflammation, genetic susceptibilities, and insufficient angiogenesis [1], have been discussed as important pathogenetic factors [2]. Poor angiogenesis detected in PEA tissue specimens also implies a poor prognosis in CTEPH patients [3]. In addition, disordered angiogenesis which leads to the delayed resolution of thrombus may be a potential etiological factor underlying the development of CTEPH [4]. However, it remains to be elucidated whether endothelial cells (ECs) are involved in the pathogenesis of this disease because of the limited number of investigations that have been reported.

* Correspondence: sakaos@faculty.chiba-u.jp
†Akira Naito and Seiichiro Sakao contributed equally to this work.
[1]Department of Respirology, Graduate School of Medicine, Chiba University, 1-8-1 Inohana, Chuo-Ku, Chiba City 260-8670, Japan
Full list of author information is available at the end of the article

Hepatocyte growth factor (HGF) and its receptor Mesenchymal-epithelial transition factor (Met), which was originally found to be a potent mitogen that promotes hepatocyte growth and liver regeneration [5, 6], are now proposed to have prominent roles in the cardiovascular diseases. It is reported that HGF has pleiotropic functions, including proliferation, angiogenesis, anti-apoptosis, anti-autophagy, anti-inflammation and anti-fibrosis in the vascular ECs, myocardial cells, and other types of cells [7], however, the precise role of HGF- Met signaling in the etiology of CTEPH remains unknown.

Here we wish to elucidate the angiogenesis-related characteristics of ECs harvested from PEA specimens from a viewpoint of HGF.

Methods

Study population

CTEPH patients who underwent PEA from June 2014 to October 2015 were enrolled. PEA specimens were obtained from CTEPH patients during PEA performed by Dr. Ishida at Chiba University Hospital. The process by which CTEPH was diagnosed has been described previously [8]. During the same period, pulmonary arteries were obtained at Chiba University Hospital from lung lobectomy specimens of patients with stage I peripheral lung cancer. The diagnosis of stage I lung cancer was confirmed by chest enhanced computed tomography, brain magnetic resonance imaging and histological examination of the lung tissue. No patients received chemotherapy or radiotherapy prior to surgery, and patients with evident chronic obstructive pulmonary disease or pulmonary fibrosis were excluded from the study.

Tissue collection

At the time of PEA, pieces of PEA specimens contained in the segmental pulmonary arteries were collected. Segmental pulmonary artery samples of approximately 1.5 cm in length were collected from lung lobectomy specimens; these arteries were located far from the primary tumor and did not show macroscopic or microscopic malignant cell invasion. These arteries were collected for primary cell culture and histopathological examination in the same manner as PEA specimens.

Isolation of CTEPH-ECs and control-ECs

The PEA specimens and pulmonary arteries from lung lobectomy specimens were washed in sterile phosphate buffered saline (PBS), minced, and incubated in Dulbecco's Modified Eagle Medium (DMEM) with 1% bovine serum albumin, 0.2% collagenase (Wako, Tokyo, Japan), 10 mg/ml DNaseI (Wako, Tokyo, Japan), 250 mg/ml dispase (Roche, Tokyo, Japan) for 1 h. The obtained cell suspensions were seeded into a 6-cm-petri dish coated with fibronectin (Corning, Corning, NY, USA) and incubated in an endothelial growth medium™-2 microvascular BulletKit™ (EGM; Lonza, Basel, Switzerland) until they reached approximately 80% confluence (7–10 days) at 37 °C in 5% CO_2 in an humidified air incubator. At the first passage, CD 31-positive ECs were isolated using CD31 MicroBeads (Miltenyi Biotec, Tokyo, Japan), as described previously [9]. The cells were incubated in EGM, and all of the experiments were carried out using cells that had been passaged less than 6 times.

Immunocytochemistry

The cells were fixed in 4% paraformaldehyde for 10 min followed by blocking with PBS-T (PBS with Tween-20, 0.1%) containing 2% normal goat serum for 30 min, and incubated with a primary antibody overnight at 4 °C and with a secondary antibody for 1 h at room temperature. The stained cells were washed with 4 μg/ml DAPI in PBS for 5 min, embedded in 50% glycerin and examined with a Fluoview FV10i-LIV (Olympus, Tokyo, Japan).

The cell growth curve, permeability assay and three-dimensional culture

To assess the proliferative potential, 5×10^4 ECs were seeded in a 6-cm Petri dish. At each indicated day, the cells were trypsinized and counted. We also evaluated the permeability of each EC cell line with CultreCoat® In Vitro Vascular Permeability Assay (Trevigen, Inc. MD, USA) according to the manufacturer's instructions. Matrigel™ Basement Membrane Matrix (Corning, Corning, NY, USA) was used for the three-dimensional culture in accordance with the manufacturer's instructions. Additional details have been described previously [10]. The total tube lengths in the microscopic fields (taken a Nikon ECLIPSE Ti-S, Tokyo, Japan; capture magnification, ×40) were calculated using the Image J software program (ver. 1.48, National Institutes of Health, Bethesda, MD; http://imagej.nih.gov/ij/).

Total RNA isolation from ECs and the PCR-based angiogenesis-related gene analysis

Total RNA was extracted from CTEPH-ECs and Control-ECs with RNeasy Mini Kit (Qiagen, Tokyo, Japan) according to the manufacturer's instruction. RT2-Profiler™ PCR Arrays (Qiagen, Tokyo, Japan) were used to analyze the expression of a focused panel of genes involved in various biological processes. The Human Angiogenesis (PAHS-024Z) 96-well plate, which profiles the expression of 84 key genes that are involved in angiogenesis, was selected to detect the differential expression of genes between CTEPH-ECs and Control-ECs. The detailed method has been described previously [9].

HGF inhibition in proliferating CTEPH-ECs and three-dimensional culture

To investigate the effects of HGF inhibition in cultured CTEPH-ECs, we used tivantinib, a selective HGF/MET inhibitor (Selleck, Houston, TX, USA) [11]. Similarly to the studies that examine the cell growth curve and the three-dimensional culture experiments that are detailed above, 5×10^4 CTEPH-ECs were seeded in a 6-cm Petri dish with EGM containing 1 μM tivantinib or 0.1% DMSO (vehicle). At each indicated day, the cells were trypsinized and counted. Furthermore, 5×10^4 of CTEPH-ECs were seeded on Matrigel™ Basement Membrane Matrix with EGM containing 1 μM tivantinib or 0.1% DMSO (vehicle) and incubated at 37 °C for 24 h, as described above.

Total RNA isolation from PEA specimens and control pulmonary arteries and the PCR-based angiogenesis-related gene analysis

Total RNA was extracted from PEA specimens and control pulmonary arteries with RNeasy Fibrous Tissue Mini Kit (Qiagen, Tokyo, Japan) according to the manufacturer's instruction. RT^2 qPCR Primer Assays (Qiagen, Tokyo, Japan) were used to analyze the expression of HGF and other inflammatory molecules.

Protein extraction from PEA specimens and Western blotting

The extraction and quantification of the protein from tissues (PEA specimens and pulmonary arteries) [12] have been described previously. Protein samples (10 μg) were separated on NuPAGE® Novex 10% Bis-Tris Gel (Invitrogen, Tokyo, Japan) and transferred to nitrocellulose membranes (Invitrogen, Tokyo, Japan). Membranes were blocked with 5% non-fat dried milk in PBS containing 0.5% Tween20 for 1 h at room temperature, and were then incubated with primary antibodies overnight at 4 °C. The membranes were incubated with peroxidase-conjugated secondary antibodies for 1 h at room temperature. Chemiluminescence was detected using a LAS-4000 (Fuji Film, Tokyo, Japan). The blots were scanned and a densitometry analysis was conducted using the Image J software program.

Immunohistochemistry

Samples were fixed in 10% buffered formalin, paraffinized and cut into 3 μm-thick slices. Deparaffinized sections were washed with PBS and blocked with PBS-T containing 2% normal goat serum for 30 min at room temperature. They were then incubated with the primary antibodies overnight at 4 °C and with secondary antibodies for 1 h at room temperature. Stained slices were washed with 4 μg/ml DAPI in PBS for 5 min, embedded in 50% glycerin and examined with a Fluoview FV10i-LIV.

Reagents

The following antibodies (Abs) were used in immunocytometry and immunohistochemistry: rabbit anti-von Willebrand factor (Factor VIII) (1:200, DAKO, Carpinterria, CA, USA), mouse anti-CD31 Ab (1:200, Abcam, Tokyo, Japan), mouse anti-Vimentin (1:200, Dako, CA, USA), mouse anti-Desmin (1:100, DAKO, Carpinterria, CA, USA), rabbit anti-hepatocyte growth factor (HGF) Ab (1:200, Abcam, Tokyo, Japan), rabbit anti-Met Ab (1:200, Abcam, Tokyo, Japan), normal Rabbit IgG isotype control (1:200, R&D Systems, Minneapolis, MN, USA), goat anti-rabbit IgG conjugated with Alexa-488 fluorescent dye (1:200, Thermofisher Scientific, Tokyo, Japan) and goat anti-mouse IgG conjugated with Alexa-594 fluorescent dye (1:200, Thermofisher Scientific, Tokyo, Japan). These antibodies were dissolved in PBS-T.

The following Abs were used in Western blotting: rabbit anti-βactin (1:1000, Biolegend, Tokyo, Japan), rabbit anti-HGF (1:1000, Abcam, Tokyo, Japan) and Goat anti-Rabbit IgG HRP conjugate (1:1000, Thermoscientific, Tokyo, Japan). These antibodies were dissolved with blocking solution (5% non-fat dried milk in PBS containing 0.5% Tween20).

Blood samples

Blood serum samples were collected from CTEPH patients at the time of their diagnostic right heart catheterization from August 2013 to June 2017. Control serum samples were obtained from pulmonary thromboembolism (PTE) survivors without evidence of pulmonary hypertension during a routine medical consultation more than 3 months after the acute PTE episode. The serum level of HGF was measured by enzyme immunoassay method (LSI Medience Inc.; Tokyo, Japan).

Statistical analysis

The PCR-array data were analyzed by the RT^2 profiler PCR array Data Analysis web-based software program (https://www.qiagen.com/jp/shop/genes-and-pathways/data-analysis-center-overview-page/), and the fold regulations are expressed as the mean and the 95% confidence interval. Other statistical analyses were performed with commercially available software (GraphPad Prism, version 6.0.2, San Diego, CA) and the results are expressed as mean ± standard deviation (SD) unless otherwise described. Serum HGF levels were analyzed using Welch's t-test and paired t-test. Other statistical analyses were compared using Mann-Whitney test. *P* values of < 0.05 were considered to indicate statistically significant differences.

Results

Cell culture and characterization of EC

Endothelial cells from five CTEPH patients and three lung cancer patients were isolated (We were unable to purify ECs from the other specimens because of contamination by fibroblast-like cells). Immunocytochemistry revealed that the CTEPH-ECs and control-ECs were positive for CD31, Factor VIII, vimentin and negative for desmin (Fig. 1).

The high proliferative and angiogenic potential of CTEPH-ECs

Each CTEPH-EC line showed a greater degree of proliferation than the control-ECs in the cell growth curve analysis (day 9; $p = 0.035$) (Fig. 2a) and CTEPH-ECs had lower permeability compared to Control-ECs ($p = 0.035$) (Fig. 2b). In the three-dimensional culture experiments, the CTEPH-ECs showed a greater degree of tube formation (Fig. 2c), and the total tube lengths were statistically longer in comparison to the control-ECs ($p = 0.035$) (Fig. 2d).

The high expression of HGF in CTEPH-ECs

The PCR array revealed that the RNA expression of HGF in CTEPH-ECs was higher than that in the control-ECs (Fold regulation 22.60, $p = 0.016$) (Fig. 3). Entire data of the PCR array is presented in Additional file 1. In response to this result, we also evaluated the mRNA expression of c-MET, RhoA, STAT3, ROCK1, ROCK2, COX-2 by qPCR analysis. CTEPH-ECs had slight increased expression of these molecules although there was no statistical difference (data not shown).

Inhibition of HGF and Met *in vitro*

The addition of 1 μmol/L of tivantinib to the medium significantly suppressed the cellular proliferation (day 7, $p = 0.0079$) (Fig. 4a) and also appeared to suppress the tube formation of CTEPH-ECs (Fig. 4b).

In vivo expression of HGF and Met

Immunohistochemical analysis of PEA specimens revealed that HGF and its receptor Met were expressed on the surface of thrombus vessels (Fig. 5a), while the internal lumens of the control pulmonary arteries were rarely positive for HGF and Met (Fig. 5b). The mRNA expression of HGF was higher in the PEA specimens, however, there were not significant mRNA upregulations of IL-1β, IL-6, TNF-αin PEA specimens (Fig. 6a). The HGF expression in extracted proteins from PEA specimens was also higher than that from the control pulmonary arteries (Fig. 6b, c).

The serum HGF level

Serum samples were collected from 61 additional CTEPH patients (include the patients who donated tissues) and 12 PTE survivors without evidence of pulmonary hypertension. The characteristics of these patients are listed in Table 1. The HGF serum level in the CTEPH group was higher than that in the control group (0.43 ± 0.44, vs 0.25 ± 0.04, $p = 0.003$) (Fig. 7a). In the

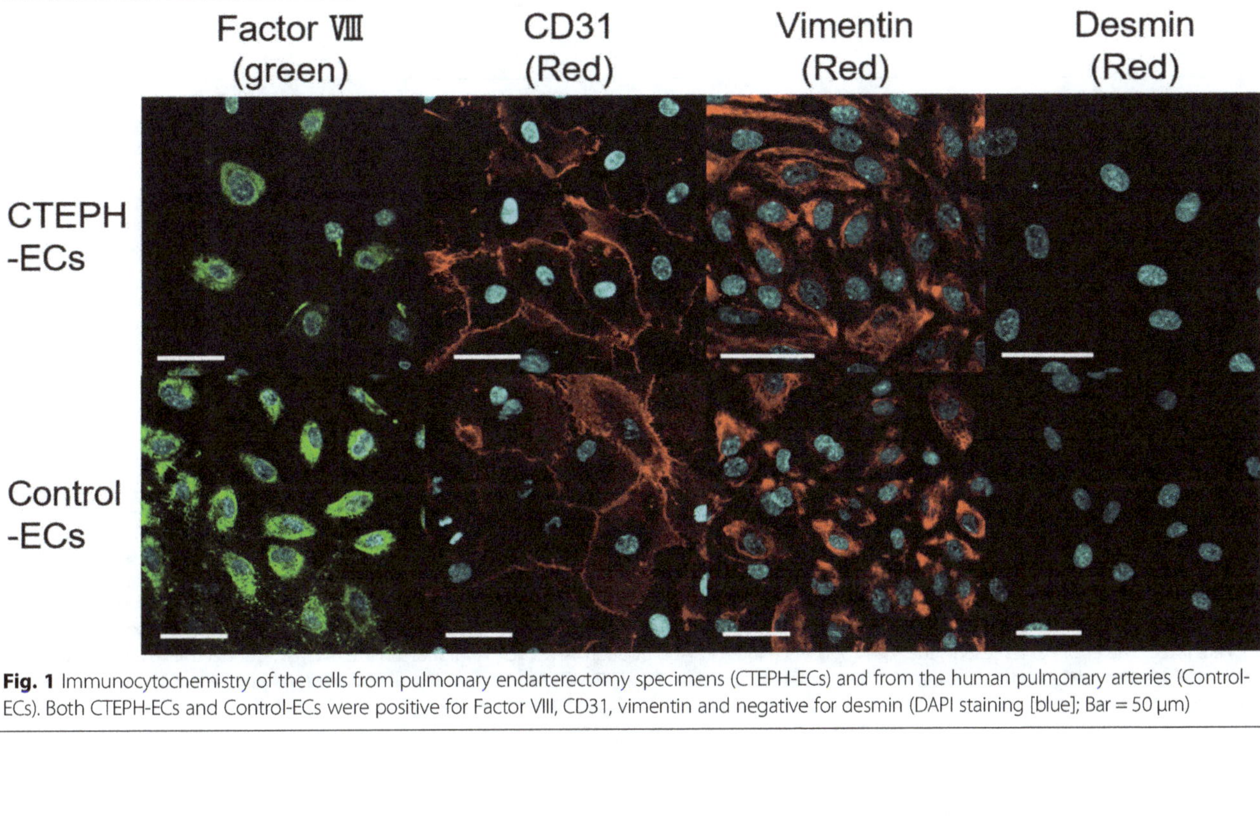

Fig. 1 Immunocytochemistry of the cells from pulmonary endarterectomy specimens (CTEPH-ECs) and from the human pulmonary arteries (Control-ECs). Both CTEPH-ECs and Control-ECs were positive for Factor VIII, CD31, vimentin and negative for desmin (DAPI staining [blue]; Bar = 50 μm)

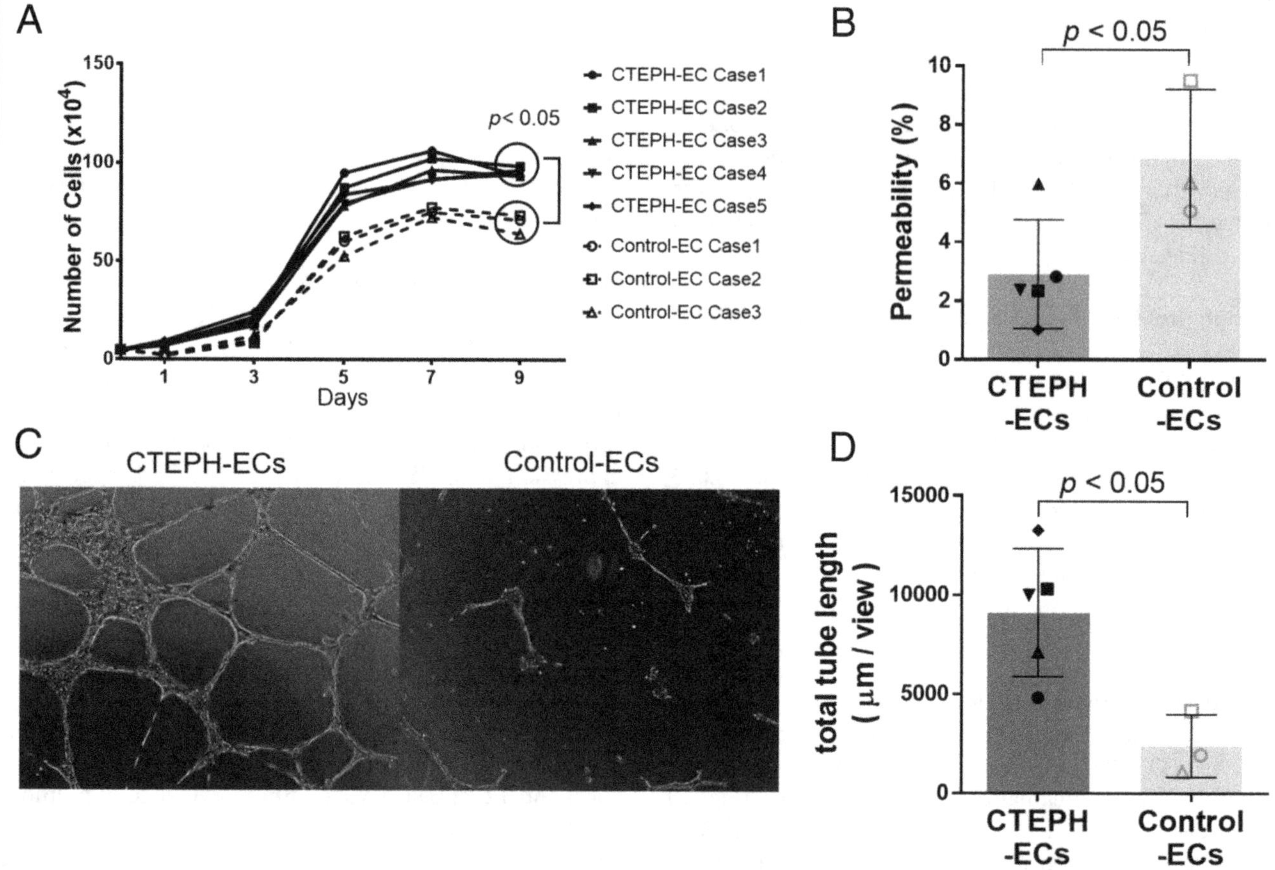

Fig. 2 The proliferation and angiogenic potential of CTEPH-ECs. **a** The cell growth curve showed the greater proliferative potential of CTEPH-ECs. **b** Permeability assay of each cell line. The value is expressed as a percentage to the well without cells (100% permeability). **c, d** Three-dimensional culture showed that CTEPH-ECs made much more tubes than Control-ECs

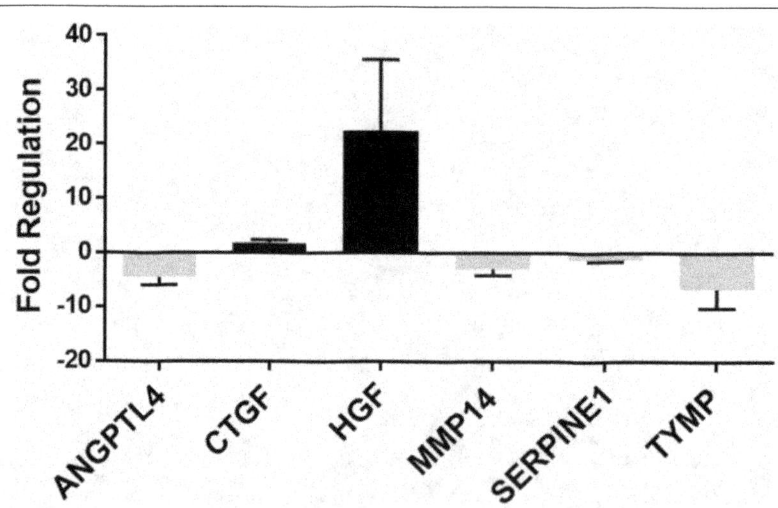

Fig. 3 PCR-Array analysis of CTEPH-ECs and Control-ECs. The fold regulation of the mRNA expression of CTEPH-ECs in comparison to Control-ECs from the angiogenesis PCR array (Qiagen, Human Angiogenesis [PAHS-024Z]). The genes that showed significantly increased or decreased expression ($p < 0.05$) are listed. The error bar represents the 95% confidence interval. Abbreviation: ANGPTL4; Angiopoietin-like 4, CTGF; Connective tissue growth factor, HGF; Hepatocyte growth factor, MMP14; Matrix metallopeptidase 14, SERPINE1; Serpin peptidase inhibitor 1 (plasminogen activator inhibitor-1), TYMP; Thymidine phosphorylase

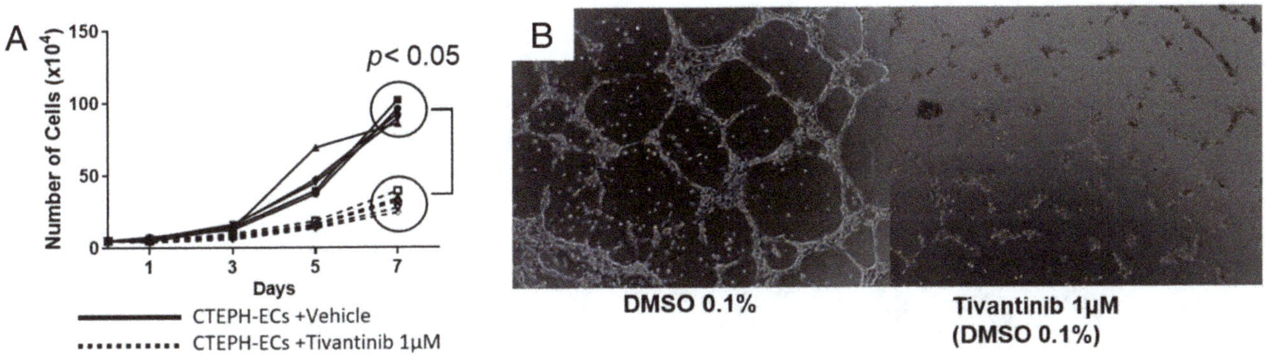

Fig. 4 The assessment of the HGF/Met signal inhibition in CTEPH-ECs. **a** Cell culture in a 6-mm fibronectin-coated Petri dish, **b** Three dimensional culture. A selective HGF/Met inhibitor, tivantinib, suppressed cellular proliferation, and clearly inhibited tube formation

CTEPH group, there was no correlation between the serum HGF level and the hemodynamic parameters (pulmonary artery pressure/resistance, the cardiac output, the oxygen level, and the plasma brain natriuretic peptide level) (data not shown). HGF levels 1 year after PEA was also determined in those 23 patients. There was slight decrease of serum HGF level (Pre PEA HGF; 0.44 ± 0.34 ng/ml, Post PEA HGF; 0.31 ± 0.28 ng/ml, $p =$ 0.013) after PEA (Fig. 7b), while remarkable decrease of PVR (Pre PVR; 782.2 ± 254.0 dyne.sec.cm^{-5}, Post PVR; 317.4 ± 132.0 dyne.sec.cm^{-5}, $p <$ 0.0001). The difference between pre and post serum HGF level did not correlate with the improvement degree of PVR. (Fig. 7c).

Additionally, plasma levels of representative inflammatory and angiogenic molecules, which were associated with HGF (IL-1β, TNF-α, VEGF-A, AngiotensinII), were measured in 26 CTEPH patients and 12 PTE survivors from the above patients. However, there was no significant difference in plasma levels of these molecule between the two groups (Additional file 2).

Discussion

Here we showed that CTEPH-ECs had a greater proliferative and angiogenic potential than control-ECs (Fig. 2a, c-d). We also showed that the expression levels of HGF were higher in CTEPH-ECs (Fig. 3), and that the inhibition

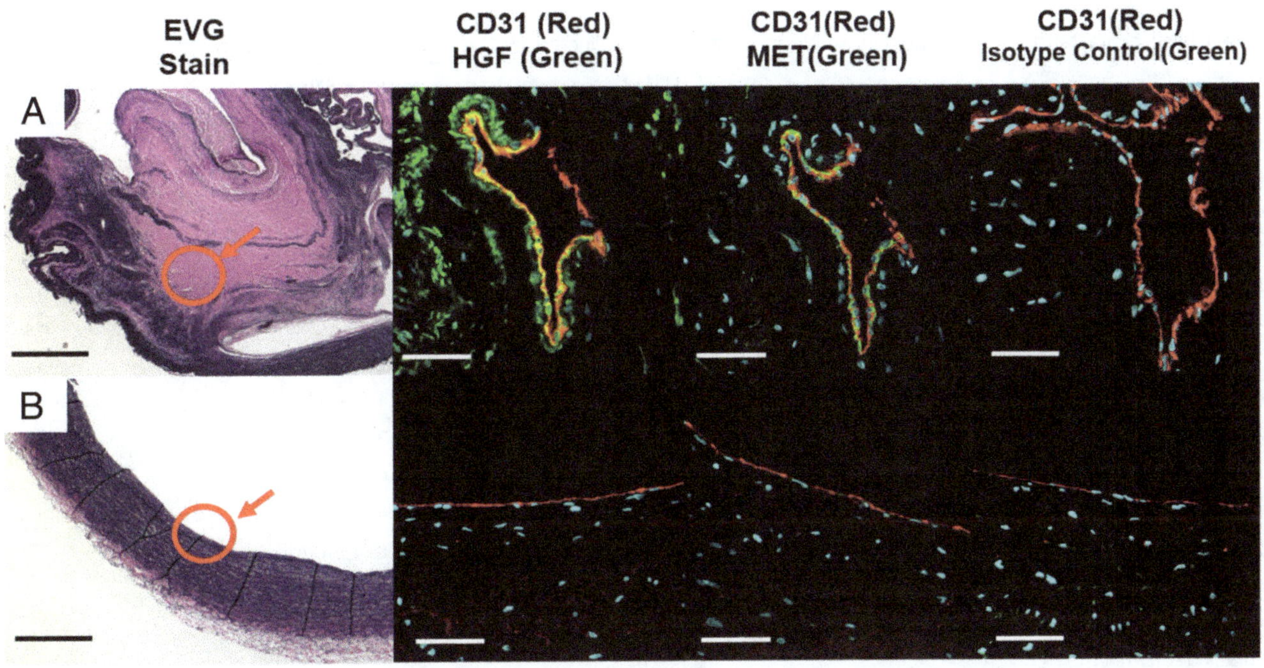

Fig. 5 The immunohistochemical analysis of (**a**) thrombus vessels in pulmonary endarterectomy specimens and (**b**) control pulmonary arteries. The internal lumen of the thrombus vessels of the pulmonary endarterectomy specimens were positive for HGF and Met. Black Bar = 500 μm, White Bar = 50 μm

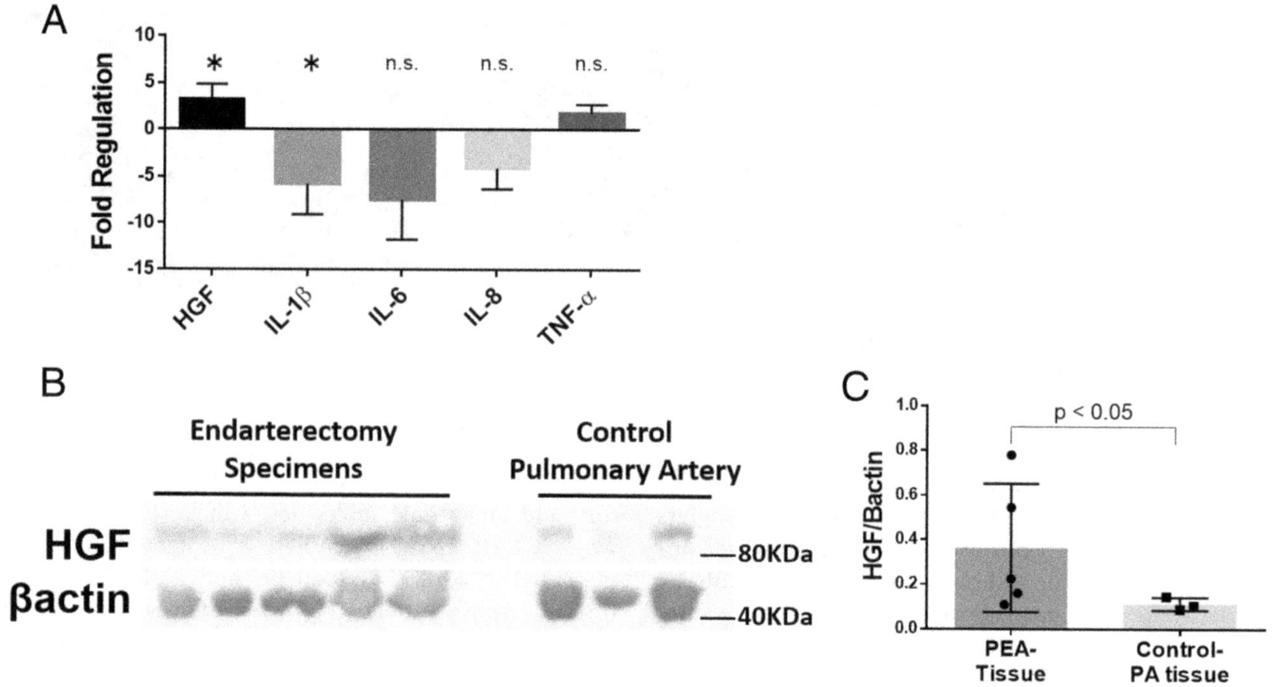

Fig. 6 **a** PCR-Array analysis compairing the mRNA expression of HGF and inflammatory cytokines between pulmonary endarterectomy tissues and control pulmonary arteries. *: $p < 0.05$. The error bar represents the 95% confidence interval. Abbreviation: HGF; Hepatocyte Growth Factor, IL-1β; Interleukin-1β, IL-6; Interleukin-6, IL-8; Interleukin-8, TNF-α; Tumor Necrosis Factor-α. **b** The Western blotting of proteins extracted from pulmonary endarterectomy specimens and control pulmonary arteries. **c** The band signal strength of HGF is expressed as the ratio to beta-actin. The error bar represents the standard deviation. The expression of HGF protein from the pulmonary endarterectomy specimens was higher than that from the control pulmonary arteries

Table 1 Basic characteristics of patients whose blood sample were collected for the analysis of serum HGF in Fig. 7a

	CTEPH group	PTE survivors (Control group)	*p* value
Number of patients	61	12	
Age (y)	62.1 ± 10.6	71.0 ± 12.4	< 0.01
Sex (M:F)	14:47	0:12	n.s.
Systolic blood pressure (mmHg)	121.9 ± 21.5	135.4 ± 10.8	< 0.05
Diastolic blood pressure (mmHg)	73.9 ± 14.3	71.2 ± 10.0	n.s.
Total cholesterol (mg/dl)	192.6 ± 33.8	197.5 ± 24.9	n.s.
ALT (U/l)	25.9 ± 10.2	24.5 ± 6.1	n.s
AST (U/l)	20.5 ± 11.7	19.9 ± 6.93	n.s.
γ-GTP (U/l)	48.6 ± 49.9	39.5 ± 49.8	n.s.
C-Reactive Protein (mg/dl)	0.18 ± 0.33	0.11 ± 0.16	n.s.
BNP (pg/ml)	147.2 ± 264.5	40.1 ± 34.4	n.s.
Disease duration (month)[a]	32.1 ± 36.6	89.4 ± 42.6	< 0.01
Mean Pulmonary artery pressure (mmHg)	41.8 ± 10.3	–	–
Pulmonary artery resistance (dyne.sec.cm^{-5})	661.6 ± 287.7	–	–
Cardiac Index (L/min/m^2)	2.74 ± 0.68	–	–
NYHA(I:II:III:IV)	0:42:18:1	–	–

Data are presented as either mean ± SD or actual value
[a]Time from the onset of symptom to the blood sampling

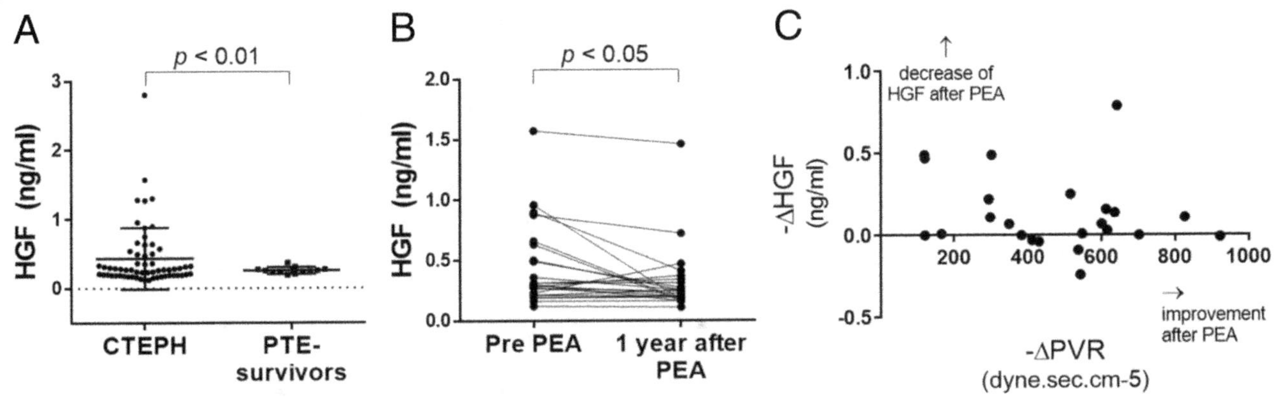

Fig. 7 The serum levels of HGF in chronic thromboembolic pulmonary hypertension (CTEPH) patients' ($n = 61$) and pulmonary thromboembolism (PTE) survivors without evidence of pulmonary hypertension (control group, $n = 12$). **a** The HGF serum level in the CTEPH group was higher than that in the control group (0.43 ± 0.25 ng/ml, 0.25 ± 0.04 ng/ml, respectively, $p = 0.003$). **b** HGF levels 1 year after PEA was also determined in those 23 patients. There was slight decrease of serum HGF level after PEA. **c** The difference between pre and post serum HGF level did not correlate with the improvement degree of PVR

of HGF action suppressed the proliferation and angiogenesis of CTEPH-EC (Fig. 4). Each cell line's permeability was less in CTEPH-ECs than in Control-ECs, which also suggests the higher HGF activity [13] in CTEPH-ECs in vitro (Fig. 2c). In vivo experiments and immunohistochemical staining demonstrated the expression of HGF in the thrombus vessel lumens of PEA specimens (Fig. 5), while RT-PCR and western blotting demonstrated that the expression of HGF was higher in PEA specimens than in the control pulmonary arteries (Fig. 6). We also demonstrated the expression of Met (HGF receptor) on the surface of thrombus vessels. In the clinical setting, we showed that CTEPH patients had higher concentrations of serum HGF in comparison to PTE survivors without evidence of pulmonary hypertension (Fig. 7), although there were no correlation between serum HGF concentration and EC phenotype in vitro described in Figs. 2, 3. Our results showed that there were ECs with high angiogenic potential, which was driven at least in part by increased activity of the autocrine, paracrine and endocrine HGF-Met signaling pathway in the thrombus vessels of the PEA specimens (Fig. 8).

There are several basic reports about the impairment of angiogenesis in CTEPH patients. Alias et al. reported that vascular endothelial growth factor receptor-2 (KDR) had an important role in the resolution of venous thrombi, and that the mRNA expression of KDR in white thrombi was reduced in comparison to that in the non-thrombosed pulmonary arteries [4]. Zabini et al. reported that homogenized PEA specimen contained several cytokines that inhibited angiogenesis [14]. On the other hand, Belik et al. reported that the plasma microparticles of CTEPH patients facilitated angiogenesis in human pulmonary artery ECs [15]. These data suggested that deficient angiogenesis in organized thrombi might be associated with an imbalance between anti-angiogenic factors (the decreased mRNA expression of angiogenetic factor-like KDR and local anti-angiogenic cytokines) and pro-angiogenic factors (plasma microparticles). Our result that ECs in PEA specimen possessed high angiogenic potential may reflect the involvement of pro-angiogenic factors.

VEGF gene therapy has previously been reported to enhance venous thrombus recanalization and resolution [16, 17], and the endothelial cell-specific deletion of KDR abated the formation of vessel thrombosis and inhibited the resolution of thrombosis [4]. In the clinical setting, the findings of low levels of angiogenesis [3] and a small number of recanalized vessels [18] in PEA specimen predicts a poor prognosis in CTEPH patients. Complementing the above reports, the high angiogenic potential associated with HGF described here in the CTEPH-ECs may point towards a positive role in the resolution of thrombosis. In addition, numerous preclinical studies have recently examined the use of HGF as a pro-angiogenic and cardio-protective agent in the treatment of myocardial infarction, heart failure, and limb ischemia [7]. Together with our results, the targeted proper induction of HGF or HGF mimetics, which may lead to angiogenesis, may have a positive role in the treatment of obstructive and/or stenotic pulmonary vascular lesions in CTEPH patients.

Our pathobiological investigations also demonstrated that the internal surface of PEA specimen was rarely positive for CD31 (Additional file 3). This may suggest that most parts of the endothelial cell layers of the neointima were damaged before the PEA procedure. Furthermore, it suggests that the isolated CTEPH-ECs might have been derived from the microvascular ECs within the thrombus vessels, which may differ from the ECs on the internal surface of thrombus. If so, the

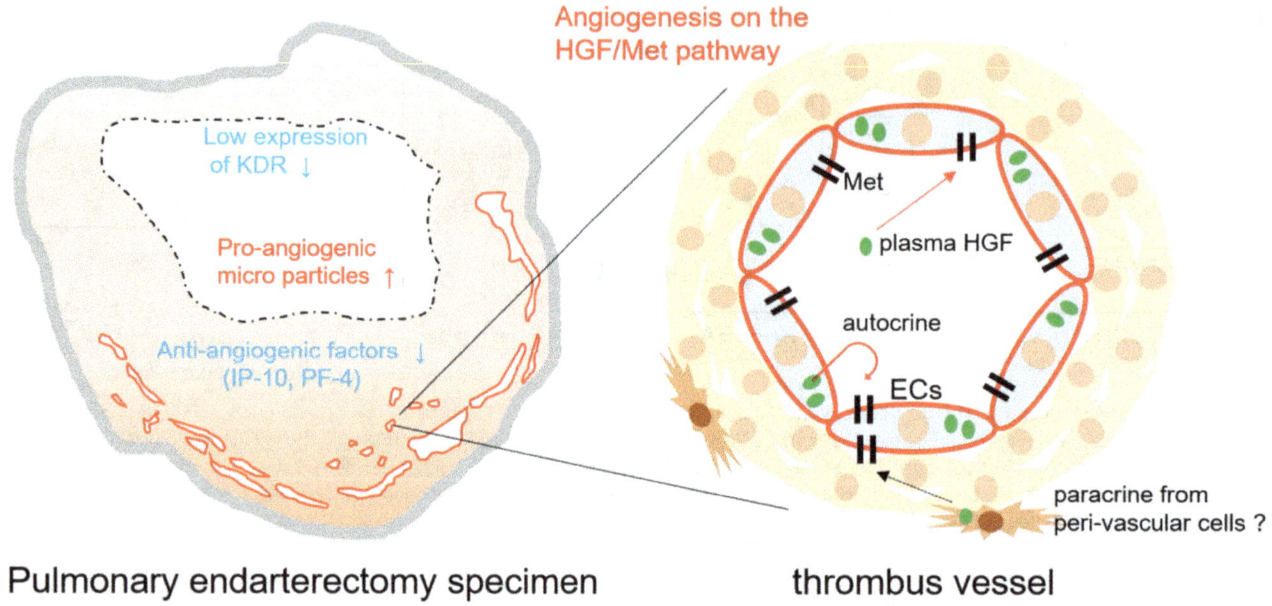

Fig. 8 The hypothesized etiology of insufficient angiogenesis in pulmonary endarterectomy specimens. Insufficient angiogenesis in the organized thrombi might consist of complex conflicts between anti-angiogenic factors (decreased mRNA expression of angiogenetic factor like KDR, loscal anti-angiogenic cytokines) and pro-angiogenic factors (plasma microparticles). The finding of pro-angiogenic factors in the thrombus vessels in the present study (endothelial cells with high angiogenic potential) may represent the latter

pro-angiogenic expression of mRNA in white thrombi could depend on the number of thrombus vessels in the specimen, which was difficult to estimate without a pathological analysis of the same specimen. This hypothesis may be able to explain the difference between our results and the results of Alias et al. [4], which showed that the angiogenesis in white thrombi was deficient in comparison to the non-thrombosed pulmonary artery. Although, and this is a speculation, if the neointima was damaged prior to PEA, the ECs of the damaged neointima might have low angiogenic potential and might play some role in the organization of thrombosis.

The mechanism of HGF production in PEA tissue is undetermined in our study. It is reported that HGF is secreted by stromal cells when they are stimulated by IL-1, IL-6, TNF-α [19], and that the levels of inflammatory cytokines (such as IL-6) are upregulated in the PEA tissues [20] and serum [21]. So we had assumed that the inflammatory cytokines in PEA specimens and the serum may stimulate ECs to secrete HGF. In this study, however, there is no increase of these inflammatory cytokines mRNA in the PEA specimens (Fig. 6a) and of these protein expression in serum (Additional file 2). Although it remains unknown whether the relationship between HGF protein and these inflammatory cytokines, increased expression of HGF mRNA and protein has been confirmed in patients with CTEPH. It is supposed that there might be other stimulators for HGF production instead of these cytokines.

Actually, it is not sure how an increased expression of serum HGF has a role in the development of organized thombus. However, it is reported that the serum HGF levels increase in patients with venous thrombosis [22] [23], pulmonary hypertension [24] as well as older age [25] and hypertension [26]. In this study, we showed that CTEPH patients had higher concentrations of serum HGF despite the younger age and lower systolic blood pressure in comparison to PTE survivors, while the decrease of HGF after successful PEA was slight in operated patients. It is currently unclear whether the increased serum level of HGF is a consequence of thrombosis itself or of other factors that are involved in the cardiovascular burden including pulmonary hypertension, but further investigation may provide us the unknown information on the etiology of PH.

The present study has several limitations. First, the number of CTEPH patients and control subjects was extremely small, and the differences between the CTEPH-ECs and the Control-ECs may not reflect the entire disease etiology. In addition, regarding histological analysis, we could not see the "whole thrombus", but only the part of the removed specimens. There could be a heterogeneity in PEA specimens and this could have introduced a selection bias. Second, passaged cells in vitro assume a different phenotype compared with ECs in vivo. EGM medium which contains several growth factors (including VEGF and FGF) was used to isolate the ECs; this could have influenced the results of comprehensive PCR-array analysis of CTEPH-ECs in Fig. 3, especially about the molecules associated with VEGF and FGF. Third, there are likely complex interactions between ECs and other cells (fibroblast, smooth muscle cells, and others) in organized thrombi which are not occurring in EC monocultures. Such interactions need to be considered when interpreting our results. Forth, although it has been reported that there are stem-like cells in PEA specimens [27] and it has been speculated that those cells might affect angiogenesis of thrombus vessels; here we did not investigate stem-like cells. Despite those limitations, however, we believe that a detailed comparison between the CTEPH-ECs and the Control-ECs, which were isolated under the identical conditions, may be helpful for understanding the disease etiology and the development of novel targeted therapies for the disease.

Conclusions

The results of our study demonstrate that there are ECs with pro-angiogenetic character and high expression of HGF in PEA specimens. It remains to be investigated how these results relate to chronic thromboembolus formation, however, further investigations focusing on HGF/ Met may provide novel diagnostic and therapeutic tools that may be used in the treatment of patients with CTEPH.

Additional files

Additional file 1: The whole data of PCR-array analysis of CTEPH-ECs. The whole data of PCR-array analysis, which compaired the mRNA expression of CTEPH-ECs and Control-ECs (Fig. 3). (DOCX 21 kb)

Additional file 2: The serum levels of representative inflammatory and angiogenic cytokines in chronic thromboembolic pulmonary hypertension (CTEPH) patients ($n = 26$) and pulmonary thromboembolism (PTE) survivors without evidence of pulmonary hypertension (control group, $n = 12$). A) Interleukin-1β, B) Tumor Necrosis Factor-α, C) Vascular Endothelial Growth Factor-A, D)Angiotensin-2. There are no significant differences between two groups in these cytokine levels. (PDF 24 kb)

Additional file 3: CD31 staining of pulmonary endarterectomy (PEA) specimens. A~D): Immunohistochemical staining of CD31 in PEA specimens from different CTEPH patients. The thrombus vessels were clearly positive for CD31, while the internal surface of PEA specimens were rarely positive for CD31. Bar = 1 mm.

Abbreviations

CTEPH: Chronic thromboembolic pulmonary hypertension; HGF: Hepatocyte growth factor; Met: Mesenchymal-epithelial transition factor

Acknowledgements

None.

Funding

The present study was supported by research grants from the Respiratory Failure Research Group (H26-Intractable diseases-General-076) from the Ministry of Health, Labour and Welfare, Japan; a grant to the Pulmonary Hypertension Research Group (15ek0109127h0001) from the Japan Agency for Medical Research and Development (AMED); and a Grant-in-Aid for Scientific Research (JSPS KAKENHI Grant Number 15 K09210) from the Japanese Ministry of Education and Science.

Authors' contributions

AN and SS conceived and designed the study. IM and VN participated in the design of the study. AN conducted the studies, and statistical analysis. AN, SS, TJ, IK, TS drafted the manuscript. IM, VN, GM, IY, NT, KT revised the manuscript. All authors have read and approved the manuscript.

Consent for publication

Not applicable.

Competing interests

Dr.Naito is a member of endowed department from Teijin Pharma ltd. and Ono Pharmaceutical Co. ltd. outside the submitted work. Dr. Sakao received honoraria for lectures from Nippon Shinyaku Co., Ltd., GlaxoSmithKline, Actelion Pharmaceuticals, and Pfizer. Dr. Tanabe is a member of endowed department from Actelion Pharmaceuticals Japan, has received grants from Nipponshinyaku, personal fees from Bayer, personal fees from Niiponshinyaku, personal fees from Pfizer, personal fees from GSK, personal fees from Actelion Pharmaceuticals Japan, outside the submitted work. Dr. Jujo is a member of endowed department from Actelion Pharmaceuticals Japan.

Author details

[1]Department of Respirology, Graduate School of Medicine, Chiba University, 1-8-1 Inohana, Chuo-Ku, Chiba City 260-8670, Japan. [2]Department of Advancing Research on Treatment Strategies for respiratory disease, Graduate School of Medicine, Chiba University, 1-8-1, Inohana, Chuo-Ku, Chiba City 260-8670, Japan. [3]Department of Internal Medicine II, Cardiology, Medical University of Vienna, Spitalgasse 23, 1090 Vienna, Austria. [4]Victoria Johnson Center for Obstructive Lung Disease, Virginia Commonwealth University, 1101 East Marshall Street, Sanger Hall, Richmond, VA 23298-0565, USA. [5]Department of Advanced Medicine in Pulmonary Hypertension, Graduate School of Medicine, Chiba University, 1-8-1 Inohana, Chuo-Ku, Chiba City 260-8670, Japan. [6]Department of Cardiovascular Surgery, Graduate School of Medicine, Chiba University, 1-8-1 Inohana, Chuo-Ku, Chiba City 260-8670, Japan. [7]Department of Thoracic Surgery, Graduate School of Medicine, Chiba University, 1-8-1 Inohana, Chuo-Ku, Chiba City 260-8670, Japan.

References

1. Lang IM, Pesavento R, Bonderman D, Yuan JX. Risk factors and basic mechanisms of chronic thromboembolic pulmonary hypertension: a current understanding. Eur Respir J. 2013;41:462–8.
2. Altmann J, Sharma S, Lang IM. Advances in our understanding of mechanisms of venous thrombus resolution. Expert Rev Hematol. 2016;9: 69–78.
3. Quarck R, Wynants M, Verbeken E, Meyns B, Delcroix M. Contribution of inflammation and impaired angiogenesis to the pathobiology of chronic thromboembolic pulmonary hypertension. Eur Respir J. 2015;46:431–43.
4. Alias S, Redwan B, Panzenbock A, Winter MP, Schubert U, Voswinckel R, Frey MK, Jakowitsch J, Alimohammadi A, Hobohm L, et al. Defective angiogenesis delays thrombus resolution: a potential pathogenetic mechanism underlying chronic thromboembolic pulmonary hypertension. Arterioscler Thromb Vasc Biol. 2014;34:810–9.
5. Nakamura T, Nawa K, Ichihara A. Partial purification and characterization of hepatocyte growth factor from serum of hepatectomized rats. Biochem Biophys Res Commun. 1984;122:1450–9.

6. Naldini L, Weidner KM, Vigna E, Gaudino G, Bardelli A, Ponzetto C, Narsimhan RP, Hartmann G, Zarnegar R, Michalopoulos GK, et al. Scatter factor and hepatocyte growth factor are indistinguishable ligands for the MET receptor. EMBO J. 1991;10:2867–78.
7. Gallo S, Sala V, Gatti S, Crepaldi T. Cellular and molecular mechanisms of HGF/Met in the cardiovascular system. Clin Sci (Lond). 2015;129:1173–93.
8. Jujo T, Sakao S, Ishibashi-Ueda H, Ishida K, Naito A, Sugiura T, Shigeta A, Tanabe N, Masuda M, Tatsumi K. Evaluation of the microcirculation in chronic thromboembolic pulmonary hypertension patients: the impact of pulmonary arterial remodeling on postoperative and follow-up pulmonary arterial pressure and vascular resistance. PLoS One. 2015;10:e0133167.
9. Sakao S, Hao H, Tanabe N, Kasahara Y, Kurosu K, Tatsumi K. Endothelial-like cells in chronic thromboembolic pulmonary hypertension: crosstalk with myofibroblast-like cells. Respir Res. 2011;12:109.
10. Jujo T, Sakao S, Tsukahara M, Kantake S, Maruoka M, Tanabe N, Masuda M, Tatsumi K. The role of matrix metalloproteinase in the intimal sarcoma-like cells derived from endarterectomized tissues from a chronic thromboembolic pulmonary hypertension patient. PLoS One. 2014;9:e87489.
11. Porta C, Giglione P, Ferrari A, Reversi F, Liguigli W, Imarisio I, Ganini C. Tivantinib (ARQ197) in hepatocellular carcinoma. Expert Rev Anticancer Ther. 2015;15:615–22.
12. Yasuda T, Tada Y, Tanabe N, Tatsumi K, West J. Rho-kinase inhibition alleviates pulmonary hypertension in transgenic mice expressing a dominant-negative type II bone morphogenetic protein receptor gene. Am J Phys Lung Cell Mol Phys. 2011;301:L667–74.
13. Chen QH, Liu AR, Qiu HB, Yang Y. Interaction between mesenchymal stem cells and endothelial cells restores endothelial permeability via paracrine hepatocyte growth factor in vitro. Stem Cell Res Ther. 2015;6:44.
14. Zabini D, Nagaraj C, Stacher E, Lang IM, Nierlich P, Klepetko W, Heinemann A, Olschewski H, Balint Z, Olschewski A. Angiostatic factors in the pulmonary endarterectomy material from chronic thromboembolic pulmonary hypertension patients cause endothelial dysfunction. PLoS One. 2012;7:e43793.
15. Belik D, Tsang H, Wharton J, Howard L, Bernabeu C, Wojciak-Stothard B. Endothelium-derived microparticles from chronically thromboembolic pulmonary hypertensive patients facilitate endothelial angiogenesis. J Biomed Sci. 2016;23:4.
16. Waltham M, Burnand K, Fenske C, Modarai B, Humphries J, Smith A. Vascular endothelial growth factor naked DNA gene transfer enhances thrombus recanalization and resolution. J Vasc Surg. 2005;42:1183–9.
17. Modarai B, Humphries J, Burnand KG, Gossage JA, Waltham M, Wadoodi A, Kanaganayagam GS, Afuwape A, Paleolog E, Smith A. Adenovirus-mediated VEGF gene therapy enhances venous thrombus recanalization and resolution. Arterioscler Thromb Vasc Biol. 2008;28:1753–9.
18. Hosokawa K, Ishibashi-Ueda H, Kishi T, Nakanishi N, Kyotani S, Ogino H. Histopathological multiple recanalized lesion is critical element of outcome after pulmonary thromboendarterectomy. Int Heart J. 2011;52:377–81.
19. Sakai K, Aoki S, Matsumoto K. Hepatocyte growth factor and Met in drug discovery. J Biochem. 2015;157:271–84.
20. Zabini D, Heinemann A, Foris V, Nagaraj C, Nierlich P, Balint Z, Kwapiszewska G, Lang IM, Klepetko W, Olschewski H, Olschewski A. Comprehensive analysis of inflammatory markers in chronic thromboembolic pulmonary hypertension patients. Eur Respir J. 2014;44:951–62.
21. von Haehling S, von Bardeleben RS, Kramm T, Thiermann Y, Niethammer M, Doehner W, Anker SD, Munzel T, Mayer E, Genth-Zotz S. Inflammation in right ventricular dysfunction due to thromboembolic pulmonary hypertension. Int J Cardiol. 2010;144:206–11.
22. Hata N, Matsumori A, Yokoyama S, Ohba T, Shinada T, Yoshida H, Tokuyama K, Imaizumi T, Mizuno K. Hepatocyte growth factor and cardiovascular thrombosis in patients admitted to the intensive care unit. Circ J. 2004;68:645–9.
23. Mosevoll KA, Lindas R, Tvedt TH, Bruserud O, Reikvam H. Altered plasma levels of cytokines, soluble adhesion molecules and matrix metalloproteases in venous thrombosis. Thromb Res. 2015;136:30–9.
24. Farha S, Asosingh K, Xu W, Sharp J, George D, Comhair S, Park M, Tang WH, Loyd JE, Theil K, et al. Hypoxia-inducible factors in human pulmonary arterial hypertension: a link to the intrinsic myeloid abnormalities. Blood. 2011;117:3485–93.
25. Bancks MP, Bielinski SJ, Decker PA, Hanson NQ, Larson NB, Sicotte H, Wassel CL, Pankow JS. Circulating level of hepatocyte growth factor predicts incidence of type 2 diabetes mellitus: the Multi-Ethnic Study of Atherosclerosis (MESA). Metabolism. 2016;65:64–72.
26. Morishita R, Moriguchi A, Higaki J, Ogihara T. Hepatocyte growth factor (HGF) as a potential index of severity of hypertension. Hypertens Res. 1999; 22:161–7.
27. Yao W, Firth AL, Sacks RS, Ogawa A, Auger WR, Fedullo PF, Madani MM, Lin GY, Sakakibara N, Thistlethwaite PA, et al. Identification of putative endothelial progenitor cells (CD34+CD133+Flk-1+) in endarterectomized tissue of patients with chronic thromboembolic pulmonary hypertension. Am J Phys Lung Cell Mol Phys. 2009;296:L870–8.

25

Sleep-disordered breathing in patients with newly diagnosed lung cancer

Michael Dreher[1*], Stefan Krüger[2], Susanne Schulze-Olden[2], András Keszei[3], Jan Hendrik Storre[4,5], Holger Woehrle[6], Michael Arzt[7] and Tobias Müller[1,5*]

Abstract

Background: There are currently no data on the prevalence of sleep-disordered breathing (SDB) in patients with newly-diagnosed lung cancer. This might be of interest given that SDB is associated with increased cancer incidence and mortality. Furthermore, intermittent hypoxia has been linked with tumor growth and progression. The aim of the current study was to investigate the prevalence of SDB in patients with newly-diagnosed lung cancer.

Methods: Patients with newly-diagnosed lung cancer from three centers in Germany were screened for SDB using a two-channel screening system (ApneaLink™). SDB was defined as an apnea-hypopnea index of > 5/h, and was classified as mild if the AHI was 5–15/h whereas an AHI ≥15/h was classified as severe SDB. The presence of SDB-related symptoms was assessed using the Epworth Sleepiness Scale (ESS) and the Pittsburgh Sleep Quality Index (PSQI).

Results: A total of 100 patients were included. The overall prevalence of SDB was 49%; 32 patients (32%) had mild SDB with a median AHI of 7.7/h (quartile [Q1 5.4/h, Q3 10.4/h]) and a median oxygen desaturation index of 8.5 [Q1 4.2/h; Q3 13.4/h] and seventeen patients (17%) had moderate to severe SDB with a median AHI of 25.2 [Q1 18/h, Q3 45.5/h] and a median oxygen desaturation index of 20.6/h [Q1 9.6/h, Q3 36.6/h]. Patients with moderate to severe SDB had mild daytime sleepiness (ESS score 8.24 ± 3.96 vs. 5.74 ± 3.53 in those without SDB vs. 6.22 ± 2.72 in those with mild SDB; $p = 0.0343$). The PSQI did not differ significantly between the three groups ($p = 0.1137$).

Conclusions: This study showed a high prevalence of SDB in patients with newly-diagnosed lung cancer. In these patients SDB was associated with intermittent hypoxia and increased daytime sleepiness. Additional research is needed to determine whether SDB influences prognosis and morbidity in patients with lung cancer.

Keywords: Lung neoplasm, sleep-related disorders, sleep-related hypoxaemia, Lung cancer, Sleep apnea, Sleep disorders

Background

Sleep-disordered breathing (SDB) is a common public health problem with a prevalence of 5–20% in the general population, [1, 2] although many patients remain undiagnosed. Obstructive sleep apnea is the most common form of SDB, and has been linked to a number of adverse clinical outcomes including increased cardiovascular and all-cause mortality [3].

* Correspondence: mdreher@ukaachen.de; tobmueller@ukaachen.de
[1]Division of Pneumology, University Hospital RWTH Aachen, Aachen, Germany
Full list of author information is available at the end of the article

The association between SDB and cancer remains to be clearly defined, although previous studies have shown SDB to be associated with increased cancer incidence and cancer mortality. [4–7] Furthermore, it has been shown that sleep time with oxygen saturation below 90% has the strongest association with cancer mortality, highlighting the importance of hypoxemia. [4] This is supported by animal studies showing that intermittent hypoxia, as occurs in patients with obstructive sleep apnea, was associated with tumor growth and progression. [8] Underlying mechanisms include angiogenesis, epithelial-mesenchymal transition, migration/invasion, maintenance of cancer stem cells, metastasis, and immune surveillance, as well as resistance to chemotherapy and radiotherapy. As a result, hypoxemia has been linked with poor prognosis in different malignancies [9, 10].

To the best of our knowledge, there is currently no published data on the prevalence of undiagnosed SDB in patients with newly-diagnosed lung cancer. This is relevant because the presence of SDB might influence morbidity and mortality in lung cancer patients and the treatment of intermittent hypoxia could therefore influence the outcome or response to therapy. This study investigated the prevalence of SDB in patients with newly-diagnosed lung cancer.

Methods

The study received approval from the Institutional Review Board for Human Studies at the University Hospital RWTH Aachen, Germany (EK 312/13). Written informed consent was provided by each subject before participation. All procedures conformed to the standards set by the Declaration of Helsinki in its latest revision.

Patients

From 5th August 2014 until 24th February 2017 consecutive patients with newly-diagnosed lung cancer from three different study centres (University Hospital RWTH - Aachen, Florence-Nightingale-Hospital - Düsseldorf, Cologne-Merheim Hospital - Cologne) were included. Inclusion into the study was done before any treatment for lung cancer (surgery, radiotherapy, or chemotherapy) was initiated. Also excluded were patients with a history of any malignancy or previously diagnosed sleep apnea.

Study design

Patient demographic data, smoking history, and co-morbidities were assessed. Screening for SDB was performed during hospital stay or at home. Daytime sleepiness was assessed using the Epworth Sleepiness Scale (ESS) and Sleep Quality was assessed using the Pittsburgh Sleep Quality Index (PSQI) [11, 12].

Assessing sleep-disordered breathing

SDB screening was performed using a two-channel screening system (ApneaLink Oxi™; ResMed Ltd., Sydney, Australia) which has been validated previously. [13, 14] The ApneaLink™ measures nasal flow via a cannula and records pulse oximetry; further details are described elsewhere. [14] Default device settings were used to define apnea, hypopnea and desaturation as follows: apnea was defined as a decrease of at least 80% in airflow for ≥10 s; hypopnea was defined as a decrease in airflow by 50–80% for ≥10 s; desaturation was defined as a ≥ 4% decrease in oxygen saturation. Mild SDB was defined as AHI of 5 to < 15/h and moderate to severe SDB as an AHI of ≥15/h. [15] The screening device was read out by one investigator at the University Hospital Aachen who was blinded to the patients' status.

Statistical analysis

Continuous data are presented as mean ± standard deviation and categorical data are tabulated as frequencies and percentages. Groups of patients defined based on cutoff values of AHI were compared using ANOVA, Kruskal-Wallis rank sum test and Chi-square test. Nominal p-values are presented for each comparison. Linear models were built using the logarithmic transformed AHI. The following variables were used as independent variables in the models: age (linear effect), sex and body mass index (BMI; linear) were included in all models, and Union for International Cancer Control (UICC) tumor stage (4 categories), arterial hypertension (yes/no), chronic obstructive pulmonary disease (COPD; yes/no) and coronary artery disease (yes/no) were added to the models using all subsets. We present results for the model with the highest adjusted r squared. In additional analyses, AHI was modeled using a generalized linear model with Poisson family and logarithmic link function (data not shown). The prevalence of SDB was estimated from the sample proportions and exact binomial 95% confidence interval (CI) values were calculated.

Results

Patient characteristics

During the study period 625 patients were newly diagnosed with lung cancer at the three study centers. Data from 100 patients who fulfilled the inclusion criteria and consented to take part in the study were included. Patient demographic data are shown in Table 1. The most common form of lung cancer was adenocarcinoma, followed by squamous cell carcinoma and small cell lung cancer (Table 1). Sleep and respiratory parameters for the total population are presented in Table 2.

SDB prevalence

The overall prevalence of SDB (AHI > 5/h) in the study population was 49% (95% CI 38.9–59.2%) and was higher in men (55%) versus women (36%). The median sleep time with oxygen saturation below 90% was 33.0 min for patients with SDB. Moderate to severe SDB was present in 17% (95% CI 10.2–25.8%), whereas mild SDB (AHI 5 to < 15/h) was present in 32% (95% CI 23.0–42.1%) of the patients. There were several statistically significant differences between patients who had mild or moderate to severe SDB and those who did not, including AHI, and ODI (Table 3). Patients with moderate to severe SDB showed mild daytime sleepiness (ESS score 8.24 ± 3.96), and were more sleepy than those without SDB or mild SDB (Table 3). Sleep quality (PSQI), BMI, tumor histology and tumor stage were not significantly different between the three groups (Table 3). The prevalence of distinct comorbidities

Table 1 Patient demographic data

	Patients (n = 100)
Age, years	68.1 ± 8.6
Male, *n*	67
BMI, kg/m^2	26.0 ± 4.6
Histology, *n*	
Small cell lung cancer	23
Non-small cell lung cancer	77
- Adenocarcinoma	45
- Squamous cell carcinoma	24
- Other	8
Tumor stage (UICC), *n*	
I	9
II	13
III	28
IV	50
Smoking history, *n*	
Current smoker	48
Ex-smoker	36
Never smoked	16
Comorbidities, *n*	
Hypertension	56
Diabetes	14
Coronary artery disease	22
Chronic heart failure	8
COPD	29

Values are mean ± standard deviation, or number of patients
BMI body mass index, *COPD* chronic obstructive pulmonary disease, *UICC* Union for International Cancer Control

Table 2 Sleep-disordered breathing analysis, daytime sleepiness and sleep quality

	Patients (n = 100)
ESS score	6.3 ± 3.5
PSQI score	7.0 ± 3.2
AHI, /h	4.9 [2.0, 10.4]
ODI, /h	5.3 [3.0, 10.1]
Mean SpO_2, %	91.3 ± 2.4
Lowest SpO_2, %	78.2 ± 8.2
Time with SpO_2 < 90%, min	34.5 [9.8, 78.0]
Heart rate, beats/min	72.7 ± 11.8
Respiration rate, breaths/min	17.7 ± 4.9
Snoring, /h	66.6 [22.7, 130.3]

Values are mean ± standard deviation, or median [first quartile, third quartile]
AHI apnea-hypopnea index, *ESS* Epworth Sleepiness Scale, *ODI* oxygen desaturation index, *PSQI* Pittsburgh Sleep Quality Index, *SpO_2* oxygen saturation

was similar in the three groups. However, there was a trend towards a higher prevalence of COPD in patients without or with mild SDB compared to patients with moderate to severe SDB (29.4 and 37.5% vs. 11.8%) (Table 3).

Comparing AHI across different tumor stages showed a lower AHI in stage III compared with earlier stages (median 5.1/h, 5.0/h, 2.3/h, and 5.1/h for stages I, II, III, and IV, respectively; $p = 0.04$) (Fig. 1). There were no significant differences in AHI by histologic tumor type (Fig. 2). Median sleep time spent with oxygen saturation below 90% was 14, 24, 45, and 33 min in stages I, II, III, and IV, respectively (Fig. 3a), and time with oxygen saturation below 90% also did not differ between different histological tumor types (Fig. 3b).

Clinical predictors for SDB

The best fitting regression model for the prediction of SDB included age, sex, BMI, and UICC categories II, III, and IV, with estimated regression coefficients of 0.03 (95% CI −0.01, 0.06), 0.57 (− 0.03, 1.17), 0.02 (− 0.05, 0. 08), 0.14 (− 1.05,1.34), − 1.03 (− 2.09, 0.04), and − 0.29 (− 1.30, 0.73), respectively. The adjusted r-squared was 0. 11, indicating that the model had weak predictive value.

Discussion

This study reports the prevalence of SDB in patients with newly-diagnosed lung cancer for the first time and showed that nearly half of all patients had any SDB (AHI > 5/h) and that the prevalence of moderate to severe SDB in this population was 17%.

The reported prevalence of SDB is dependent on the AHI cutoff value used. [13, 14] The 17% prevalence rate for moderate to severe SDB in our cohort with newly-diagnosed lung cancer lies within the estimated prevalence range in the general population (5 to 20%). [1, 2] When an AHI cutoff value of 5/h was used, the estimated prevalence of SDB in patients with newly-diagnosed lung cancer rose markedly to 49%. Of note the average BMI was in the normal range and not significantly different between the groups. Hence one could speculate that the prevalence of SDB is even increased in lung cancer patients. However, as we do not have a control group with similar anthropometric characteristics not suffering from lung cancer this cannot be deducted from the results of the current study.

The exact prevalence of SDB in patients with lung cancer may be less important than the fact that our study shows that a high proportion of patients with newly-diagnosed lung cancer have undiagnosed SDB. This might be particularly relevant given that previous studies have shown that SDB is associated with both increased cancer incidence and increased cancer mortality. [4–7] If this is also the case for patients with lung cancer, screening for SDB in these patients is likely to be clinically important.

Table 3 Comparison of patients without (AHI < 5/h), with mild (AHI 5–15/h)or moderate to severe (AHI > 15/h) sleep-disordered breathing

	AHI < 5/h	AHI 5–15/h	AHI > 15/h	*p*-value
n	51	32	17	N/A
Age, years	66.31 ± 8.48	69.16 ± 8.06	71.35 ± 8.775	0.0736
Male, *n* (%)	30 (58.8)	24 (75.0)	13 (76.5)	0.2062
BMI, kg/m^2	25.53 ± 4.45	26,67 ± 4,95	26.41 ± 4.14	0.5133
AHI, /h	2 [1, 3]	7.7 [5.4, 10.4]	25.2 [18, 45.5]	< 0.0001
ODI, /h	3.1 [1.5, 5.1]	8.5 [4.2, 13.4]	20.6 [9.6, 36.6]	< 0.0001
Mean SpO_2, %	91.47 ± 2.56	91.09 ± 2.36	91.35 ± 2.14	0.7900
Time with SpO_2 < 90%, min	36 [8, 84]	25.5 [8.3, 92.3]	41 [10.5,63]	0.9999
ESS score	5.74 ± 3.53	6.22 ± 2.72	8.24 ± 3.96	0.0343
PSQI score	6.49 ± 2.69	7.97 ± 3.97	6.71 ± 2.62	0.1137
Snoring, /h	69 [19.6, 148]	61.2 [26.8, 156.4]	69 [30.5,89.7]	0.9343
Histology, *n* (%)				
SCLC	14 (27.5)	4 (12.5)	5 (29.4)	0.2280
NSCLC	37 (72.5)	28 (87.5)	12 (70.6)	
- Adenocarcinoma	22 (43.1)	18 (56.3)	5 (29.4)	0.7034
- Squamous cell carcinoma	12 (23.5)	7 (21.9)	5 (29.4)	
- Other	3 (5.9)	3 (9.4)	2 (11.8)	
Tumor stage (UICC), *n* (%)				
I	3 (5.9)	4 (12.5)	2 (11.8)	0.1556
II	5 (9.8)	3 (9.4)	5 (29.4)	
III	19 (37.3)	7 (21.9)	2 (11.8)	
IV	24 (47.1)	18 (56.3)	8 (47.1)	
Smoking history, *n* (%)				
Current smoker	27 (52.9)	14 (43.8)	7 (41.2)	0.8782
Ex-smoker	16 (31.4)	13 (40.6)	7 (41.2)	
Never smoked	8 (15.7)	5 (15.6)	3 (17.6)	
Comorbidities, *n* (%)				
Hypertension	26 (50.1)	21 (65.6)	9 (52.9)	0.4088
Diabetes	4 (7.8)	6 (18.8)	4 (23.5)	0.1749
Coronary artery disease	9 (17.6)	7 (21.9)	6 (35.3)	0.3144
Chronic heart failure	4 (7.8)	3 (9.4)	1 (5.9)	0.9105
COPD	15 (29.4)	12 (37.5)	2 (11.8)	0.1670
Pulmonary function				
FEV1 (% predicted)	64.69 ± 17.88	67.51 ± 18.65	77.09 ± 20.02	0.0926
PaO_2 (mmHg)	67.62 ± 12.44	66.69 ± 9.01	69.34 ± 17.69	0.9264

Values are mean ± standard deviation, median [first quartile, third quartile], or number of patients (%)

AHI apnea-hypopnea index, *BMI* body mass index, *COPD* chronic obstructive pulmonary disease, *ESS* Epworth Sleepiness Scale, *FEV1* Forced Expiratory Volume in 1 s, *NSCLC* non-small cell lung cancer, *ODI* oxygen desaturation index, *PaO_2* capillary partial pressure of oxygen, *PSQI* Pittsburgh Sleep Quality Index, *SpO_2* oxygen saturation, *SCLC* small cell lung cancer, *UICC* Union for International Cancer Control

Both increased cancer incidence and increased cancer mortality have been shown to be dependent on the severity of hypoxemia occurring during SDB,[4,6] and animal data demonstrated an association between intermittent hypoxia and tumor growth and progression. [8] The mean ODI in the present study was 9 ± 12/h overall and 25 ± 20/h in patients with moderate to severe SDB. Although intermittent hypoxia was present in our cohort we did not find any correlation between the severity of SDB and cancer type or tumor stage. Furthermore, sleep time with oxygen saturation below 90% was not correlated with cancer type or tumor stage. However, this was not the

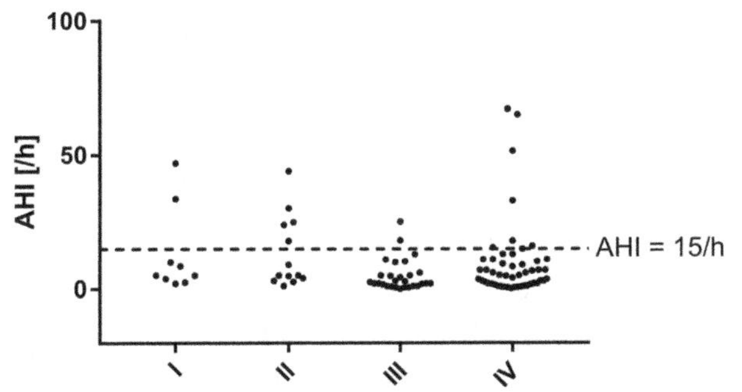

Fig. 1 Relationship between the apnea-hypopnea index (AHI) and UICC tumor stage

goal of the current study and the trial was not powered for these analyses. Nevertheless, our results might stimulate research to assess clinical outcomes in lung cancer patients with underlying SDB. Continuous positive airway pressure is the standard of care for patients with obstructive sleep apnea, improving both the AHI and ODI. [16] Therefore, studies investigating the impact of treating intermittent hypoxia in patients with lung cancer on the clinical course of the disease would be of high clinical interest.

Sleep apnea is associated with impaired health-related quality of life due to symptoms such as reduced sleep quality, daytime sleepiness, and fatigue. [16] Chronic fatigue is a common problem in patients with lung cancer, [17] which might be aggravated in the presence of SDB or, in some instances, may even be caused by SDB. Although sleep quality measured using the PSQI was not different in patients with and without SDB, daytime sleepiness based on the ESS score, was significantly higher in newly-diagnosed lung cancer patients who also had SDB. Therefore, treating SDB in patients with lung cancer might have the potential to improve SDB symptoms and thus also health-related quality of life. However, this remains speculative and should be evaluated in a prospective clinical trial.

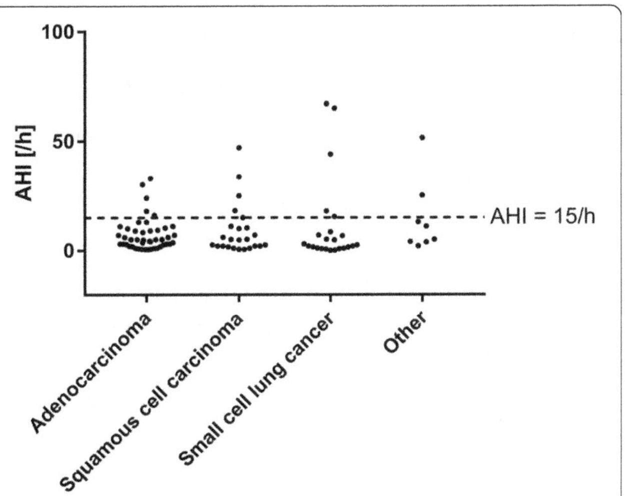

Fig. 2 Relationship between the apnea-hypopnea index (AHI) and different subtypes of lung cancer

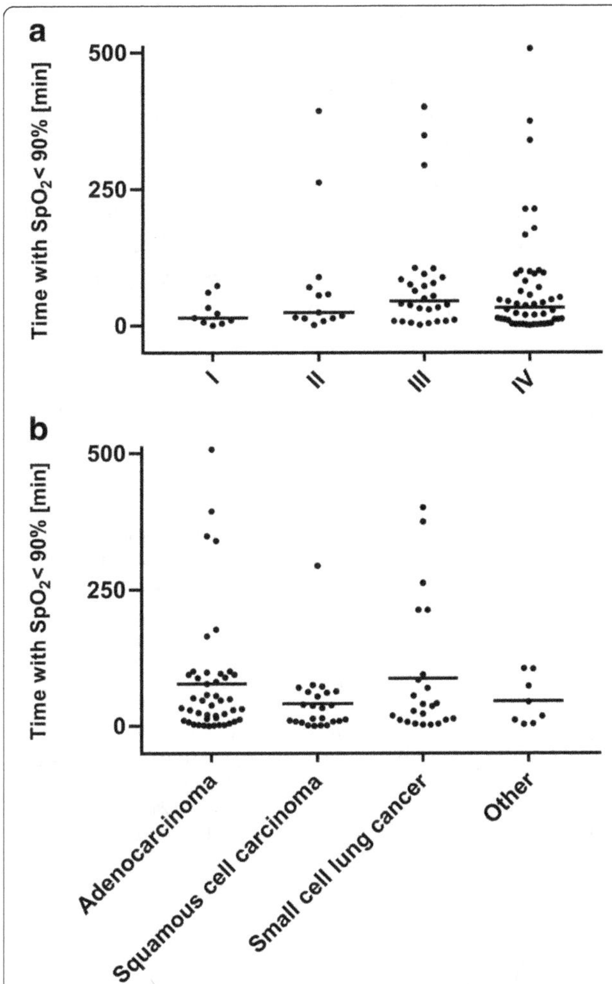

Fig. 3 Relationship between sleep time with oxygen saturation < 90% (T < 90%) and different tumor stages (**a**) or tumor histology (**b**)

In our cohort of patients with newly-diagnosed lung cancer, age, BMI, sex, and tumor stage did not predict SDB, but this may be due to a lack of statistical power for the analyses.

Our study has several limitations which have to be addressed: Firstly, the device used to screen for SDB has limited diagnostic abilities, e. g. it does not allow to distinguish obstructive from central sleep apnea. Secondly, the proportion of screening failures was high, and we did not collect data about the prevalence of SDB in a matched control group without lung cancer. Thirdly, SDB was assessed both at home and in hospital which might have yielded different results.

Conclusions

In conclusion, the rate of moderate to severe SDB in patients with newly-diagnosed lung cancer was 17% and nearly half of all patients had any SDB. Moderate to severe SDB in this cohort was associated with intermittent hypoxia and increased daytime sleepiness. Since previous studies have linked pathophysiological features of SDB, such as intermittent hypoxia, with tumor growth and progression, further research is warranted to determine whether SDB influences the outcome of patients with lung cancer and whether treatment of SDB can improve health-related quality of life, slow disease progression, or even increase survival in lung cancer patients.

Abbreviations

AHI: Apnea hypopnea index; ESS: Epworth sleepiness scale; ODI: Oxygen desaturation index; SDB: Sleep disordered breathing

Acknowledgements

The authors thank the staff of the Center for Translational & Clinical Research Aachen (CTC-A) for their help with data collection. English language editing support was provided by Nicola Ryan, independent medical writer.

Authors' contributions

Conception of the study was done by MD, MA, HW, and TM. Recruitment of patients was done by MD, SK, SSO, JHS and TM. The first draft of the manuscript was prepared by MD and TM, who had unrestricted access to the data. Statistical analysis was done by APK. The manuscript was reviewed and edited by MA, HW and SK. All authors made the decision to submit the manuscript for publication. MD and TM assume responsibility for the accuracy and completeness of the analyses and for the fidelity of this report to the trial protocol. The final version of the manuscript was read and approved by all authors.

Competing interests

MD received honoraria from Linde AG, ResMed, Respironics, Weinmann, Heinen und Löwenstein, Hamilton for participations in advisory boards and lectures. JHS received research grants, speaking fees and travel funding from different companies producing or selling devices and consumables for mechanical ventilation and oxygen therapy. HW was employed by ResMed until 2016, received lecture fees from Astra Zeneca, GSK, Vital Air, Weinmann, Boehringer Ingelheim, ResMed and research support from Weinmann and ResMed. MA received grant support and lecture fees from ResMed, Philips and Respironics. SK, SSO, APK and TM have no competing interests to declare.

Author details

[1]Division of Pneumology, University Hospital RWTH Aachen, Aachen, Germany. [2]Department of Pneumology, Florence-Nightingale-Hospital, Düsseldorf, Germany. [3]Department of Medical Informatics, University Hospital RWTH Aachen, Aachen, Germany. [4]Department of Intensive Care, Sleep Medicine and Mechanical Ventilation, Asklepios Fachkliniken Munich-Gauting, Gauting, Germany. [5]Department of Pneumology, University Medical Hospital, Freiburg, Germany. [6]Sleep and Ventilation Center Blaubeuren, Lung Center Ulm, Ulm, Germany. [7]Center of Sleep Medicine, Department of Internal Medicine II, University Hospital Regensburg, Regensburg, Germany.

References

1. Heinzer R, Vat S, Marques-Vidal P, Marti-Soler H, Andries D, Tobback N, et al. Prevalence of sleep-disordered breathing in the general population: the HypnoLaus study. Lancet Respir Med. 2015;3:310–8. Available from: http://www.ncbi.nlm.nih.gov/pubmed/25682233
2. Peppard PE, Young T, Barnet JH, Palta M, Hagen EW, Hla KM. Increased prevalence of sleep-disordered breathing in adults. Am J Epidemiol. 2013;177:1006–14. Available from: http://www.ncbi.nlm.nih.gov/pubmed/23589584
3. Loke YK, Brown JWL, Kwok CS, Niruban A, Myint PK. Association of obstructive sleep apnea with risk of serious cardiovascular events: a systematic review and meta-analysis. Circ Cardiovasc Qual Outcomes. 2012;5:720–8. Available from: http://www.ncbi.nlm.nih.gov/pubmed/22828826
4. Nieto FJ, Peppard PE, Young T, Finn L, Hla KM, Farré R. Sleep-disordered breathing and cancer mortality: results from the Wisconsin sleep cohort study. Am J Respir Crit Care Med. 2012;186:190–4. Available from: http://www.ncbi.nlm.nih.gov/pubmed/22610391
5. Martínez-García MÁ, Campos-Rodríguez F, Almendros I, Farré R. Relationship between sleep apnea and cancer. Arch Bronconeumol. 2015;51:456–61. Available from: http://www.ncbi.nlm.nih.gov/pubmed/25843225
6. Campos-Rodriguez F, Martinez-Garcia MA, Martinez M, Duran-Cantolla J, de La Peña M, Masdeu MJ, et al. Association between obstructive sleep apnea and cancer incidence in a large multicenter Spanish cohort. Am J Respir Crit Care Med. 2013;187:99–105. Available from: http://www.ncbi.nlm.nih.gov/pubmed/23155146
7. Palamaner Subash Shantha G, Kumar AA, Cheskin LJ, Pancholy SB. Association between sleep-disordered breathing, obstructive sleep apnea, and cancer incidence: a systematic review and meta-analysis. Sleep Med. 2015;16:1289–94. Available from: http://www.ncbi.nlm.nih.gov/pubmed/26212231
8. Almendros I, Montserrat JM, Torres M, Bonsignore MR, Chimenti L, Navajas D, et al. Obesity and intermittent hypoxia increase tumor growth in a mouse model of sleep apnea. Sleep Med. 2012;13:1254–60. Available from: http://www.ncbi.nlm.nih.gov/pubmed/23149216
9. Lévy P, Godin-Ribuot D, Pepin J-L. Sleep apnoea and cancer: the new challenge. Eur Respir J. 2014;43:1567–70. Available from: http://erj.ersjournals.com/cgi/doi/10.1183/09031936.00065714
10. McDonald PC, Chafe SC, Dedhar S. Overcoming hypoxia-mediated tumor progression: combinatorial approaches targeting pH regulation, angiogenesis and immune dysfunction. Front. Cell Dev Biol. 2016;4:27. Available from: http://www.pubmedcentral.nih.gov/articlerender.fcgi?artid=4814851&tool=pmcentrez&rendertype=abstract
11. Johns MW. A new method for measuring daytime sleepiness: the Epworth sleepiness scale. Sleep. 1991;14:540–5. Available from: http://www.ncbi.nlm.nih.gov/pubmed/1798888
12. Buysse DJ, Reynolds CF, Monk TH, Berman SR, Kupfer DJ. The Pittsburgh sleep quality index: a new instrument for psychiatric practice and research. Psychiatry Res. 1989;28:193–213. Available from: http://www.ncbi.nlm.nih.gov/pubmed/2748771
13. Chen H, Lowe AA, Bai Y, Hamilton P, Fleetham JA, Almeida FR. Evaluation of a portable recording device (ApneaLink) for case selection of obstructive sleep apnea. Sleep Breath. 2009;13:213–9. Available from: http://www.ncbi.nlm.nih.gov/pubmed/19052790
14. Erman MK, Stewart D, Einhorn D, Gordon N, Casal E. Validation of the ApneaLink for the screening of sleep apnea: a novel and simple single-channel recording device. J Clin Sleep Med. 2007;3:387–92. Available from: http://www.ncbi.nlm.nih.gov/pubmed/17694728
15. Arzt M, Woehrle H, Oldenburg O, Graml A, Suling A, Erdmann E, et al. Prevalence and predictors of sleep-disordered breathing in patients with stable chronic heart failure: the SchlaHF registry. JACC Hear Fail. 2016;4:116–25. Available from: http://www.ncbi.nlm.nih.gov/pubmed/26682790
16. Giles TL, Lasserson TJ, Smith BJ, White J, Wright J, Cates CJ. Continuous positive airways pressure for obstructive sleep apnoea in adults. Cochrane Database Syst. Rev. 2006;CD001106. Available from: http://www.ncbi.nlm.nih.gov/pubmed/16437429.
17. Pearman T. Psychosocial factors in lung cancer: quality of life, economic impact, and survivorship implications. J Psychosoc Oncol. 2008;26:69–80. Available from: http://www.ncbi.nlm.nih.gov/pubmed/18077263

26

Occupational risk factors for idiopathic pulmonary fibrosis in Southern Europe

Giulia Paolocci[1], Ilenia Folletti[1], Kjell Torén[2], Magnus Ekström[2], Marco Dell'Omo[1], Giacomo Muzi[1] and Nicola Murgia[1,2*]

Abstract

Background: Idiopathic pulmonary fibrosis (IPF) is a chronic, progressive fibrosing interstitial pneumonia of unknown cause associated with the histopathologic and/or radiologic pattern of usual interstitial pneumonia (UIP). Occupational risk factors have been proposed to be associated with UIP. The aim of this case-control study is to evaluate the relationship between UIP pattern and occupational exposure in Southern Europe.

Methods: Sixty nine cases with a UIP radiological pattern at CT-scan were selected from a clinical database of the University Hospital of Perugia, Umbria, between January 2010 and December 2013. Controls ($n = 277$) not reporting doctor diagnosed pulmonary fibrosis, were ascertained casually among general population from the same catching area of cases. Data were collected by a questionnaire used previously in a similar study. Logistic regression models, adjusted for gender, age and smoking, were performed to evaluate the association between UIP and occupational exposure.

Results: Farmers, veterinarians and gardeners (OR = 2.73, 95%CI = 1.47–5.10), metallurgical and steel industry workers (OR = 4.80, 95%CI = 1.50–15.33) were occupations associated with UIP. Metal dust and fumes and organic dust were risk factors for UIP. Increasing the length of occupational exposure in jobs at risk of pulmonary fibrosis, increased the risk of having UIP.

Conclusions: This case control study confirm partially the results from previous similar studies. Some discrepancies could be explained by the different geographical origins of the population under study, reflecting also different occupational exposures.

Keywords: Occupational, Workers, UIP, Pulmonary fibrosis

Background

Idiopathic pulmonary fibrosis (IPF) is a chronic, progressive, fibrosing interstitial lung disease of unknown cause with a high risk of rapid progression and mortality, the median survival after diagnosis is approximately 2 years [1].

The diagnosis of IPF requires exclusion of other known causes of idiophatic lung diseases, the presence of a usual interstitial pneumonia (UIP) pattern on high resolution CT-scan (HRCT) in patients not subjected to surgical lung biopsy (SLB) and specific combinations of HRCT and SLB patterns in patients subjected to SLB [2].

While several key cellular and molecular events have been identified in the pathogenesis of IPF, such as age-associated telomerase dysfunction [3], incidence of IPF has increased in the last years with regional differences suggesting the pathogenic role of various environmental and occupational exposures [4].

Mechanisms governing the relationship between smoking, gender, occupational exposure and the development of severe pulmonary fibrosis are unknown but likely involve complex interactions between different environmental factors in genetically predisposed individuals [5].

* Correspondence: nicola.murgia@unipg.it
[1]Section of Occupational Medicine, Respiratory Diseases and Toxicology, University of Perugia, Piazzale Gambuli, 06100 Perugia, Italy
[2]Department of Occupational and Environmental Medicine, Sahlgrenska University Hospital, Göteborg, Sweden

In similar studies made in America [6], Northern Europe [7] and Japan [8] occupational risk factors, including metal, stone and wood dust have been linked to higher risk of developing pulmonary fibrosis, but to date, the consistency of epidemiological evidence is suggestive but not sufficient to infer a causal relationship between several environmental exposure and IPF.

The aim of this study is to evaluate the relationship between UIP pattern and occupational exposure in Southern Europe.

Methods

The design was a case-control study of the adult population in Perugia, Umbria, Central Italy. 69 consecutive cases were included from the Perugia University Hospital clinical database between January 2010 and December 2013 and a random sample of 308 controls was selected among inhabitants of the same catchment area (Region Umbria). The diagnosis of UIP was based on clinical history, UIP pattern at CT scan and, when available, on open lung biopsy. All cases were consecutively included. Exclusion criteria were: laboratory testing compatible with autoimmune diseases, lung irradiation (radiotherapy), current or previous intake of medication known to cause lung fibrosis, compensation for occupational lung diseases resembling clinically and radiologically UIP (e.g asbestosis). Furthermore, cases with high suspicion, based on medical records and exposure history, of an occupational disease, even if not-compensated, were excluded.

All this information were gathered through the UIP patients medical records available at the Section of Occupational Medicine, Respiratory Diseases and Toxicology of the University Hospital of Perugia. The study protocol was approved by the Regional Ethical Committee (CEAS UMBRIA) and all the participants gave their informed verbal consent to the study. Due to the specific design of the study (telephone questionnaire), the informed consent was verbal. To approve the study, the ethical committee (CEAS UMBRIA) required the presence of a witness during questionnaire administration.

Questionnaire and definitions

Data were collected through an extensive telephonic questionnaire with items about occupations, duration of this occupations, specific self-reported occupational exposure, smoking habits and diagnosis of pulmonary fibrosis with information on atopy, rhinitis, family autoimmunity and family history of pulmonary fibrosis. The questionnaire has been described in detail elsewhere [7]. The response rate was 100% among cases and 90% among controls. Thus, the final number of controls enrolled in the study was 277.

Occupational exposure was ascertained by the answers to the self-reported questions. Self-reported exposures were lumped in 5 larger categories, metal dust and fumes, mineral dust, organic dust, vapour gas and non-metal fumes, environmental tobacco smoke. To be classified as exposed, a subject had to report an occupation or an exposure lasting for at least 5 years and for cases, starting 5 years or more before the diagnosis of IPF, based on UIP pattern at CT scan.

Another measure of exposure was based on self-reported occupations: job titles were grouped into 12 job categories and of these, 5 have been considered at risk to cause UIP. The selection of the 5 job categories at risk to develop UIP was made through a review of the literature (Additional file 1). The search was conducted in the PubMed electronic database using the following search phrase: *"Idiopathic pulmonary fibrosis" or "usual interstitial pneumonia" AND (occupation* OR work* OR environment)* considering only review articles, in English language and human studies. Therefore, of 68 studies, 11 were selected and based on these 11 review articles, construction, wood, metallurgical and steel and chemical workers, as well as farmers, veterinarians (vets) and gardeners were considered professions at risk to generate the disease.

Statistical analysis

Significance of differences in prevalence were calculated by Chi-square test, and Fisher's exact test, when appropriate. Significance of differences in means were calculated using t-test. To evaluate different risk factors, logistic regression models have been built for occupation at risk of UIP and for self-reported exposure to occupational hazards, adjusting for gender, age, and smoking (ever and never). Specific models stratifying for gender and adjusting for age and smoking were also build. Associations were expressed as OR with 95% CI, statistical significance was defined as a double-sided $p < 0.05$. Only exposure categories with five or more exposed cases were considered in the final analysis. Statistical analyses were performed using SPSS statistical software, version 20.0 (SPSS, IBM Corporation, New York, NY, USA).

Results

The study comprises 69 consecutive patients with UIP radiological pattern and 277 controls. The mean age was 75 years for cases and 71 for controls, 72.5% of cases and 54.2% of controls were males. Cases and controls had the same smoking exposure. No differences were found in distribution of family history pulmonary fibrosis as well as in atopy and rhinitis history between the two groups. Baseline characteristics are shown in Table 1.

Subjects with any occupational exposure to agents known to cause UIP had an increased risk for UIP (OR 4.1 95% CI 2.3–7.55) (Table 2).

Table 1 Characteristics of the population

	UIP cases ($n = 69$)	Controls ($n = 277$)	p
Males, n (%)	50 (72.5)	150 (54. 2)	< 0.01
Age, mean ± SD	75 (± 14)	71 (± 13)	0.02
Smoking			
No smokers	27 (39.1)	110 (39.7)	NS
Eversmokers	42 (60.9)	167 (60.3)	
Atopy, n (%)	5 (7.2)	25 (9.0)	NS
Rhinitis, n (%)	22 (31.9)	75 (27.1)	NS
Family history of pulmonary fibrosis, n (%)	3 (4.5)	3 (1.1)	0.09
Family autoimmunity, n (%)	7 (10.1)	33 (11.9)	NS
Work duration (years), mean ± SD	38.6 (± 10.6)	35.4 (± 10.5)	0.02
Job title			
Legislators, entrepreneurs, scientific and intellectual professions	4 (5.8)	21 (7.6)	NS
Technical, social and health professions	9 (13)	62 (22.4)	NS
Office workers	11 (15.9)	48 (17.3)	NS
Dealers and service workers	11 (15.9)	63 (22.7)	NS
Drivers or operatives of vehicles and installations	6 (8.7)	42 (15.2)	NS
Construction workers	14(20.3)	26 (9.4)	0.02
Food industry workers	5 (7.2)	30 (10.8)	NS
Textile industry workers	9 (13)	36 (13)	NS
Wood industry workers	6 (8.7)	15 (5.4)	NS
Metallurgical and steel industry	8 (11.6)	6 (2.2)	0.02
Farmers, vets and gardeners	30 (43.5)	51 (18.4)	< 0.01
Chemical industry	2 (2.9)	0 (0)	0.04

To have worked in a metallurgical and steel industry (OR 4.8 95% CI 1.5–15.3) and to be a farmer, vet or gardener (OR 2.7 95% CI 1.5–5.1) increased the risk of UIP (Table 2). There was an association between a longer occupational exposure in any job at risk of UIP and the risk of UIP (Table 3).

The self-reported exposure confirmed the findings obtained from the job title analysis underlying an excess of risk if the subject reported the exposure to metal dust and fumes or organic dust. In this latter analysis a self-reported exposure to environmental tobacco smoke doubled the risk of UIP (Table 4).

When the analysis was made considering also those who have reported shorter exposure (< 5 years) the results did not change (data not shown).

Discussion

The main finding of this study was the increased risk of UIP among those with a job known to be at risk of UIP. In detail, farmers, veterinarians, gardeners, metal and

Table 2 Job at risk for UIP in the whole sample, in men and women, adjusted for age and smoking

	All[a]	Men	Women
Exposure	OR (95% CI)	OR (95% CI)	OR (95% CI)
None	1	1	1
Any job at risk of UIP	*4.14 (2.27–7.53)*	*4.40 (2.13–9.05)*	*3.91 (1.18–12.86)*
Costruction workers	1.31 (0.58–2.98)	1.37 (0.60–3.12)	–
Wood industry workers	1.36 (0.46–3.97)	1.35 (0.46–3.95)	–
Metallurgical and steel industry	*4.80 (1.50–15.33)*	*4.76 (1.50–15.15)*	–
Farmers, vets and gardeners	*2.73 (1.47–5.10)*	*2.42 (1.14–5.11)*	*3.91 (1.18–12.86)*

Significant risk estimates in italic
[a]the whole sample also adjusted for gender

Table 3 Effect of the length of the occupation in a job at risk of UIP and the risk of UIP, adjusted for sex, age and smoking

Exposure	OR	95% CI
None	1	
1–9 years	*3.32*	*1.06–10.33*
10–19 years	*3.41*	*1.30–8.95*
≥ 20 years	*5.01*	*2.55–9.84*

Significant risk estimates in italic

steel workers were at risk of UIP. Self-reported exposure to metal dust, fumes and organic dust was confirmed as a risk factor for UIP. This association provided support for the hypothesis that pulmonary fibrosis may be a heterogeneous disorder caused by a number of environmental and occupational exposures. The same risk factors have been found in observational studies from different countries [9]. Agricultural workers, veterinarians and gardeners are exposed to organic dust and aerosolized particulates from a variety of sources, including feed grains, bedding and cattle fecal material. The contribution of this exposure to the pathogenesis of lung fibrosis is not completely clear, but, even if all the cases were negative for common serum precipitins, the presence of end-stage unrecognized chronic hypersensitivity pneumonitis can not be excluded. In fact, chronic hypersensitivity pneumonitis could have an UIP radiological pattern [10] and can be confused with idiopathic pulmonary fibrosis, also by experienced physicians [11]. Moreover, veterinarians are usually less exposed to organic dust than agricultural workers and gardener, in this study the contribution of this job title (veterinarians) to the risk of UIP was quite low, since we had just one controls doing this job and his exclusion from the study did not change significantly the results.

The association between metal exposure and lung fibrosis is demonstrated in original studies [6] and review [12]. Metal-related lung fibrosis could be explained by the transition of alveolar cells to mesenchymal cells, caused by reactive oxygen species [13], where some metals are well established inducers of reactive oxygen species [14]. However, asbestos exposure in steel and metallurgy, as well in construction industry, can not be excluded [15], especially in those working in steel mills before '90s.

Table 4 Self-reported exposure and risk for UIP, adjusted for age, gender and smoking

Occupational exposure	Cases n	Controls n	OR (95%CI)
Metal Dust or metal fumes	9	9	*3.8 (1.2–12.2)*
Mineral Dust	23	39	1.7 (0.8–3.6)
Organic Dust	37	104	*2.4 (1.3–4.3)*
Vapours, gas, fumes	25	85	0.9 (0.5–1.7)
Environmental tobacco smoke at work	43	116	*2.2 (1.2–4.0)*

Significant risk estimates in italic

In a previous similar study an association between severe pulmonary fibrosis and wood exposure was found; in this study wood dust exposure did not affect significantly the risk of IPF. This finding could be explained by the different geographical origins of the population considered, reflecting also different economic and productive situation and thus occupational exposures. As a matter of fact, in the present study, the number of subjects exposed to wood dust was rather low compared to the previous study [7].

The association with occupational exposure was time-dependent: the risk of IPF increases with the duration of exposure. The finding of a dose-response relationship between years of potential exposure and risk of disease confirmed previous findings [16, 17]. The exposure assessment in this study was not based only on self-reported exposure, easily prone to recall bias by IPF patients, but also on a job exposure matrix, grounded on previous studies merged in reviews. The reason to consider just reviews was to have a more homogeneous source of information. Anyway, to avoid misclassification, an a posteriori literature search among original articles was performed, confirming the same results obtained with reviews- restricted search. Anyway, we can not exclude exposure misclassification, beside the possibile asbestos exposure in steel and metallurgy, carpenters, classified as wood workers could have been also exposed to asbestos, as well many construction workers.

In this study, we do not perform matching and gender distribution was not similar among cases and controls. Nevertheless, stratified analysis for gender led to the same results in men and women (data not shown), even if women did not report to work or have worked in some occupations (construction, wood and metal).

In the International Consensus Statement regarding the diagnosis and treatment of IPF, Costabel et al. cited cigarette smoking as a potential risk factor for IPF [18] and it have shown in previous studies a dose-related association with increased risk of severe pulmonary fibrosis [19]. Our findings do not support this association, maybe because ever-smoking prevalence, despite the recent introduction of restrictions, is still rather high in Southern Europe, compared to other western countries from where the majority of previous studies were coming. The high prevalence of smokers could be one of the reason of a very high prevalence of self-reported exposure to environmental tobacco smoke in this study among UIP patients (62. 3%), although a recall bias or same artifact in the statistical analysis cannot be excluded.

One of the strengths of the present study is the case definition, which includes cases with a medical diagnosis of UIP based on medical records with rather strict exclusion criteria, lung CT-scan UIP radiological pattern and, when available, histological data. In previous studies, case definition by medication registry (e.g. liquid oxygen therapy registry) could yield to misclassification and survivor bias [20]. Moreover, the recruitment of controls from the general population of the same catchment area should avoid bias related to the presence of shared risk factors (smoking, occupation) in an hospital-based case-control design. Not having imaging from control subjects could lead to a classification bias, if some of the controls has a not yet diagnosed pulmonary fibrosis; however, the very low prevalence of UIP in the general population (8.2 cases/100000) [21] could reduce the risk of this bias.

The reason to exclude exposure in the five years before the diagnosis is based on the nature of IPF which is chronic and progressive and a minimum lag time of five years was considered reasonable, based on previous studies dealing with occupational exposures to a known fibrogenic agent, such as silica, and the occurrence of non-malignant fibrotic lung diseases, such as silicosis [22]. However, in a case-control study design, the criterion of temporality, with exposure preceding the onset of UIP, cannot be established safely, because exposure and disease are measured, unlike cohort study, simultaneously [23] and UIP, as other chronic diseases, could also have been diagnosed later than the real onset.

A possible limitation of this study is the low number of cases, but other previous [23] and more recent studies, even if multicenter, have considered similar numbers [24].

Lack of matching for gender and age could be seen as another potential limitation, but the homogeneity of the sample, recruited in the same area and the results after adjustment for age and gender in the whole model and stratification for gender, could contribute to reduce the burden of this limitation on risk estimates. Moreover, it is not clear whether gender is a strong confounder (e.g. for hormone-related issues or for some protective effect of pregnancy on UIP) or an intermediate factor because the exposure to some occupational or environmental risk factor for UIP is more likely to occur in men. Therefore, to avoid underestimation, we decide to not match for gender.

Another possible drawback of a case-control design is the risk of recall bias regarding the exposure assessment. However, in this study, the use of a job exposure matrix would reduce significantly the risk of recall bias in cases and controls.

Another limitation, difficult to overcome given this study design, is the change in exposure intensity over years [25], it is plausible that younger participants underwent to a lighter exposure than the older ones. A larger number of cases could have allowed a stratified analysis for age, which could take into account this aspect.

Finally, some important risk factor for UIP, such as acid microaspiration in gastroesophageal reflux (GER), have not been taken into account in this study. However, GER have been found frequently in UIP patients but its role in causation is still rather unclear, furthermore, diagnostic tools to evaluate the occurrence of GER prior the diagnosis of UIP are still lacking [26].

Conclusions

Despite some potential limitations, this study confirm data from previous epidemiological studies and overall stress the importance of occupational and environmental factors in UIP pathogenesis. A better understanding of the risk factors for UIP is still needed to prevent its occurrence and, in order to assess the real impact of occupational exposure, further studies are required in larger population samples.

Abbreviations

GER: Gastro esophageal reflux; HRCT: High resolution CT-scan; IPF: Idiopathic pulmonary fibrosis; SLB: Surgical lung biopsy; UIP: Usual interstitial pneumonia

Funding

The Italian National Institute for Insurance against Accidents at Work (INAIL) supported the study.

Authors' contributions

GP contribute to plan the study, perform the survey, contribute to write the manuscript, contribute to data analysis; IF contribute to plan the study, contribute to write the manuscript, contribute to data analysis; KT contribute to plan the study, review the manuscript; ME contribute to plan the study, contribute to write the manuscript; MDO contribute to perform the survey, contribute to write the manuscript; GM contribute to recruit cases, review the manuscript; NM contribute to plan the study, contribute to recruit cases, contribute to data analysis, contribute to write and review the manuscript. All authors have read and approved the manuscript.

Competing interests

All the authors declare that they have no competing interests about the subject and the content of this article.

References

1. Raghu G, Collard HR, Egan JJ, et al. An official ATS/ERS/JRS/ALAT statement: idiopathic pulmonary fibrosis: evidence –based guidelines for diagnosis and management. Am J Respir Crit Care Med. 2011;183:788–824.
2. An official American Thoracic Society/European Respiratory Society Statement. Update of the international multidisciplinary classification of the idiopathic interstitial pneumonias. Am J Respir Crit Care Med Sep. 2013;188: 733–48.

3. King TE Jr, Pardo A, Selman M. Idiopathic pulmonary fibrosis. Lancet. 2011; 378:1949–61.
4. Navaratnam V, Fleming KM, West J, et al. The rising incidence of idiopathic pulmonary fibrosis in the U.K. Thorax. 2011;66:462–7.
5. Macneal K, Schwartz DA. The genetc and environmental causes of pulmonary fibrosis. ProcAmThorac Soc. 2012;9:120–5.
6. Baumgartner KB, Samet JM, Coultas DB, et al. Occupational and environmental risk factors for idiopathic pulmonary fibrosis: a multicentre case-control study. Collaborating centers. Am J Epidemiol. 2000;152(4):307–15.
7. Gustafson T, Dahlman-Höglund A, Nilsson K, et al. Occupational exposure and severe pulmonary fibrosis. Respir Med. 2007;101(10):2207–12. Epub 2007 Jul 12
8. Awadalla NJ, Hegazy A, Elmetwally RA, et al. Occupational and environmental risk factors for idiopathic pulmonary fibrosis in Egypt: a multicenter case-control study. Int J Occup Environ Med. 2012;3(3):107–16.
9. Taskar VS, Coultas DB. Is idiopathic pulmonary fibrosis an environmental disease? Proc Am Thorac Soc. 2006;3(4):293–8.
10. Vasakova M, Morell F, Walsh S, et al. Hypersensitivity pneumonitis: perspectives in diagnosis and management. Am J Respir Crit Care Med. 2017;196(6):680–9.
11. Morell F, Villar A, Montero MÁ, et al. Chronic hypersensitivity pneumonitis in patients diagnosed with idiopathic pulmonary fibrosis: a prospective case-cohort study. Lancet Respir Med. 2013;1(9):685–94.
12. Fontenot AP, Amicosante M. Metal-induced diffuse lung disease. Semin Respir Crit Care Med. 2008;29(6):662–9.
13. Wu CH, Tang SC, Wang PH, et al. Nickel-induced epithelial-mesenchymal transition by reactive oxygen species generation and E-cadherin promoter hypermethylation. J Biol Chem. 2012;287(30):25292–302.
14. Barchowsky A, O'Hara KA. Metal-induced cell signaling and gene activation in lung diseases. Free Radic Biol Med. 2003;34(9):1130–5.
15. Nesti M, Marinaccio A, Gennaro V, et al. ReNaM working group. Epidemiologic surveillance for primary prevention of malignant mesothelioma: the Italian experience. Med Lav. 2005;96(4):338–46.
16. Hubbard R. Occupational dust exposure and the aetiology of cryptogenic fibrosing alveolitis. Eur Respir J Suppl. 2001;32:119s–21s.
17. Garantziotis S, Schwartz DA. Host-environment interactions in pulmonary fibrosis. Semin Respir Crit Care Med. 2006;27(6):574–80. Review
18. Costabel U, King TE. International consensus statement on idiopathic pulmonary fibrosis. Eur Respir J. 2001;17(2):163–7.
19. Coultas DB, Zumwalt RE, Black WC, et al. The epidemiology of interstitial lung diseases. Am J Respir Crit Care Med. 1994;150(4):967–72.
20. Ekström M, Gustafson T, Boman K, et al. Effects of smoking, gender and occupational exposure on the risk of severe pulmonary fibrosis: a population-based case-control study. BMJ Open. 2014;4(1):e004018. https://doi.org/10.1136/bmjopen-2013-004018.
21. Duchemann B, Annesi-Maesano I, Jacobe de Naurois C, et al. Prevalence and incidence of interstitial lung diseases in a multi-ethnic county of greater Paris. Eur Respir J. 2017;50(2):1602419. [https://doi.org/10.1183/13993003.02419-2016].
22. Kreuzer M, Sogl M, Brüske I, et al. Silica dust, radon and death from non-malignant respiratory diseases in German uranium miners. Occup Environ Med. 2013;70(12):869–75.
23. Hubbard R, Cooper M, Antoniak M, et al. Risk of cryptogenic fibrosing alveolitis in metal workers. Lancet. 2000;355(9202):466–7.
24. Koo JW, Myong JP, Yoon HK, et al. Occupational exposure and idiopathic pulmonary fibrosis: a multicentre case-control study in Korea. Int J Tuberc Lung Dis. 2017;21(1):107–12.
25. Peters S, Kromhout H, Portengen L, et al. Sensitivity analyses of exposure estimates from a quantitative job-exposure matrix (SYN-JEM) for use in community-based studies. Ann Occup Hyg. 2013;57(1):98–106.
26. Lee JS. The role of gastroesophageal reflux and microaspiration in idiopathic pulmonary fibrosis. Clin Pulm Med. 2014;21(2):81–5.

Underlying and immediate causes of death in patients with idiopathic pulmonary fibrosis

Miia Kärkkäinen[1,2,7*], Hanna Nurmi[1,3], Hannu-Pekka Kettunen[4], Tuomas Selander[5], Minna Purokivi[3] and Riitta Kaarteenaho[6]

Abstract

Background: The most common cause of death of patients with idiopathic pulmonary fibrosis (IPF) has been reported to be the lung disease itself and mortality from IPF appears to be increasing. However, the causes of death in patients with IPF taking into account differences between genders and smoking histories as well as disease progression, have not been previously explored.

Methods: Retrospective data from hospital register and death certificates from national database of IPF patients treated in Kuopio University Hospital (KUH) from 2002 to 2012 were collected. Mortality was also explored from the death registry database via ICD-10 code J84 revealing the numbers of deaths from pulmonary fibrosis in Finland from 1998 to 2015.

Results: Out of 117 deaths, 26.5% were females and 73.5% males in KUH. The most common underlying causes of death were IPF 67.5% and ischemic heart diseases 14.8%. More males died for reasons other than IPF (39.5%) compared to females (12.9%) ($p = 0.007$). Pneumonia as the immediate cause of death was more common in males (27.9%) than in females (3.2%) ($p = 0.004$) and in ex-smokers (32.7%) compared to non-smokers (9.3%) ($p = 0.007$). Death register based mortality from pulmonary fibrosis is increasing in Finland.

Conclusions: Even though the overall mortality was higher in males with IPF, the disease-specific mortality for IPF was higher in females i.e. in males, comorbidities were more often the underlying causes of death. Pneumonia-triggered acute exacerbations of IPF may be associated with smoking and gender since females and non-smokers were less likely to succumb to pneumonia. We conclude that disease progression at the end of life may vary depending on smoking habits and gender.

Keywords: Cause of death, Idiopathic pulmonary fibrosis, Mortality, Acute exacerbation

Background

Idiopathic pulmonary fibrosis (IPF) is the most common form of the idiopathic interstitial lung diseases [1]. The most common cause of death in IPF patients has been reported to be the disease itself followed by cardiac disorders and lung cancer [2–5]. A rapid deterioration of the disease may be caused by pulmonary embolism, pneumothorax, infections or heart failure [6]. Nearly half of all patients (47%) dying primarily from IPF had experienced a deterioration of their lung disease prior to their death [7]. A new definition and revised diagnostic criteria for acute exacerbation of IPF have been proposed recently; exclusion of infection or other potential triggers is no longer required, the only qualifier is that the clinician should determine that cardiac failure or fluid overload does not fully explain the radiological findings of new bilateral ground glass opacification or consolidation [8].

Global mortality from IPF has been increasing, with males being reported to have higher mortality than

* Correspondence: miia.karkkainen@kuh.fi
[1]Division of Respiratory Medicine, Institute of Clinical Medicine, School of Medicine, Faculty of Health Sciences, University of Eastern Finland, P.O. Box 1627, 70211 Kuopio, Finland
[2]Kuopio City Home Care, Rehabilitation and Medical Services for Elderly, Tulliportinkatu 37E, 70100 Kuopio, Finland
Full list of author information is available at the end of the article

females [9–12]. It seems that mortality varies between countries depending on the definition and diagnosis codes used [9]. In the years 2011–2013 in the European Union (EU), the highest IPF mortality rates were reported in the United Kingdom while the lowest rates were in Lithuania [12]. In Finland, the median mortality rate for males was 7.36 per 100,000 and 3.62 per 100,000 for females, these values being the second highest in the EU [12].

The aim of this study was to examine the mortality rates of patients with IPF in the Kuopio University Hospital (KUH) area located in eastern Finland. The underlying and immediate causes of death from the patients' death certificates were gathered. All data was explored in the whole study group as well as separately for females and males. Smoking history, disease progression categorized according to the life span into rapid (0–2 years), moderate (2–5 years) and slow (> 5 years) as well as gender-age-physiology (GAP) stage were taken into account. Furthermore, the total numbers of deaths due to pulmonary fibrosis (PF) according to the ICD-10 code J84 were investigated in Finland between the years 1998–2015 from the national registry database of Statistics Finland and this data was compared to that from the local area served by KUH.

Methods

Patients and data collection

A total of 223 patients (91 female, 132 male) with PF treated in KUH between 1st January 2002 and 31st December 2012 were collected from the hospital's medical records by using ICD-10 codes J84.1, J84.8 and J84.9. Clinical, radiological and histological information of each patient was transferred from medical records to special forms designed for the present study. PF with a known etiology i.e. associated with rheumatoid arthritis or connective-tissue disease and asbestosis, were excluded. The data concerning causes of death and places of death was updated on 14th December 2016.

Smoking history was assessed such that the individual was defined as a non-smoker, ex-smoker or current smoker. Pulmonary function tests included results of forced vital capacity (FVC), forced expiratory volume in 1 sec (FEV1), FEV1 / FVC ratio and diffusion capacity of carbon monoxide (DLco). Information was collated from histological samples from surgical lung biopsies or autopsy.

Death causes were obtained from the death certificates using ICD-10 codes and registered as underlying and immediate causes of death. Places of death were also registered. The overall death rates due to PF according to ICD-10 code J84 and ischemic heart diseases (ICD-10 codes I21–25) were obtained from the open national database of Statistics Finland, in which the ICD-10 codes are available only at a 3-character level, and therefore data with more specific codes, such as J84.1, was not available "http://www.stat.fi/til/ksyyt/2015/ksyyt_2015_2016-12-30_tau_001_en.html". In Finland, the disease classification of the death certificates was altered in the years 2005–2006. Subsequently, pneumonia was no longer accepted as the underlying cause of death if some other chronic disease had weakened the patient prior to the development of pneumonia. In such cases, the weakening chronic illness is recorded as the underlying cause of death "http://www.stat.fi/til/ksyyt/2015/ksyyt_2015_2016-12-30_tau_001_en.html".

Acute exacerbation was defined using diagnostic criteria with 1) a previous diagnosis of IPF 2) acute worsening or development of dyspnea typically of less than 1 month duration 3) computed tomography with new bilateral ground-glass opacity and/or consolidation superimposed on a background pattern consistent with UIP and 4) a deterioration not fully explained by cardiac failure or fluid overload [8]. If computed tomography was not available, the designation of suspected acute exacerbation of IPF was used.

No consents for the inclusion into this study were collected since it was retrospective, with the majority of the patients already deceased. The study protocol was approved by the Research Ethics Committee of the Northern Savo Hospital District (statement 17/2013) and from the National Institute for Health and Welfare (Dnro THL/1052/5.05.01/2013). Permission to use data from death certificates was given by Statistics Finland (Dnro: TK-53-911-13). This study was conducted in compliance with the Declaration of Helsinki.

Assessment of the data

The findings of the first and last high resolution computed tomography (HRCT) of each patient were reevaluated by an experienced radiologist according to the recent statement of the American Thoracic Society (ATS) and the European Respiratory Society (ERS) and re-classified as usual interstitial pneumonia (UIP), possible UIP and not UIP [1, 13]. All the patients whose re-analyses were categorized as not definite UIP in HRCT or histology were evaluated during a multidisciplinary discussion with a radiologist, a pathologist and a pulmonologist before inclusion into the present study.

The patients were categorized into classes according to the observed time elapsing until their death: 1) rapid (0–2 years), 2) moderate (2–5 years) and 3) slow (> 5 years). Those patients that were still alive and with a follow-up time less than 5 years were not included into the categorization. The GAP stage was calculated using gender, age and results of FVC and DLco (physiology) at the time of IPF diagnosis to obtain a total points score, which was then used to classify patients into stages I (0–3 points), II (4–5 points), or III (6–8 points) [14].

Statistical analysis

Statistical analysis was performed with IBM SPSS Statistics version 21. Group differences were tested by Chi-square testing or Fisher exact test with categorical variables. Data is presented as mean with standard deviation for continuous variables or frequencies with percentages when variables are categorical. The survival was estimated by the Kaplan-Meier method using the time of diagnosis as the starting-point and death or lung transplantation as the end-point. The median survival time is presented. Multivariate survival analyses were computed using Cox regression models and results are shown in the form of a hazard ratio (HR) with 95% confidence intervals. *P*-value < 0.05 was considered as statistically significant.

Results

Patient characteristics

After re-analyses of radiological, histological and clinical data from a total of 223 patients, 89 cases were excluded due to diagnoses other than IPF, i.e. 132 patients with IPF were included in this study. Four patients had missing data of their smoking histories. Out of 128 patients, 45 (35.2%) were non-smokers, 66 (51.6%) were ex-smokers and 17 (13.3%) were current smokers. A total of 117 deaths had occurred by 14th December 2016. Three male patients, two current smokers and one ex-smoker, had undergone lung transplantation; one of them was a current smoker and had subsequently died. We calculated the following mean ages; the time of diagnosis, 70.5 years (SD 9.78); at death, 74.8 years (SD 8.98) and at lung transplantation, 53.3 years (SD 8.08). At the time of diagnosis, mean FVC was 76.7% predicted (SD 18.51), mean FEV1 77.0% predicted (SD 16.99), mean FEV1/FVC 101.4% predicted (SD 9.68) and mean DLco 56.1% predicted (SD 17.51) (Table 1.)

The median survival was 42.0 months. Fifty (43.5%) patients died in a tertiary hospital; 4 of them (8.0%) in an intensive care unit; 50 (43.5%) in a community hospital, 16 (13.9%) at home and 1 (0.9%) in a nursing home.

Mortality

In the KUH district, which was serving 248,000 citizens at the end of year 2012, the 5 year overall mortality rate between the years 2003–2007 was 2.5 per 100,000 whereas between the years 2008–2012, it was 4.7 per 100,000. When including only patients with IPF (ICD-10 code J84.1) as the underlying cause of death i.e. disease-specific mortality, the 5 year mortality rates were 1.7 per 100,000 and 3.1 per 100,000 in 2011 and 2012, respectively. The total numbers of PF deaths (ICD-10 code J84) in Finland from 1998 to 2015 are presented in Fig. 1 "http://www.stat.fi/til/ksyyt/2015/ksyyt_2015_2016-12-30_tau_001_en.html". There were 280 PF deaths in the year 2015 in Finland; from these values, one can calculate a mortality rate of 5.1 per 100,000, when the official total population of Finland at the end of the year 2015 was 5,487,308 "http://www.stat.fi/til/ksyyt/2015/ksyyt_2015_2016-12-30_tau_001_en.html; http://www.stat.fi/til/vaerak/2015/vaerak_2015_2016-04-01_tie_001_en.html?ad=notify".

The 5 year mortality rates in KUH district between years 2003–2007 were 0.7 and 1.9 per 100,000 for females and males, respectively; between the years 2008–2012, the mortality rates were 1.85 per 100,000 for females and 3.3 per 100,000 for males.

Table 1 Demographic characteristics of the patients

	Total	Male	Female	*p*-value[a]
N (%)	132 (100)	97 (73.5)	35 (26.5)	
Age years (SD)	70.5 (9.78)	70.2 (10.34)	71.3 (8.17)	0.562
Median survival (Mo)	42.0	36.0	60.0	0.045
Non-smokers n (%)	45 (35.2)	21 (22.1)	24 (72.7)	< 0.001
Former smokers n (%)	66 (51.6)	60 (63.2)	6 (18.2)	< 0.001
Current smokers n (%)	17 (13.3)	14 (14.7)	3 (9.1)	< 0.001
Pulmonary function test results at the time of diagnosis[b]				
FVC % predicted (SD)	76.7 (18.51)	75.7 (18.91)	79.2 (17.39)	0.354
FEV1% predicted (SD)	77.0 (16.99)	75.3 (17.22)	81.6 (15.66)	0.065
FEV1/FVC % predicted	101.4 (9.68)	100.3 (9.45)	104.2 (9.88)	0.049
DLCO % predicted (SD)	56.1 (17.51)	55.8 (18.02)	56.7 (16.33)	0.803

p-values calculated using Fisher test, Chi-squared test or Kaplan-Meier log-rank test
[a]Between genders
[b]Spirometry results were missing from 6 patients and diffusion capacity results from 8 patients
N number, *Mo* months, *FVC* forced vital capacity, *FEV1* forced expiratory volume in one second, *DLco* diffusion capacity of carbon monoxide

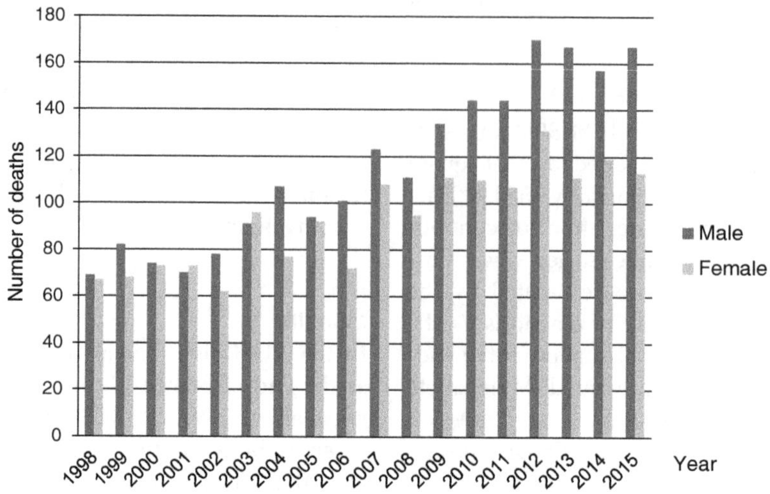

Fig. 1 The number of pulmonary fibrosis deaths in Finland between the years 1998–2015 "http://www.stat.fi/til/ksyyt/2015/ksyyt_2015_2016-12-30_tau_001_en.html". Underlying cause of death according to J84 (ICD-10, 3-character level): The data of this time series is otherwise comparable, but the classification of pneumonia was altered in 2005 and 2006. From that time onwards, an international guideline was adopted. Accordingly, pneumonia is not accepted as the underlying cause of death if a chronic disease which has weakened the individual, is mentioned in the death certificate. In such cases, the disease in question is recorded as the person's underlying cause of death. The revision of the classification was gradually taken into use in 2005 and 2006 "http://www.stat.fi/til/ksyyt/2015/ksyyt_2015_2016-12-30_tau_001_en.html"

Exacerbations and causes of death

The main underlying causes of death were IPF, ischemic heart disease and lung cancer. The most common immediate causes of death were IPF, pneumonia and ischemic heart disease (Table 2). An acute exacerbation was observed in 10 (12.7%) and a suspected acute exacerbation of IPF in 28 (35.4%) patients with IPF as the underlying cause of death. An acute exacerbation was observed in 7 (12.9%) and a suspected acute exacerbation in 18 (33.3%) patients with IPF as the immediate causes of death. Sixty (52.2%) patients had coronary artery disease (CAD) as a comorbidity from which 28.3% had ischemic heart disease as the underlying cause of death and 25.0% as the immediate causes of death. Compared to males, a higher percentage of females died from IPF. In contrast, more males than females had pneumonia as the immediate cause of death (Table 2).

Ex-smokers and current smokers had more often lung cancer as the underlying cause of death compared to non-smokers ($p = 0.045$ and 0.016, respectively). Non-smokers had more often IPF and less often pneumonia mentioned as the immediate cause of death compared to ex-smokers ($p = 0.043$ and $p = 0.007$, respectively). A trend towards a statistically significant difference was observed when comparing the underlying causes of death between non-smokers and current smokers ($p = 0.062$ for IPF and $p = 0.091$ for pneumonia). No statistically significant differences were observed in the causes of death between ex-smokers and current smokers (Table 3).

A multivariate analysis was performed to investigate whether differences in deaths between genders could potentially be explained by smoking status or vice versa. It was found that both gender and smoking status were independent predictors of mortality; for males, the HR was 1.7 (1.05–2.90) compared to females ($p = 0.033$) and for ex-smokers, the HR was 2.0 (1.10–3.60) compared to current smokers ($p = 0.024$).

There were significantly more deaths (100%) in the rapid disease progression group compared to slow disease progression (80%) ($p = 0.006$). More patients with a slow disease progression had IPF as the underlying cause of death compared to patients with a moderate disease progression ($p = 0.033$). More patients with a rapid disease progression died from an acute exacerbation compared to their counterparts with a moderate and slow disease progression (Table 4). No statistically significant differences were detected in the causes of death in the different GAP stages (Table 5).

Discussion

As far as we are aware, this is the first detailed clarification of the causes of death in patients with IPF taking into account differences between genders and smoking histories as well as disease progression. Even in this relatively small patient cohort, differences in the causes of death were detected between females and males. Moreover, by examining the smoking histories, we observed that more males and ex-smokers as well as more current smokers died of triggered exacerbations of IPF. Furthermore, more patients with a rapid disease progression died from an acute exacerbation compared to the other disease progression subtypes.

Table 2 Causes of death in the patients with IPF in the Kuopio University Hospital area

	Total ($n = 132$)	Female ($n = 35$)	Male ($n = 97$)	p-value[a]
Deaths N (%)	117 (88.6)	31 (88.6)	86 (90.7)	0.774
Underlying cause of death				
IPF	79 (67.5)	27 (87.1)	52 (60.5)	0.007
Pneumonia	3 (2.3)		3 (3.1)	0.292
Ischemic heart disease	17 (14.5)	3 (9.7)	14 (16.3)	0.371
Lung cancer	7 (6.0)		7 (8.1)	0.101
Pulmonary embolism	2 (1.7)	1 (3.2)	1 (1.2)	0.447
Colon cancer	2 (1.7)		2 (2.3)	0.392
COPD	1 (0.9)		1 (1.2)	0.547
Other[b]	6 (5.2)		6 (7.1)	
Immediate cause of death				
IPF	54 (47.0)	23 (74.2)	31 (36.0)	< 0.001
Pneumonia	25 (21.4)	1 (3.2)	24 (27.9)	0.004
Ischemic heart disease	15 (12.8)	2 (6.5)	13 (15.1)	0.216
Heart failure[c]	8 (6.8)	2 (6.5)	6 (7.0)	0.921
Lung cancer	5 (4.3)		5 (5.8)	0.170
Pulmonary embolism	2 (1.7)	1 (3.2)	1 (1.2)	0.447
Colon cancer	2 (1.7)		2 (2.4)	0.392
Other[d]	6 (5.2)	1 (3.2)	5 (6.0)	
Exacerbations preceding death				
Acute exacerbation	11 (9.4)	3 (9.7)	8 (9.3)	0.932
Suspected acute exacerbation[e]	31 (26.5)	7 (22.6)	24 (27.9)	0.609

p-values calculated using Fisher test
IPF idiopathic pulmonary fibrosis, *COPD* chronic obstructive pulmonary disease;
[a]Between genders
[b]Sick sinus syndrome ($N = 1$), cerebral infarction ($N = 1$), aortic rupture ($N = 1$), ileum strangulation ($N = 1$), heart failure ($N = 1$), drowning ($N = 1$)
[c]For any reason, including cor pulmonale
[d]Cerebral infarction ($N = 1$), aortic arteriosclerosis ($N = 1$), ileum strangulation ($N = 1$), hypotension ($N = 1$), respiratory failure due to COPD ($N = 1$), drowning ($N = 1$)
[e]No HRCT confirmation

Depending on the methods and diagnostic codes used, the mortality rates have been shown to vary globally and in different countries in the EU [9, 12]. Data from death certificates using ICD-10 codes J84 mortality in 2012 have been reported to be 4.25 per 100,000 in Sweden, 8.88 per 100,000 in Scotland and 8.22 per 100,000 in England and Wales [15]. In Finland, the mortality rate was 5.1 per 100,000 in 2012, being rather similar to the value from Sweden. When classified according to code J84.1, mortality in England and Wales was reported to be 6.90 per 100,000 in 2012 which is higher than our value i.e. 4.7 per 100,000 in the period from 2008 to 2012 [15]. A recent publication based on World Health Organization (WHO) mortality data revealed that the median IPF mortality rate has been rising between the years 2001 and 2013 in 10 out of 17 EU countries, being highest in the United Kingdom (12.01 and 5.63 per 100,000 for males and females, respectively) [12]. The mortality rates in Finland were the second highest i.e. 7.36 and 3.62 per 100,000 for males and females, respectively [12]. Our results are in line with the above-mentioned study revealing that mortality of PF and IPF has risen during the twenty-first century in Finland [12].

The number of PF deaths in Finland has doubled in the last 15 years; in addition, a gender difference has become more apparent since currently more males than females die from PF "http://www.stat.fi/til/ksyyt/2015/ksyyt_2015_2016-12-30_tau_001_en.html". It could be argued that the changes in the death certificates' disease classification in the years 2005–2006 may have had some effect on the rising number of PF deaths in Finland "http://www.stat.fi/til/ksyyt/2015/ksyyt_2015_2016-12-30_tau_001_en.html". This argument, however, was not supported by the results of our study on KUH patient cohort, since the numbers of the patients with pneumonia as the underlying cause of death have not changed after the year 2006; in fact, only three patients had pneumonia as the underlying cause of death during the complete study period. However, the diagnostic methods have improved in the past 10–20 years after the

Table 3 Causes of death according to smoking history

	Non-smokers ($n = 45$)	Ex-smokers ($n = 66$)	Current smoker ($n = 17$)	p-value[a]
Total N of deaths (%)	43 (95.5)	55 (83.3)	15 (88.2)	0.153
Underlying cause of death				
IPF	34 (79.1)	35 (63.6)	8 (53.3)	0.111
Pneumonia		2 (3.6)	1 (6.7)	0.315
Ischemic heart disease	6 (14.0)	6 (10.9)	3 (20.0)	0.646
Lung cancer		5 (9.1)	2 (13.3)	0.084
Pulmonary embolism	2 (4.7)			0.191
Colon cancer		2 (3.6)		0.342
COPD			1 (6.7)	0.133
Other[b]	1 (2.3)	5 (9.1)		
Immediate cause of death				
IPF	27 (60.5)	21 (38.2)	6 (40.0)	0.076
Pneumonia	4 (9.3)	18 (32.7)	3 (20.0)	0.021
Ischemic heart disease	5 (11.6)	6 (10.9)	3 (20.0)	0.627
Heart failure[c]	4 (9.3)	2 (3.6)	1 (6.7)	0.512
Lung cancer		4 (7.3)	1 (6.7)	0.200
Pulmonary embolism	2 (4.8)			0.191
Colon cancer		2 (3.6)		0.342
Other[d]	1 (2.3)	3 (5.5)	1 (7.1)	
Exacerbations preceding death				
Acute exacerbation	5 (11.6)	6 (10.7)		0.370
Suspected acute exacerbation[e]	11 (25.6)	16 (28.6)	4 (25.0)	0.929

p-values calculated using Fisher test
IPF idiopathic pulmonary fibrosis, *COPD* chronic obstructive pulmonary disease;
[a]p-value between different smoking histories
[b]Sick sinus syndrome ($N = 1$), cerebral infarction ($N = 1$), aortic rupture ($N = 1$), ileum strangulation ($N = 1$), heart failure ($N = 1$), drowning ($N = 1$)
[c]For any reason, including cor pulmonale
[d]Cerebral infarction ($N = 1$), aortic arteriosclerosis ($N = 1$), ileum strangulation (N = 1), hypotension ($N = 1$), respiratory failure due to COPD ($N = 1$), drowning ($N = 1$)
[e]No HRCT confirmation

appearance of ATS guidelines for IPF in 2000 [16]. It is possible that more of the other types of interstitial lung diseases such as non-specific interstitial pneumonia were included with IPF at the beginning of the twenty-first century. Since IPF is the most common form of idiopathic PF, the numbers of deaths for PF coded as J84 are likely to reflect the actual number of IPF deaths. The rising trend was also seen in the mortality rate in the KUH cohort. This proposal is supported by the recent data from the WHO mortality database, from which it can be estimated that in the year 2001 the mortality rates in males were 4.7 and 5.0 per 100,000 for the narrow (ICD-10 code J84.1) and the broad (ICD-10 code J84) definitions, respectively, while in females, the rates were around 3.0 per 100,000 with both definitions [12]. In the year 2013, the estimated mortality rates were 7.9 and 8.6 per 100,000 for males, and 3.5 and 3.9 per 100,000 for females, with the narrow and broad definitions, respectively [12]. Thus, it can be concluded that most of the cases coded as J84 represented code J84.1. Moreover, since 30% of IPF patients in the KUH area died for reasons other than IPF, one can estimate from the statistics that approximately 350–400 IPF patients die every year in Finland.

A previous study reported that most IPF patients with CAD die from IPF and only 12% from CAD [17]. Here, the number of ischemic heart disease deaths among IPF patients with CAD was higher (28. 3%) probably due to the large disease burden of CAD and other cardiovascular diseases in Finland "http://urn.fi/URN:NBN:fi-fe2016111829194". However, the total proportion of ischemic heart disease deaths was in line with published reports [3, 5]. In our previous study, we determined that 72.7% of the patients had one or more cardiovascular diseases (hypertension, CAD, cerebral infarction) as a comorbidity and CAD was diagnosed in 49.2% of the patients [13]. Lung cancer accounted for approximately 6% of the deaths in this study, which is somewhat less common than in the previous studies [4, 18].

Table 4 Causes of death in different types of disease progression

	Rapid ($n = 40$)	Moderate ($n = 42$)	Slow ($n = 45$)	p-value[a]
Total N of deaths (%)	40 (100)	41 (97.6)	36 (80.0)	< 0.001
Underlying cause of death				
IPF	29 (72.5)	22 (53.7)	28 (77.8)	0.056
Pneumonia	2 (5.0)	1 (2.4)		0.387
Ischemic heart disease	5 (12.5)	9 (22.0)	3 (8.3)	0.216
Lung cancer	1 (2.5)	4 (9.8)	2 (5.6)	0.384
Pulmonary embolism	1 (2.5)		1 (2.8)	0.575
Colon cancer		1 (2.4)	1 (2.8)	0.586
COPD		1 (2.4)		0.393
Other[b]	1 (2.0)	3 (4.9)	1 (2.8)	
Immediate cause of death				
IPF	20 (50.0)	16 (39.0)	18 (50.0)	0.524
Pneumonia	10 (25.0)	9 (22.0)	6 (16.7)	0.672
Ischemic heart disease	5 (12.5)	7 (17.1)	3 (8.3)	0.518
Heart failure[c]	1 (2.5)	3 (7.3)	4 (11.1)	0.328
Lung cancer	1 (2.5)	2 (4.9)	2 (5.6)	0.783
Pulmonary embolism	1 (2.5)		1 (2.8)	0.575
Colon cancer		1 (2.4)	1 (2.8)	0.586
Other[d]	2 (4.1)	3 (7.3)	1 (2.8)	
Exacerbations preceding death				
Acute exacerbation	8 (20.0)	1 (2.4)	2 (5.4)	0.014
Suspected acute exacerbation[e]	15 (37.5)	6 (14.3)	10 (27.0)	0.056

p-values calculated using Fisher test
Rapid = survival ≤2 years, moderate = survival 2–5 years, slow = survival ≥5 years
IPF idiopathic pulmonary fibrosis, *COPD* chronic obstructive pulmonary disease
[a] p-value between the groups of different disease progression
[b] Sick sinus syndrome ($N = 1$), cerebral infarction ($N = 1$), aortic rupture ($N = 1$), ileum strangulation ($N = 1$), heart failure ($N = 1$), drowning ($N = 1$)
[c] For any reason, including cor pulmonale
[d] Cerebral infarction ($N = 1$), aortic arteriosclerosis ($N = 1$), ileum strangulation ($N = 1$), hypotension ($N = 1$), respiratory failure due to COPD ($N = 1$), drowning ($N = 1$)
[e] No HRCT confirmation

One can speculate on the reasons for the relatively high number of pneumonias and the low number of acute exacerbations. The data of the current study was collected from the IPF patients diagnosed in KUH between the years 2002–2012 i.e. during the period when the first international perspectives including diagnostic criteria for acute exacerbation of IPF were published (2007) [19]. Since then, Finnish physicians specializing in respiratory medicine have gradually become aware of the exacerbation phenomenon. Since nearly 60% of the patients in our study died outside of tertiary centers, most of the death certificates had been prepared by primary health care physicians. Thus, it is possible that the acute exacerbations were not correctly identified due to the time point of the study and the places of death. Furthermore, HRCT, which would have been needed for diagnosing an acute exacerbation of IPF, is usually not available in the community hospitals in which most of the deaths occurred.

Never-smokers have been claimed to possess a higher risk for acute exacerbation of IPF, although this finding has not been confirmed in all studies [20–22]. A recent study revealed no gender difference in the numbers of acute exacerbations [22]. We observed that few death certificates reported acute exacerbations whereas pneumonias were reported to be the second most common immediate cause of death. Pneumonias are likely to represent triggered acute exacerbations as defined in the recent statement [8]. Since we found significantly less mentions of pneumonia as the immediate cause of death in females than in males and in non-smokers than ex-smokers, it seems that males and ex-smokers experienced more acute pneumonia-triggered exacerbation-linked deaths than females and non-smokers. If that is the case, the exacerbation may be associated with smoking since non-smokers were also less likely to suffer pneumonia than current smokers.

A recently published study, which investigated causes of death associated with GAP scoring (using GAP points), detected no differences between the groups with different scores [23]. In our study, more patients in GAP

Table 5 Causes of death according to the GAP stage

	GAP I ($n = 67$)	GAP II ($n = 47$)	GAP III ($n = 12$)	p-value[a]
Deaths N (%)	57 (85.1)	42 (93.3)	12 (100)	0.455
Underlying cause of death				
IPF	41 (71.9)	24 (57.1)	10 (83.3)	0.140
Pneumonia		3 (7.1)		0.079
Ischemic heart disease	10 (17.5)	6 (14.3)	1 (8.3)	0.703
Lung cancer	3 (5.3)	3 (7.1)	1 (8.3)	0.888
Pulmonary embolism	1 (1.8)			0.620
Colon cancer	2 (3.5)			0.381
COPD		1 (2.4)		0.437
Other[b]		5 (11.9)		
Immediate cause of death				
IPF	28 (49.1)	17 (40.5)	7 (58.3)	0.487
Pneumonia	10 (17.5)	11 (26.2)	3 (25.0)	0.561
Ischemic heart disease	3 (5.3)	3 (7.1)		0.440
Heart failure[c]	4 (7.1)	3 (7.1)		0.636
Lung cancer	2 (3.5)	2 (4.8)	1 (8.3)	0.761
Pulmonary embolism	1 (1.8)			0.620
Colon cancer	2 (3.5)			0.381
Other[d]		4 (9.5)		
Exacerbations preceding death				
Acute exacerbation	6 (10.2)	3 (7.1)	2 (16.7)	0.610
Suspected acute exacerbation[e]	10 (16.9)	14 (33.3)	5 (41.7)	0.072

p-values calculated using Fisher test
GAP Gender-Age-Physiology stage, *IPF* idiopathic pulmonary fibrosis, *COPD* chronic obstructive pulmonary disease
[a]*p*-value between different GAP-stages
[b]Sick sinus syndrome ($N = 1$), cerebral infarction ($N = 1$), aortic rupture ($N = 1$), ileum strangulation ($N = 1$), heart failure ($N = 1$), drowning ($N = 1$)
[c]For any reason, including cor pulmonale; [d] Cerebral infarction ($N = 1$), aortic arteriosclerosis ($N = 1$), ileum strangulation ($N = 1$), hypotension ($N = 1$), respiratory failure due to COPD ($N = 1$), drowning ($N = 1$)
[e]No HRCT confirmation

stage III (GAP score 6) died from IPF (83.0% vs 46.2%) and fewer from infections (0 vs 30.8%). The other GAP stages are more difficult to compare due to their different study approach. However, our study confirms that acute exacerbation leading to death may develop at any stage of the disease. We also found that IPF patients living less than 2 years suffered from lethal acute exacerbations more often than patients with longer survival times.

The limitations of the study mainly result from the relatively small number of patients and the retrospective study protocol. Our data is, however, comparable with those of other studies and moreover, it was very thoroughly collected and re-evaluated. Since histological data was available from only a minority of patients, the diagnoses are mostly based on clinical and radiological investigations which reflect diagnostic procedures of true clinical practice. The percentage of histological diagnoses in this study, however, was comparable with most of the previous studies. Nevertheless, the radiological data of all patients has been carefully re-evaluated and re-classified. The decision to utilize the national death registry base of Finland and its ICD-10 code at the 3 character level i.e. J84, may mean that it includes other fibrotic lung diseases in addition to IPF. We aimed to reduce this potential inaccuracy by investigating the same ICD-codes in our local KUH cohort.

Conclusions

The mortality determined in this study population reflects the demographics of IPF since there has been a year-on-year increase in the numbers of males and smokers with IPF dying from this disease. Even though the overall mortality was higher in males, the disease-specific mortality for IPF was higher in females, with males having more commonly comorbidities as the underlying cause of death. An acute exacerbation of IPF may be associated with smoking and gender since females and non-smokers were less likely to develop pneumonia, an illness that is known to trigger acute exacerbations. Thus, we conclude that disease progression at the end of life may vary depending on smoking habits and gender in IPF patients.

Abbreviations

ATS: American Thoracic Society; CAD: Coronary artery disease; DLco: Diffusion capacity of carbon monoxide; ERS: European Respiratory Society; EU: European Union; FEV1: Forced expiratory volume in one second; FVC: Forced vital capacity; GAP: Gender-age-physiology index; HR: Hazard ratio; HRCT: High resolution computed tomography; ICD-10: International Classification of Diseases version 10; IPF: Idiopathic pulmonary fibrosis; KUH: Kuopio University Hospital; PF: Pulmonary fibrosis; UIP: Usual interstitial pneumonia; WHO: World Health Organization

Acknowledgements

The authors wish to thank Ewen MacDonald for providing assistance with the language.

Funding

M. K. Has received grants for scientific work from the Foundation of the Finnish Anti-Tuberculosis Association, the Organization for Respiratory Health in Finland, Väinö and Laina Kivi Foundation, the Kuopio region respiratory foundation and Jalmari and Rauha Ahokas foundation; H.N. Has received grants for scientific work from the Foundation of the Finnish Anti-Tuberculosis Association, the Organization for Respiratory Health in Finland, Väinö and Laina Kivi Foundation, the North Savo Regional Fund of the Finnish Cultural Foundation, the Kuopio region respiratory foundation, Jalmari and Rauha Ahokas foundation and the state subsidy of the Kuopio University Hospital; M.P. Received grants for scientific work from research director of Kuopio University Hospital, Foundation of the Finnish Anti-Tuberculosis Association, the Kuopio region respiratory foundation and the Jalmari and Rauha Ahokas foundation; R. K. Has received grants for scientific work and for the research team from the state subsidy of Kuopio University Hospital, the Foundation of the Finnish Anti-Tuberculosis Association and the Kuopio Region Respiratory Foundation.

Authors' contributions

MK collected the study material, analyzed the data and takes responsibility for the integrity of the data and accuracy of the data analysis and prepared the draft of the manuscript. HN participated in the interpretation of the data and the presentation of the results. H-PK planned the radiological data collection form and performed the radiological analyses. TS participated in the statistical analyses. MP contributed to the study design, planning of the data collection form and data interpretation. RK managed and designed the study, planned the data collection form and interpreted the data. All authors participated in the preparation of the manuscript, read and have approved the final manuscript.

Competing interests

M.K. has received congress travel grants from Intermune, Boehringer-Ingelheim, Orion Pharma and Roche; lecture fee from Boehringer-Ingelheim; H. N. has received congress travel grants from Boehringer-Ingelheim, Lilly Oncology, Novartis, Orion Pharma and GlaxoSmithKline; Consulting fees from Boehringer-Ingelheim and Roche Oy; H-P.K. received consulting fees from Roche Oy; M. P. has received travel grants from Boehringer-Ingelheim Finland Ltd., Takeda Leiras Ltd., Roche, personal fees from Boehringer-Ingelheim Finland Ltd., Chiesi, Intermune, Orion Pharma Ltd., Roche, Takeda Leiras Ltd.; T.S. has no conflicts of interest, R.K. has received congress and meeting travel costs from Orion Pharma, Roche and Boehringer-Ingelheim, consulting fees from GSK and lecture fees from Roche and Ratiopharm.

Author details

[1]Division of Respiratory Medicine, Institute of Clinical Medicine, School of Medicine, Faculty of Health Sciences, University of Eastern Finland, P.O. Box 1627, 70211 Kuopio, Finland. [2]Kuopio City Home Care, Rehabilitation and Medical Services for Elderly, Tulliportinkatu 37E, 70100 Kuopio, Finland. [3]Center of Medicine and Clinical Research, Division of Respiratory Medicine, Kuopio University Hospital, P.O. Box 100, 70029 KYS Kuopio, Finland. [4]Department of Clinical Radiology, Kuopio University Hospital, P.O. Box 100, 70029 KYS Kuopio, Finland. [5]Science Services Center, Kuopio University Hospital, P.O. Box 100, 70029 KYS Kuopio, Finland. [6]Respiratory Medicine, Research Unit of Internal Medicine, University of Oulu and Medical Research Center Oulu, Oulu University Hospital, P.O. Box 20, 90029 Oulu, Finland. [7]Kuopio University Hospital and University of Eastern Finland, Puijonlaaksontie 2, 70210, P.O. Box 100, 70029 KYS Kuopio, Finland.

References

1. Raghu G, Collard HR, Egan JJ, Martinez FJ, Behr J, Brown KK, et al. An official ATS/ERS/JRS/ALAT statement: idiopathic pulmonary fibrosis: evidence-based guidelines for diagnosis and management. Am J Respir Crit Care Med. 2011; 183(6):788–824.
2. Mannino DM, Etzel RA, Parrish RG. Pulmonary fibrosis deaths in the United States, 1979-1991. An analysis of multiple-cause mortality data. Am J Respir Crit Care Med. 1996;153(5):1548–52.
3. King TE Jr, Albera C, Bradford WZ, Costabel U, du Bois RM, Leff JA, et al. All-cause mortality rate in patients with idiopathic pulmonary fibrosis. Implications for the design and execution of clinical trials. Am J Respir Crit Care Med. 2014;189(7):825–31.
4. Kreuter M, Ehlers-Tenenbaum S, Palmowski K, Bruhwyler J, Oltmanns U, Muley T, et al. Impact of comorbidities on mortality in patients with idiopathic pulmonary fibrosis. PLoS One. 2016;11(3):e0151425.
5. Rajala K, Lehto JT, Saarinen M, Sutinen E, Saarto T, Myllarniemi M. End-of-life care of patients with idiopathic pulmonary fibrosis. BMC Palliat Care. 2016;15(1):85.
6. Panos RJ, Mortenson RL, Niccoli SA, King TE Jr. Clinical deterioration in patients with idiopathic pulmonary fibrosis: causes and assessment. Am J Med. 1990;88(4):396–404.
7. Martinez FJ, Safrin S, Weycker D, Starko KM, Bradford WZ, King TE Jr, et al. The clinical course of patients with idiopathic pulmonary fibrosis. Ann Intern Med. 2005;142(12 Pt 1):963–7.
8. Collard HR, Ryerson CJ, Corte TJ, Jenkins G, Kondoh Y, Lederer DJ, et al. Acute exacerbation of idiopathic pulmonary fibrosis. An international working group report. Am J Respir Crit Care Med. 2016;194(3):265–75.
9. Hutchinson J, Fogarty A, Hubbard R, McKeever T. Global incidence and mortality of idiopathic pulmonary fibrosis: a systematic review. Eur Respir J. 2015;46(3):795–806.
10. Swigris JJ, Olson AL, Huie TJ, Fernandez-Perez ER, Solomon J, Sprunger D, et al. Ethnic and racial differences in the presence of idiopathic pulmonary fibrosis at death. Respir Med. 2012;106(4):588–93.
11. Olson AL, Swigris JJ, Lezotte DC, Norris JM, Wilson CG, Brown KK. Mortality from pulmonary fibrosis increased in the United States from 1992 to 2003. Am J Respir Crit Care Med. 2007;176(3):277–84.
12. Marshall DC, Salciccioli JD, Shea BS, Akuthota P. Trends in mortality from idiopathic pulmonary fibrosis in the European Union: an observational study of the WHO mortality database from 2001-2013. Eur Respir J. 2018;51(1) https://doi.org/10.1183/13993003.01603-2017. Print 2018 Jan
13. Karkkainen M, Kettunen HP, Nurmi H, Selander T, Purokivi M, Kaarteenaho R. Effect of smoking and comorbidities on survival in idiopathic pulmonary fibrosis. Respir Res. 2017;18(1):160. 017-0642-6
14. Ley B, Ryerson CJ, Vittinghoff E, Ryu JH, Tomassetti S, Lee JS, et al. A multidimensional index and staging system for idiopathic pulmonary fibrosis. Ann Intern Med. 2012;156(10):684–91.
15. Hutchinson JP, McKeever TM, Fogarty AW, Navaratnam V, Hubbard RB. Increasing g lobal mortality from idiopathic pulmonary fibrosis in the twenty-first century. Ann Am Thorac Soc. 2014;11(8):1176–85.
16. American Thoracic Society. Idiopathic pulmonary fibrosis: diagnosis and treatment. International consensus statement. American Thoracic Society (ATS), and the European Respiratory Society (ERS). Am J Respir Crit Care Med. 2000;161(2 Pt 1):646–64.

17. Kim WY, Mok Y, Kim GW, Baek SJ, Yun YD, Jee SH, et al. Association between idiopathic pulmonary fibrosis and coronary artery disease: a case-control study and cohort analysis. Sarcoidosis Vasc Diffuse Lung Dis. 2015;31(4):289–96.
18. Lee SH, Kim SY, Kim DS, Kim YW, Chung MP, Uh ST, et al. Comparisons of prognosis between surgically and clinically diagnosed idiopathic pulmonary fibrosis using gap model: a Korean National Cohort Study. Medicine (Baltimore). 2016;95(11):e3105.
19. Collard HR, Moore BB, Flaherty KR, Brown KK, Kaner RJ, King TE Jr, et al. Acute exacerbations of idiopathic pulmonary fibrosis. Am J Respir Crit Care Med. 2007;176(7):636–43.
20. Song JW, Hong SB, Lim CM, Koh Y, Kim DS. Acute exacerbation of idiopathic pulmonary fibrosis: incidence, risk factors and outcome. Eur Respir J. 2011;37(2):356–63.
21. Kishaba T, Nagano H, Nei Y, Yamashiro S. Clinical characteristics of idiopathic pulmonary fibrosis patients according to their smoking status. J Thorac Dis. 2016;8(6):1112–20.
22. Johannson KA, Vittinghoff E, Lee K, Balmes JR, Ji W, Kaplan GG, et al. Acute exacerbation of idiopathic pulmonary fibrosis associated with air pollution exposure. Eur Respir J. 2014;43(4):1124–31.
23. Lee SH, Kim SY, Kim DS, Kim YW, Chung MP, Uh ST, et al. Predicting survival of patients with idiopathic pulmonary fibrosis using GAP score: a nationwide cohort study. Respir Res. 2016;17(1):131.

28

Radiological pleuroparenchymal fibroelastosis associated to limited cutaneous systemic sclerosis

D. Hassoun[1], S. Dirou[2], P. P. Arrigoni[3], C. Durant[1], M. Hamidou[1], A. Néel[1] and C. Agard[1*]

Abstract

Background: Pleuroparenchymal fibroelastosis (PPFE) is a very rare interstitial lung disease (ILD) characterized by progressive fibrotic lesions of the visceral pleura and the sub-pleural parenchyma, affecting predominantly the upper lobes. PPFE may occur in different contextes like bone marrow or lung transplantations, but also in the context of telomeropathy with mutations of telomerase reverse transcriptase (*TERT*), telomerase RNA component (*TERC*) or regulator of telomere elongation helicase 1 (*RTEL1*) genes. PPFE-like lesions have recently been described in patients with connective tissue disease (CTD)-related ILD. We report here the first detailed case of PPFE associated to systemic sclerosis (SSc) in a woman free of telomeropathy mutations.

Case presentation: A caucasian 46 year old woman was followed for SSc in a limited form with anti-centromere Ab since 1998, and seen in 2008 for a routine visit. Her SSc was stable, and she had no respiratory signs. Pulmonary function tests showed an isolated decreased cTLCO at 55.9% (of predicted value). Cardiac ultrasonography was normal. Thoracic CT-scan showed upper lobes predominant mild and focal pleural and subpleural thickenings, suggestive of PPFE, with a slight worsening at 8 years of follow-up. She remained clinically stable. Biology only found a moderate and stable peripheral thrombocytopenia, and sequencing analysis did not find any mutations in *TERT* and *TERC* genes.

Conclusions: ILD is frequent in SSc but isolated PPFE has never been described so far. In our case, PPFE is not related to telomeropathy, has indolent outcome and seems to have good prognosis. PPFE might be an extremely rare form of SSc-related ILD, although a fortuitous association remains possible.

Keywords: Pleuroparenchymal fibroelastosis, Systemic sclerosis, Interstitial lung disease

Background

Pleuroparenchymal fibroelastosis (PPFE) is a very rare condition characterized by progressive fibrotic lesions of the visceral pleura and the sub-pleural parenchyma, intra-alveolar and septal structures, affecting mainly the upper lobes [1, 2]. Regarding the 2013 classification of idiopathic interstitial pneumonias, PPFE is considered as a distinct entity among a heterogeneous group of rare interstitial lung diseases (ILD) [1]. Poor is known about this disease that may occur in different conditions such as transplantation or chemotherapy, while idiopathic and familial forms of PPFE are also mentioned. Moreover, PPFE has been reported in family histories of telomeropathy associated to mutations of telomerase reverse transcriptase (*TERT*), telomerase RNA component (*TERC*) or telomere elongation helicase 1 (*RTEL1*) genes [3, 4]. We report here the first case of isolated PPFE in a caucasian patient with systemic sclerosis (SSc) who does not carry *TERT* and *TERC* mutations.

Case presentation

A caucasian 46 year old woman was seen in 2008 for a follow-up visit. She had a SSc in a limited form since 1998, comprising Raynaud phenomenon, sclerodactily, digital and facial telangiectasia, and sicca syndrome, with anti-centromere antibodies (Abs). She had never developed any other specific organ involvements. She had also thyroid insufficiency since 2005. No familial medical

* Correspondence: christian.agard@chu-nantes.fr
[1]Internal Medicine Department, Hôpital Hôtel-Dieu, Centre Hospitalier Universitaire de Nantes, 1 place Alexis Ricordeau, 44093 Nantes, France
Full list of author information is available at the end of the article

history was noted. Her treatment included ocular cyclosporine, ocular vitamin A, aspirin 75 mg/d, diltiazem 240 mg/d and levothyroxine 75 µg/d. She had never smoked. No toxic occupational exposures were found.

Weight was stable at 42 kg and body mass index was at 16.4 kg/m^2 (constitutionnal thinness). Thorax morphology was normal. Skin fibrosis was stable, involving the fingers and the face, with a Rodnan modified skin score (mRSS) at 3. She did not complain of dyspnea or cough and lung auscultation was normal. Usual laboratory tests were normal. Pulmonary function tests (PFT) showed a decreased cTLCO (transfer factor of the lung for carbon monoxide, corrected for hemoglobin) at 55.9% (of predicted value), FVC (forced vital capacity) was at 2.68 L (87.8%) and total lung capacity (TLC) at 5.17 L (108.4%). FEV1/FVC ratio was at 1. Cardiac ultrasonography was normal. Thoracic CT-scan showed upper lobes predominant mild and focal pleural and subpleural thickenings without any other specific lesions (Fig. 1a). She was then followed every year without any signs of active SSc or respiratory signs, and BMI was stable. Treatment was unchanged and PFT remained stable.

In 2016, on the thoracic CT-scan, pleural thickenings appeared more pronounced, associated with bilateral subpleural foci of lung fibrosis in both upper lobes (Fig. 1b). At that time, the diagnosis of PPFE was made. 18-Fluorodeoxyglucose (FDG)-PET-scan was performed and found a mild uptake of the pleuro-parenchymal lesions without any suspicion of underlying neoplasia. Various differential diagnosis were ruled out and she did not have any signs suggesting Langerhans Cell Histiocytosis, spondylarthropathy or inflammatory bowel disease. On biologic analysis, a moderate peripheral thrombocytopenia was noted (31-75 G/L) without any other hematologic alterations: hemoglobin at 12 g/dL, leucocytes at 5.64 G/L, including 3.36 G/L neutrophils and 1.13 G/L lymphocytes. Liver tests and renal function (creatinine at 55 µMol/L) were normal. Gammaglobulins were at 9.2 g/L and albumin at 40.5 g/L. Arterial blood gas were normal. Auto-immune profile was stable, with anti-nuclear Abs (1/2560) and anti-centromere Abs, while anti-SSA/Ro, anti-SSB/La, anti-U1RNP Abs and rheumatoid factors were negative. The search for *Mycobacterium tuberculosis* was negative (culture of sputum). Otherwise sequencing analysis did not find any mutations in *TERT* and *TERC* genes. At last evaluation in 2017, patient was stable, there was a slight decrease in cTLCO (48%), FVC (83%) and TLC (88%), while lung involvement was unchanged on CT-scan (Fig. 1c).

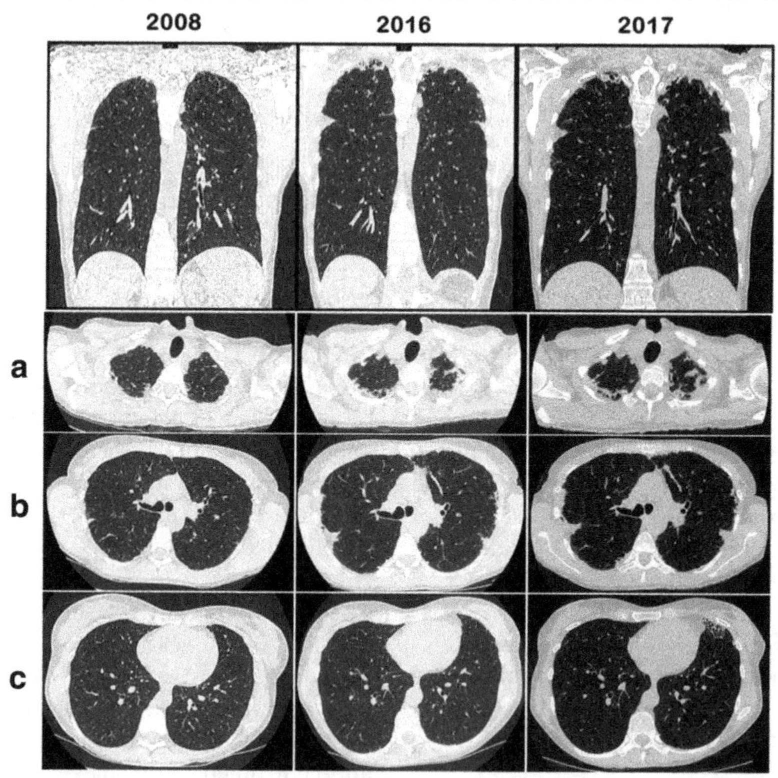

Fig. 1 Evolution of thoracic imaging by CT-scan over time. Axial images centered on **a** 2nd thoracic vertebra, **b** 5th thoracic vertebra and **c** 8th thoracic vertebra. Pleural and pulmonary injuries are characterized by fibrotic foci of the upper lobes, without any other signs of SSc-related ILD. An apico-basal gradient of lesions was found. A slow extention of the fibrosis was seen in 2016 and 2017

Discussion and conclusions

To the best of our knowledge, this is the first reported case of isolated PPFE associated with SSc in a Caucasian woman. PPFE developed progressively in the decade after initial diagnosis of limited SSc, without any other specific involvement. Imaging showed progressive alterations of lung fibrotic lesions, a slow decrease of TLC and TLCO, with mild uptake of 18-FDG on PET-scan. However, our patient had no dyspnea neither cough or chest pain, and no objective clinical signs suggestive of ILD like basilar crackles. Finally, this case of PPFE has a grumbling pattern outcome.

SSc is a rare connective tissue disease affecting predominantly women, and typically characterized by Raynaud phenomenon, dermal fibrosis, and auto-immunity. Severe organ lesions may occur, like intestinal, renal, myocardic or pulmonary involvements, mainly ILD and pulmonary arterial hypertension that are the two leading causes of mortality in SSc. ILD affects about 80% of SSc patients, but only 15-20% of them, mainly those with diffuse skin involvement and anti-topoisomerase 1 Abs, develop an extensive lung disease of bad prognosis [5]. Most SSc patients with ILD (around 3/4) have a non-specific interstitial pneumonia (NSIP) pattern whereas usual interstitial pneumonia (UIP) remains uncommon [5]. Rare patients may also develop combined pulmonary fibrosis and emphysema syndrome. Our present case raises the question whether PPFE might be considered as a potential additional pattern of ILD associated to SSc.

Recently, radiologic PPFE-like lesions have been described in 21 japanese patients with various connective tissue disease (CTD)-related ILD [6]. In this study, most of these patients had clinical signs of ILD with fine crackles on chest auscultation (17 among 19 patients evaluated). Enomoto et al. found that 6 of 14 patients with SSc-related ILD (43%) had also radiologic PPFE lesions, and this frequency was lower among patients with inflammatory myopathy (11%), rheumatoid arthritis (6%), primary Sjögren's syndrome (29%) and overlapping CTD (28%). In this original study, lung lesions were commonly progressive and associated to higher risk for respiratory death [6]. Patients with radiologic PPFE-like lesions had also higher frequency of pneumothorax and/or pneumomediastinum than those without (38% vs 15%). Interestingly, mean BMI was significantly lower in patients with PPFE-like lesions (19.8 vs 22.4 in patients without PPFE-like lesions), and this was also the case in our patient who had a BMI at 16.4.

Pathologic proof of PPFE is rarely obtained in CTD patients, and most of diagnosis has been made using CT-scan showing appearance and progression of PPFE-suggestive lesions. For our non-symptomatic patient, we decided to not perform any lung biopsy, and we finally made the diagnosis of "radiologic" PPFE. However, previous pathologic studies have shown that PPFE is typically characterized by upper lobes predominant elastin full fibrotic lesions of visceral pleura and sub-pleural intra-alveolar and septal structures [1, 2, 6, 7]. Pathophysiology of PPFE remains unknown and natural history of the disease usually consists of a progressive extent of fibrotic lesions leading to chronic respiratory failure. There are no specific treatments recommended and lung transplantation might be considered in severe patients. Clinical presentation of PPFE is not specific with predominant exertional dyspnea and chronic cough, but a flat chest and a high susceptibility to pneumothorax have been noted [7]. Around 200 cases of PPFE have been reported worldwide, and some of them occurred during various conditions like bone marrow transplantation, lung transplantation, chemotherapy, radiotherapy, but also immune diseases (spondylarthropathy, hemorrhagic recto-colitis) [7, 8]. PPFE may also be associated to heterozygous mutations in telomere-related genes like *TERT, TERC*, or *RTEL1*. In these cases, PPFE affects predominantly females [3, 4]. These telomeropathies are familial genetic disorders due to dysfunction of telomerase enzymes that are meant to reduce the shortening of telomere over time (molecular aging). They might be also associated to idiopathic pulmonary fibrosis, chronic hypersensitivity pneumonitis, but also interstitial pneumonia with autoimmune features, and even SSc-related ILD [3]. Whatever the underlying type of lung fibrosis, these mutations seem to be correlated with a progressive disease [3].

To conclude, our case suggests that PPFE could be specifically associated to SSc, as other known causes of PPFE might be ruled out, especially telomeropathy. Of course, a fortuitous association of SSc and PPFE might also be considered. It is to highlight that PPFE occurred very progressively, in a patient with low BMI and remaining asymptomatic after 10 years of follow-up.

Abbreviations

ILD: Interstitial lung disease; PPFE: Pleuroparenchymal fibroelastosis; SSc: Systemic sclerosis

Authors' contributions

DH and CA analyzed the medical file and wrote the manuscript. SD and PPA analyzed imaging data. CD, MH and AN were involved in revising the manuscript for important intellectual content. All authors read and approved the final manuscript.

Consent for publication

Patient gave consent for publication and consent for publication was written.

Competing interests

The authors declare that they have no competing interests.

Author details

[1]Internal Medicine Department, Hôpital Hôtel-Dieu, Centre Hospitalier Universitaire de Nantes, 1 place Alexis Ricordeau, 44093 Nantes, France.

[2]Pneumology Department, Institut du Thorax, Hôpital Guillaume et René Laënnec, Centre Hospitalier Universitaire de Nantes, Nantes, France.
[3]Radiology Department, Hôpital Hôtel-Dieu, Centre Hospitalier Universitaire de Nantes, Nantes, France.

References

1. Travis WD, Costabel U, Hansell DM, King TE Jr, Lynch DA, Nicholson AG, et al. An official American Thoracic Society/European Respiratory Society statement: update of the international multidisciplinary classification of the idiopathic interstitial pneumonias. Am J Respir Crit Care Med. 2013;188:733–48.
2. Kusagaya H, Nakamura Y, Kono M, Kaida Y, Kuroishi S, Enomoto N, et al. Idiopathic pleuroparenchymal fibroelastosis : consideration of a clinicopathological entity in a series of Japanese patients. BMC Pulm Med. 2012;12:72.
3. Newton CA, Batra K, Torrealba J, Kozlitina J, Glazer CS, Aravena C, et al. Telomere-related lung fibrosis is diagnostically heterogeneous but uniformly progressive. Eur Respir J. 2016;48:1710–20.
4. Armanios M, Blackburn EH. The telomere syndromes. Nat Rev Genet. 2012;13(10):693–704.
5. Cappelli S, Bellando Randone S, Camiciottoli G, De Paulis A, Guiducci S, Matucci-Cerinic M. Interstitial lung disease in systemic sclerosis: where do we stand ? Eur Respir Rev. 2015;24:411–9.
6. Enomoto Y, Nakamura Y, Colby TV, Johko T, Sumikawa H, Nishimoto K, et al. Radiologic pleuroparenchymal fibroelastosis-like lesion in connective tissue disease-related interstitial lung disease. PLoS One. 2017;12:e0180283.
7. Reddy TL, Tominaga M, Hansell DM, von der Thusen J, Rassl D, Parfrey H, et al. Pleuroparenchymal fibroelastosis: a spectrum of histopathological and imaging phenotypes. Eur Respir J. 2012;40(2):377–85.
8. Watanabe K. Pleuroparenchymal Fibroelastosis: its clinical characteristics. Curr Respir Med Rev. 2013;9:229–37.

Permissions

All chapters in this book were first published in PM, by BioMed Central; hereby published with permission under the Creative Commons Attribution License or equivalent. Every chapter published in this book has been scrutinized by our experts. Their significance has been extensively debated. The topics covered herein carry significant findings which will fuel the growth of the discipline. They may even be implemented as practical applications or may be referred to as a beginning point for another development.

The contributors of this book come from diverse backgrounds, making this book a truly international effort. This book will bring forth new frontiers with its revolutionizing research information and detailed analysis of the nascent developments around the world.

We would like to thank all the contributing authors for lending their expertise to make the book truly unique. They have played a crucial role in the development of this book. Without their invaluable contributions this book wouldn't have been possible. They have made vital efforts to compile up to date information on the varied aspects of this subject to make this book a valuable addition to the collection of many professionals and students.

This book was conceptualized with the vision of imparting up-to-date information and advanced data in this field. To ensure the same, a matchless editorial board was set up. Every individual on the board went through rigorous rounds of assessment to prove their worth. After which they invested a large part of their time researching and compiling the most relevant data for our readers.

The editorial board has been involved in producing this book since its inception. They have spent rigorous hours researching and exploring the diverse topics which have resulted in the successful publishing of this book. They have passed on their knowledge of decades through this book. To expedite this challenging task, the publisher supported the team at every step. A small team of assistant editors was also appointed to further simplify the editing procedure and attain best results for the readers.

Apart from the editorial board, the designing team has also invested a significant amount of their time in understanding the subject and creating the most relevant covers. They scrutinized every image to scout for the most suitable representation of the subject and create an appropriate cover for the book.

The publishing team has been an ardent support to the editorial, designing and production team. Their endless efforts to recruit the best for this project, has resulted in the accomplishment of this book. They are a veteran in the field of academics and their pool of knowledge is as vast as their experience in printing. Their expertise and guidance has proved useful at every step. Their uncompromising quality standards have made this book an exceptional effort. Their encouragement from time to time has been an inspiration for everyone.

The publisher and the editorial board hope that this book will prove to be a valuable piece of knowledge for researchers, students, practitioners and scholars across the globe.

List of Contributors

Kaori Sakurai, Shotaro Chubachi, Hidehiro Irie, Akihiro Tsutsumi, Naofumi Kameyama, Takashi Kamatani and Tomoko Betsuyaku
Division of Pulmonary Medicine, Department of Medicine, Keio University School of Medicine, 35 Shinanomachi, Shinjuku-ku, Tokyo 160-8582, Japan

Hidefumi Koh
Department of Medicine, Tachikawa Hospital, Tokyo, Japan

Takeshi Terashima
Division of Pulmonary Medicine, Department of Internal Medicine, Tokyo Dental College, Chiba, Japan

Hidetoshi Nakamura
Department of Respiratory Medicine, Saitama Medical University, Saitama, Japan

Koichiro Asano
Division of Pulmonary Medicine, Department of Medicine, Tokai University School of Medicine, Kanagawa, Japan

Taizou Hirano, Tadahisa Numakura, Yutaka Shishikura, Hisatoshi Sugiura and Masakazu Ichinose
Department of Respiratory Medicine, Tohoku University Graduate School of Medicine, 1-1 Seiryou-machi, Aoba-ku, Sendai 980-8574, Japan

Jun Shiihara, Taizou Hirano, Tadahisa Numakura and Yutaka Shishikura
Department of Respiratory Medicine, Hiraka General Hospital, Yokote, Japan

Hiroshi Moriyama
Department of Respiratory Medicine, Nishi-Niigata Chuo National Hospital, Niigata, Japan

Ryoko Saito
Department of Anatomic Pathology, Tohoku University Graduate School of Medicine, Sendai, Japan

Jun Shiihara
Department of Respiratory Medicine, Saitama Medical Center Jichi Medical University, Saitama, Japan

Voahangy Andrianaivoarimanana and Minoarisoa Rajerison
Plague Unit- Institut Pasteur de Madagascar, BP1274 Ambatofotsikely, 101 Antananarivo, Madagascar

Eric Bertherat
Department of Infectious Hazard Management, World Health Organization, Avenue Appia 20, CH-1211, 27 Geneva, Switzerland

Rojo Rajaonarison
Centre Hospitalier Anti-pesteux d'Ambohimiandra, 101 Antananarivo, Madagascar

Tiana Rakotondramaro
Centre Hospitalier de District de Miarinarivo, Antananarivo, Madagascar

Christophe Rogier
Institut Pasteur de Madagascar, BP1274 Ambatofotsikely, 101 Antananarivo, Madagascar
Present address: Service de Santé des Armées, Direction Centrale, Division Expertise et Stratégie Santé de Défense, 60 Boulevard du Général Martial Valin - CS21623, 75509 Paris Cedex 15, France

Gisela Hovold, Fredrik Kahn and Lisa I. Påhlman
Department of Clinical Sciences Lund, Division of Infection Medicine, BMC B14, Lund University, Skåne University Hospital, Tornavägen 10, SE-22184 Lund, Sweden

Victoria Palmcrantz
Skåne University Hospital, Clinic of Paediatrics, Lund, Sweden

Arne Egesten
Department of Clinical Sciences Lund, Respiratory Medicine & Allergology, Lund University, Lund, Sweden

Jonas K F Jakobsson, Anders Gudmundsson and Jenny Rissler Per Wollmer and Jakob Löndahl
Division of Ergonomics and Aerosol Technology, Lund University, Lund, Sweden

H Laura Aaltonen and Hanna Nicklasson
Department of Translational Medicine, Lund University, Malmö, Sweden

Jenny Rissler
Chemistry, Materials and Surfaces, SP Technical Research Institute of Sweden, Lund, Sweden

Mayra Caleffi-Pereira, Renata Pletsch-Assunção, Letícia Zumpano Cardenas, Pauliane Vieira Santana, Jeferson George Ferreira, Vinícius Carlos Iamonti, Pedro Caruso, Carlos Roberto Ribeiro de Carvalho and André Luís Pereira Albuquerque
Pulmonary Division, Heart Institute (Incor), Hospital das Clínicas da Faculdade de Medicina da Universidade de São Paulo, Av. Dr. Enéas Carvalho Aguiar, n°44. Cerqueira Cesar., São Paulo 05403-900, Brazil

Angelo Fernandez
Thoracic Surgery Division, Heart Institute (Incor), Hospital das Clínicas da Faculdade de Medicina da Universidade de São Paulo, São Paulo, Brazil

André Luís Pereira Albuquerque
Sírio-Libanês Teaching and Research Institute, São Paulo, Brazil

Keigo Kobayashi, Takanori Asakura, Makoto Ishii, Soichiro Ueda, Hidehiro Irie and Tomoko Betsuyaku
Division of Pulmonary Medicine, Department of Medicine, Keio University School of Medicine, 35 Shinanomachi, Shinjuku, Tokyo 160-8582, Japan

Hiroyuki Ozawa
Department of Otorhinolaryngology, Head and Neck Surgery, Keio University School of Medicine, 35 Shinanomachi, Shinjuku, Tokyo, 160-8582, Japan

Kohei Saitoh, Isao Kurihara and Hiroshi Itoh
Division of Endocrinology, Metabolism and Nephrology, Department of Medicine, Keio University School of Medicine, 35 Shinanomachi, Shinjuku, Tokyo, 160-8582, Japan

Hario Baskoro, Tadashi Sato, Keiko Karasutani, Yohei Suzuki, Aki Mitsui, Naoko Arano, Fariz Nurwidya, Motoyasu Kato, Fumiyuki Takahashi, Yuzo Kodama, Kuniaki Seyama and Kazuhisa Takahashi
Department of Respiratory Medicine, Juntendo University Graduate School of Medicine, 3-1-3 Hongo, Bunkyo-ku, Tokyo 113-8431, Japan

Fariz Nurwidya
Department of Pulmonology and Respiratory Medicine, Universitas Indonesia Faculty of Medicine, Jalan Persahabatan Raya No. 1, Rawamangun, Jakarta 13230, Indonesia

Caiyong Yin, Kai Li, Yanfang Yu, Huijie Huang, Youjia Yu, Zheng Li, Ding Li, Peng Chen and Feng Chen
Department of Forensic Medicine, Nanjing Medical University, Nanjing, Jiangsu 211166, People's Republic of China
MOE Key Laboratory of Contemporary Anthropology, Department of Anthropology and Human Genetics, School of Life Sciences, Fudan University, Shanghai 200438, People's Republic of China

Jinchuan Yan and Zhongqun Wang
Department of Cardiology, Affiliated Hospital of Jiangsu University, Zhenjiang, Jiangsu 212001, People's Republic of China

Yan Pu
School of Medicine, Southeast University, Nanjing, Jiangsu 210009, People's Republic of China

Feng Chen
Key Laboratory of Targeted Intervention of Cardiovascular Disease, Collaborative Innovation Center for Cardiovascular Disease Translational Medicine, Nanjing Medical University, Nanjing, Jiangsu 211166, People's Republic of China

Christian Niels Meyer
Department of Internal Medicine, Zealand University Hospital Roskilde, Sygehusvej 10, 4000 Roskilde, Denmark
Department of Clinical Medicine, University of Copenhagen, Copenhagen, Denmark

Karin Armbruster
Department of Respiratory Medicine, Copenhagen University Hospital Gentofte, Gentofte, Denmark

Michael Kemp
Department of Clinical Microbiology, Odense University Hospital, University of Southern Denmark, Odense, Denmark

Trine Rolighed Thomsen
Danish Technological Institute, Life Science, Århus and Section of Biotechnology, Aalborg University, Aalborg, Denmark

Ram Benny Dessau
Department of Clinical Microbiology, Slagelse Hospital, Slagelse, Denmark

Yaoju Tan, Biyi Su, Xingshan Cai, Shaojia Kuang, Haobin Kuang and Jianxiong Liu
Department of Clinical Laboratory, Guangzhou Chest Hospital, State Key Laboratory of Respiratory Disease, No. 62, Hengzhigang Road, Yuexiu District, Guangzhou, Guangdong Province 510095, People's Republic of China

Wei Shu and Yu Pang
National Clinical Laboratory on Tuberculosis, Beijing Key laboratory on Drug-resistant Tuberculosis Research, , Beijing Chest Hospital, Beijing Tuberculosis and Thoracic Tumor Institute, No. 9, Beiguan Street, Tongzhou District, Beijing 101149, People's Republic of China

Kia Nikoomanesh
Department of Internal Medicine, Arrowhead Regional Medical Center, Colton, California, USA

Julian Choi and Sarkis Arabian
Department of Pulmonary and Critical Care Medicine, Arrowhead Regional Medical Center, Colton, California, USA

Pietro Pirina and Elisabetta Zinellu
Department of Respiratory Diseases, University Hospital Sassari (AOU), Sassari, Italy

Viviana Marras and Alessandro G. Fois
Department of Clinical and Experimental Medicine, University of Sassari, Sassari, Italy

Salvatore Sotgia, Ciriaco Carru, Angelo Zinellu and Panagiotis Paliogiannis
Department of Biomedical Sciences, University of Sassari, Sassari, Italy

C. Addy and D. G. Downey
Centre for Experimental Medicine, Queen's University Belfast, 97 Lisburn Road, Belfast BT9 7BL, Northern Ireland

G. Doran, S. Caskey, C. Addy and D. G. Downey
Regional Respiratory Centre, Belfast City Hospital, 51 Lisburn Road, Belfast BT9 7AB, Northern Ireland

A. L. Jones
Department of Respiratory Medicine, Royal Brompton Hospitals, Sydney Street, London SW3 6NP, England

G. Wright
Department of Rheumatology, Musgrave Park Hospital, Stockmans Ln, Belfast BT9 7JB, Northern Ireland

Weiju Wang, Jie Weng, Lei Yu, Qiaobing Huang, Yong Jiang and Xiaohua Guo
Department of Pathophysiology, Guangdong Province Key Laboratory for Shock and Microcirculation Research, Guangdong Provincial Key Laboratory of Proteomics, State Key Laboratory of Organ Failure Research, Southern Medical University, Guangzhou 510515, China

Naoki Watanabe, Tomoya Ishii, Nobuyuki Kita, Nobuhiro Kanaji, Norimitsu Kadowaki and Shuji Bandoh
Department of Internal Medicine, Hematology, Rheumatology and Respiratory Medicine, Faculty of Medicine, Kagawa University, 1750-1 Ikenobe, Miki-cho, Kita-gun, Kagawa 761-0793, Japan

Hiroyuki Nakamura
Department of Respiratory Medicine, Sakaide City Hospital, 3-1-2, Kotobuki-cho, Sakaide, Kagawa 762-8550, Japan

Nobuki Nanki
Department of Respiratory Medicine, Sanuki Municipal Hospital, 387-1, Ishidahigashi-kou, Sangawa-cho, Sanuki, Kagawa 769-2393, Japan

Yutaka Ueda
Department of Respiratory Medicine, Kagawa Prefectural Central Hospital, 1-2-1, Asahimachi, Takamatsu, Kagawa 760-8557, Japan

Yasunori Tojo
Department of Respiratory Medicine, National Hospital Organization Takamatsu Medical Center, 8, Shindencho-otsu, Takamatsu, Kagawa 761-0193, Japan

Eva Verjans, Kim Ohl, Angela Schippers, Norbert Wagner and Klaus Tenbrock
Department of Pediatrics, Medical Faculty, RWTH Aachen, Aachen, Germany

Stefan Uhlig, Christian Martin, Annette D. Rieg, Nadine Ruske, Stephanie Kanzler and Eva Verjans
Institute of Pharmacology and Toxicology, RWTH Aachen, Aachen, Germany

Annette D. Rieg
Department of Anaesthesiology, Medical Faculty, RWTH Aachen, Aachen, Germany

Kohei Horiuchi, Takanori Asakura and Fumitake Saito
Department of Pulmonary Medicine, Eiju General Hospital, 2-23-16 Higashi Ueno, Taito-ku, Tokyo 110-8645, Japan

Takanori Asakura
Division of Pulmonary Medicine, Department of Medicine, Keio University School of Medicine, Tokyo, Japan
Department of Mycobacteriology, National Institute of Infectious Diseases, Tokyo, Japan

Naoki Hasegawa
Center for Infectious Diseases and Infection Control, Keio University School of Medicine, Tokyo, Japan

Yao Tong, Zhuang Yu, Renlingzi Zhang, Xibing Ding, Zhixia Chen and Quan Li
Yao Tong, Zhuang Yu and Renlingzi Zhang contributed equally to this work. Department of Anesthesiology, Shanghai East Hospital, School of Medicine, Tongji University, 150 Jimo Road, Shanghai 200120, China

Linn T. Aalstad1, Jon A. Hardie, Einar Thorsen, Per S. Bakke and Tomas M. L. Eagan
Department of Clinical Science, University of Bergen, Bergen, Norway

Birgitte Espehaug
Centre for Evidence-Based Practice, Western Norway University of Applied Sciences, Bergen, Norway

Einar Thorsen
Department of Occupational Medicine, Haukeland University Hospital, Bergen, Norway

Tomas M. L. Eagan
Department of Thoracic Medicine, Haukeland University Hospital, Bergen, Norway

Bente Frisk
Department of Health and Functioning, Western Norway University of Applied Sciences, Inndalsveien 28, 5063 Bergen, Norway
Department of Physiotherapy, Haukeland University Hospital, Bergen, Norway

Xiaoxiao Lin, Min Ye, Yuping Li, Jing Ren, Qiyan Lou and Chengshui Chen
Department of Pulmonary and Critical Care Medicine, The First Affiliated Hospital of Wenzhou Medical University, Ouhai District, Wenzhou, China

Yangyang Li
Department of Pathology, The First Affiliated Hospital of Wenzhou Medical University, Ouhai District, Wenzhou, China

Xiaohui Jin
Department of Endoscopy, The First Affiliated Hospital of Wenzhou Medical University, Ouhai District, Wenzhou, China

Ko-Pen Wang
Division of Pulmonary and Critical Care Medicine, Johns Hopkins University School of Medicine, Baltimore, USA

Azusa Tanimoto, Shinji Takeuchi, Hiroshi Kotani, Kaname Yamashita, Koushiro Ohtsubo, Hiromichi Ebi and Seiji Yano
Division of Medical Oncology, Cancer Research Institute, Kanazawa University, 13-1, Takara-machi, Kanazawa, Ishikawa 920-0934, Japan

Tadaaki Yamada
Department of Pulmonary Medicine, Graduate School of Medical Science, Kyoto Prefectural University of Medicine, Kyoto, Japan

Hiroko Ikeda
Division of Pathology, Kanazawa University Hospital, Kanazawa, Japan

Vito Terlizzi
Dipartimento di Pediatria, Centro Regionale Toscano per la Fibrosi Cistica, Azienda Ospedaliero-Universitaria Meyer, Viale Gaetano Pieraccini 24, 50139 Florence, Italy

Marco Lucarelli
Dipartimento di Biotecnologie Cellulari ed Ematologia, Istituto Pasteur Fondazione Cenci Bolognetti, Sapienza Università e Policlinico Umberto I, Rome, Italy

Donatello Salvatore
Centro Regionale Fibrosi Cistica, Centro Pediatrico Bambino Gesù Basilicata, AOR San Carlo, Potenza, Italy

Adriano Angioni
Laboratorio di Genetica Medica, Ospedale Pediatrico Bambino Gesù, Rome, Italy

Serena Quattrucci
Centro Fibrosi Cistica Regione Lazio, Dipartimento di Pediatria e Neuropsichiatria Infantile, Sapienza Università-Policlinico Umberto I, Rome, Italy

Valeria Raia
Centro Regionale Fibrosi Cistica, Sezione Pediatrica, Dipartimento di Scienze Mediche Traslazionali, Università di Napoli Federico II, Naples, Italy

Manuela Seia
Laboratorio di Genetica Medica, Fondazione IRCCS Policlinico Ca' Granda Ospedale, Milan, Italy

Lisa Termini
Ospedale dei Bambini G. Di Cristina, Centro Regionale Fibrosi Cistica, Palermo, Italy

Federica Zarrilli
Dipartimento di Bioscienze e Territorio, Università del Molise, Isernia, Italy

Akira Naito, Seiichiro Sakao, Takayuki Jujo, Toshihiko Sugiura, Nobuhiro Tanabe and Koichiro Tatsumi
Department of Respirology, Graduate School of Medicine, Chiba University, 1-8-1 Inohana, Chuo-Ku, Chiba City 260-8670, Japan

Akira Naito
Department of Advancing Research on Treatment Strategies for respiratory disease, Graduate School of Medicine, Chiba University, 1-8-1, Inohana, Chuo-Ku, Chiba City 260-8670, Japan

Irene M. Lang
Department of Internal Medicine II, Cardiology, Medical University of Vienna, Spitalgasse 23, 1090 Vienna, Austria

Norbert F. Voelkel
Victoria Johnson Center for Obstructive Lung Disease, Virginia Commonwealth University, 1101 East Marshall Street, Sanger Hall, Richmond, VA 23298-0565, USA

Takayuki Jujo
Department of Advanced Medicine in Pulmonary Hypertension, Graduate School of Medicine, Chiba University, 1-8-1 Inohana, Chuo-Ku, Chiba City 260-8670, Japan

Goro Matsumiya and Keiichi Ishida
Department of Cardiovascular Surgery, Graduate School of Medicine, Chiba University, 1-8-1 Inohana, Chuo-Ku, Chiba City 260-8670, Japan

Ichiro Yoshino
Department of Thoracic Surgery, Graduate School of Medicine, Chiba University, 1-8-1 Inohana, Chuo-Ku, Chiba City 260-8670, Japan

Michael Dreher and Tobias Müller
Division of Pneumology, University Hospital RWTH Aachen, Aachen, Germany

Stefan Krüger and Susanne Schulze-Olden
Department of Pneumology, Florence-Nightingale-Hospital, Düsseldorf, Germany

András Keszei
Department of Medical Informatics, University Hospital RWTH Aachen, Aachen, Germany

Jan Hendrik Storre and Tobias Müller
Department of Pneumology, University Medical Hospital, Freiburg, Germany
Department of Intensive Care, Sleep Medicine and Mechanical Ventilation, Asklepios Fachkliniken Munich-Gauting, Gauting, Germany

Holger Woehrle
Sleep and Ventilation Center Blaubeuren, Lung Center Ulm, Ulm, Germany

Michael Arzt
Center of Sleep Medicine, Department of Internal Medicine II, University Hospital Regensburg, Regensburg, Germany

Giulia Paolocci, Ilenia Folletti, Marco Dell'Omo, Giacomo Muzi and Nicola Murgia
Section of Occupational Medicine, Respiratory Diseases and Toxicology, University of Perugia, Piazzale Gambuli, 06100 Perugia, Italy

Kjell Torén, Magnus Ekström and Nicola Murgia
Department of Occupational and Environmental Medicine, Sahlgrenska University Hospital, Göteborg, Sweden

Miia Kärkkäinen and Hanna Nurmi
Division of Respiratory Medicine, Institute of Clinical Medicine, School of Medicine, Faculty of Health Sciences, University of Eastern Finland, 70211 Kuopio, Finland

Miia Kärkkäinen
Kuopio City Home Care, Rehabilitation and Medical Services for Elderly, Tulliportinkatu 37E, 70100 Kuopio, Finland

Minna Purokivi and Hanna Nurmi
Center of Medicine and Clinical Research, Division of Respiratory Medicine, Kuopio University Hospital, 70029 KYS Kuopio, Finland

Hannu-Pekka Kettunen
Department of Clinical Radiology, Kuopio University Hospital, 70029 KYS Kuopio, Finland

Tuomas Selander
Science Services Center, Kuopio University Hospital, 70029 KYS Kuopio, Finland

Riitta Kaarteenaho
Respiratory Medicine, Research Unit of Internal Medicine, University of Oulu and Medical Research Center Oulu, Oulu University Hospital, , 90029 Oulu, Finland

D. Hassoun, C. Durant, M. Hamidou, A. Néel and C. Agard
Internal Medicine Department, Hôpital Hôtel-Dieu, Centre Hospitalier Universitaire de Nantes, 1 place Alexis Ricordeau, 44093 Nantes, France

S. Dirou
Pneumology Department, Institut du Thorax, Hôpital Guillaume et René Laënnec, Centre Hospitalier Universitaire de Nantes, Nantes, France

P. P. Arrigoni
Radiology Department, Hôpital Hôtel-Dieu, Centre Hospitalier Universitaire de Nantes, Nantes, France

Index

www.ingramcontent.com/pod-product-compliance
Lightning Source LLC
LaVergne TN
LVHW080706210926
848485LV00003B/426